"We have all looked for a unifying framework that integrates interventions with vulnerable children regardless of setting or discipline. MISC is the most powerful pan-theoretical framework currently available as an invaluable and effective guide to support mental health interventions in social care, education or community settings. It is breathtakingly simple in implementation yet breathtaking in its scope. An inspiring contribution for all those working with vulnerable youth."

Peter Fonagy, OBE, FMedSci, FBA, FAcSS,
Chief Executive, Anna Freud Centre and Professor of
Developmental Science, University College London

"Like the MISC itself, this book is filled with care and concern about all children, especially vulnerable children. Although we, as a civilization, claim to strive for every child to reach their potential, reality, reflected in the UN's reported figure of 200,000,000 children failing to thrive, demands much more systematic effort. The MISC, and those who preach and practice it, are at the forefront of society's efforts to support every child. As long as there are children who need support, the MISC and its practitioners, including the contributors to this volume, are in high demand and deserve the highest respect."

Elena Grigorenko, Hugh Roy and Lillie Cranz Cullen
Distinguished Professor of Psychology, University of Houston

Growing Up Resilient

It is universally accepted that sensitive and responsive caregiving leads to positive cognitive and socio-emotional outcomes for children. While several intervention approaches exist, this text brings together the rationale and current evidence base for one such approach—the Mediational Intervention for Sensitizing Caregivers (MISC).

MISC integrates aspects of socio-emotional health and cognitive development as well as being less culturally intrusive than existing approaches. It is a strengths-based program complementing existing practices and cultures. Editors bring together in one volume the theory and research from the last decade supporting the MISC approach. Chapters focus on a range of topics, such as training the trainer, maternal depression and MISC, applying MISC to families reunited after migration-related separation and more. The book also focuses on several country-specific cases, such as applying MISC to HIV/AIDS-affected children in South Africa or in early childhood care settings in Israel.

This book is essential reading for those working in early educational or clinical settings tasked with developing policy to ensure optimal child developmental outcomes. The book is applicable to professionals from a wide variety of disciplines including clinical, counselling, educational, psychology, psychiatry, paediatrics, nursing, social work and public health.

Carla Sharp, PhD, is Professor in the Clinical Psychology Doctoral Program at the University of Houston (UH), and Interim Associate Dean for Faculty and Research. She is also Director of Adolescent Diagnosis Assessment Prevention and Treatment (ADAPT) Center at UH and directs the Developmental Psychopathology Lab at UH. As a developmental psychopathologist, she makes use of multiple methods across different levels of analyses to understand, detect and treat emotional and behaviour problems in children and adolescents with a specific focus on attachment, social-cognitive and socio-emotional development. As a South African citizen and a child clinical psychologist, she has a longstanding interest in addressing these issues in children in resource-limited settings where children are at high risk for developing mental health problems as a result of attachment disruption and trauma. The HIV/AIDS epidemic created a tragic natural experiment that sheds light on socio-emotional and socio-cognitive development in the context of losing a primary caregiver. Since 2008, Dr Sharp's research has been continuously funded in South Africa to study the effects of losing a parent due to HIV/AIDS. It is in this context that Dr Sharp became acquainted with the Mediational Intervention for Sensitizing Caregivers (MISC), which was evaluated in a recent trial in South Africa funded by the NICHD. She has published over 270 peer-reviewed publications (H-index 61), numerous chapters and books.

Lochner Marais, PhD, is Professor of Development Studies and Acting Director of the Centre for Development Support (University of the Free State, South Africa). Marais's research interests cover three different, though related, themes: housing policy, small urban areas and public health (including his work on OVC). He has authored, co-authored and compiled more than 250 research reports, including more than 180 refereed articles in peer-reviewed journals or books (H-index 26). He has also co-edited eight books (two previous ones with Routledge). His work on OVC includes collaborative projects with Professor Sharp funded by the NICHD and projects funded by the Bill and Melinda Gates and Huffman Foundations.

Growing Up Resilient

The Mediational Intervention for
Sensitizing Caregivers (MISC)

**Edited by Carla Sharp and Lochner
Marais**

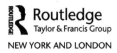

Routledge
Taylor & Francis Group

NEW YORK AND LONDON

First published 2022
by Routledge
605 Third Avenue, New York, NY 10158

and by Routledge
2 Park Square, Milton Park, Abingdon, Oxon, OX14 4RN

Routledge is an imprint of the Taylor & Francis Group, an informa business

Library of Congress Cataloging-in-Publication Data
A catalog record for this book has been requested

ISBN: 978-0-367-70360-8 (hbk)
ISBN: 978-0-367-70358-5 (pbk)
ISBN: 978-1-003-14589-9 (ebk)

DOI: 10.4324/9781003145899

Typeset in Bembo
by Apex CoVantage, LLC

This book is dedicated to my mother, Alta Sharp, who provided the first context for learning about the serve-and-return.

Carla Sharp

We also dedicate the book to the following four Community-based Organizations in Mangaung, South Africa who pioneered MISC in South Africa

Tshepong Care Centre

Tshwaraganang Community Based Organization

Heartbeat Centre for Community Development

Atlehang Multipurpose Centre

Carla Sharp and Lochner Marais

Contents

Foreword

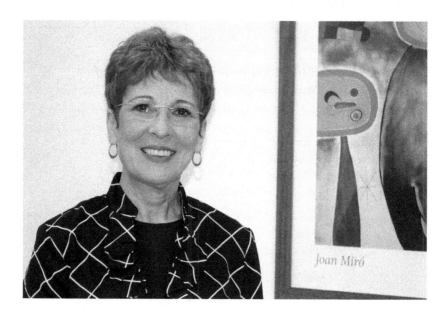

Joan Miró

A Tribute to MISC Developer Pnina Klein

Cilly Shohet and Deborah Givon
Bar Ilan University

Professor Pnina S. Klein was born in November, 1945 in Tarnów, Poland. The daughter of Holocaust survivors, she was the first baby born after the war into a family that had lost all its children. She had immigrated to Israel with her parents, who instilled in her a commitment to excel and contribute to the State of Israel. By age 16, she graduated from high school with honors and was accepted to study psychology and biology in college. During her graduate studies, she worked in educational psychological services in Tel-Aviv, where she was exposed to at-risk children and became interested in the development of early intervention programs for them.

Following Reuven Feuerstein's MLE—Mediated Learning Experience theory—an approach to help children with profound disabilities to learn and develop, Pnina translated this model in the early 1980s into intervention with young children and parents called the MISC, for enhancing the quality of communication and interactions in children and their impact on child development.

The MISC interventional model has been implemented and evaluated in various countries around the globe: **Ethiopia** (supported by Norwegian Aid to Developing Countries—NORAD-HEMIL), **Uganda** (supported by NIMH), **Indonesia** (supported by Gold Cross of the Leger Foundation), **Sri Lanka** (supported by UNICEF and Redd Barna, Norway), **Portugal** (supported by the Gulbenkian Foundation), **Israel** (supported by Government and Academic Funding), **Norway** and **Sweden** (supported by the Norwegian Research Council—HEMIL), **USA** (Hofstra U., Long Island, New York and U. of S. Florida, Tampa, Florida), and **South Africa** (supported by the NICHD). Pnina's contributions extended, throughout the years, to Zimbabwe, Kenya, Singapore, Holland, Belgium, the United Kingdom, and South America and are continuing to spread even after her passing to South Africa and DC Congo.

With her remarkable personality, in her own special way, Pnina succeeded in overcoming challenges, in crossing boundaries, cultures, educational levels, and poverty. She was always able, in a humble way, to reach into the hearts of parents, caregivers, and policymakers, seeking to advance children's development and wellbeing.

Pnina has been, for over 30 years, the head of the Child Development program at the School of Education, at the Bar-Ilan University, and the head of the Baker Center for Study of Development Disorders in Infants and Young Children. For more than 20 years, she was also head of the I. B. Harris Program, for supporting infants, toddlers, and families in Israel. Over the years, the program has become a lighthouse for research, consultation, training, intervention, and dissemination of information on infant mental health and early child educare in Israel. Her work was led by a deep belief that we can influence and change young children's lives in cross-cultural populations, and it was implemented through clinical, academic, and policy avenues of intervention.

For her remarkable work, Pnina received the ISRAEL Prize, for Research in Education, the highest honor which Israel reserves for those who make the greatest contributions to knowledge and have demonstrated excellence or broken new ground in a certain field.

Pnina smiled to the world with a gleam in her eye and brought hope and knowledge to those she reached, and she will always be remembered for how she touched the world of young children and families, opening possibilities for their future. She was a multi-talented person who published numerous professional books and articles, and was a gifted artist. Her drawings were colorful, expressing energy and zest, just like her special personality. The pearl of her crown was the family; nothing mattered for her more than her spouse, her children, and especially her grandchildren, of whom she was very proud.

Pnina left this world full of plans and new ideas for future projects. She certainly did not complete her mission, and it is up to us to do so! This volume brings together the researchers and clinicians in whose work Pnina's legacy lives on.

Cover Art by Pnina Klein

Painting title: Flakes

Painting caption:

"What are your aspirations for your child? Consider them as attainable goals that can be reached through sensitive understanding of the child's characteristics and needs"—Pnina Klein

Figures

Tables

Editor Biographies

Carla Sharp is Professor of Psychology in the clinical psychology program at the University of Houston. She directs the Developmental Psychopathology Lab and the Adolescent Diagnosis Assessment Prevention and Treatment (ADAPT) Center at the University of Houston. As a South African citizen and child clinical psychologist, she has a longstanding interest in understanding, preventing and treating mental health problems in children and adolescents in resource-limited countries. She is particularly interested in populations where attachment disruption occurs and the mechanisms and interventions that ameliorate its negative effects. She has published over 270 peer-reviewed articles, numerous chapters and books. Her research in South Africa has been funded by the National Institute of Health for more than a decade.

Lochner Marais is a professor of development studies at the Centre for Development Support at the University of the Free State (UFS). His research interests include community-based approaches to public health, housing policy and mining communities. In addition to concentrating on each of these themes separately, he focuses on integrating them. Marais has authored, co-authored and compiled more than 250 research reports, including more than 180 refereed articles in peer-reviewed journals or books. He has also co-edited eight books. He has a specific passion for creating and managing interdisciplinary projects and prefers research focusing on real-world problems in public health, housing policy and mine-community relations.

Contributors

Madeleine Allman, Department of Psychology, University of Houston, Houston, Texas, USA.

Jodi Berger Cardoso, University of Houston Graduate College of Social Work, Houston, Texas, USA.

John Bickel, University of Houston Graduate College of Social Work, and Texas Children's Hospital, Houston, Texas, USA.

Arlene Bjugstad, University of Houston Graduate College of Social Work, Houston, Texas, USA.

Michael J. Boivin, Departments of Psychiatry and Neurology & Ophthalmology, Michigan State University, East Lansing, Michigan, USA and Department of Psychiatry, the University of Michigan, Ann Arbor, Michigan, USA.

Kalina Brabeck, Department of Counseling & School Psychology, Rhode Island College, Providence, Rhode Island, USA.

Barbie Brashear, Harris County Domestic Violence Coordinating Council, Houston, Texas, USA.

Jan Cloete, Centre for Development Support, University of the Free State, Bloemfontein, South Africa.

Itziar Familiar, Michigan State University, East Lansing, Michigan, USA.

Ornit Freudenstein, Developmental Clinic Unit Director, I.B. Harris Program, Bar Ilan University.

Monica K. Gentchev, Departments of Psychiatry and Neurology & Ophthalmology, Michigan State University, East Lansing, Michigan, USA.

Deborah Givon, I.B. Harris Program, Bar Ilan University, Israel.

Jessica Hernandez Ortiz, Department of Psychology, University of Houston, Houston, Texas, USA.

Nurit Jaegermann, Developmental Clinic Unit Director, I.B. Harris Program, Bar Ilan University.

Esperance Kashala-Abotnes, Institute of Public Health, University of Bergen, Bergen, Norway.

Sophie Kerr, Department of Psychology, University of Houston, Houston, Texas, USA.

Ofra Korat, School of Education, Bar-Ilan University, Israel.

Molefi Lenka, Centre for Development Support, University of the Free State, Bloemfontein, South Africa.

Lochner Marais, Centre for Development Support, University of the Free State, Bloemfontein, South Africa.

Judith McFarlane, College of Nursing, Texas Woman's University, Houston, Texas, USA.

Veronica McLaren, Department of Psychology, University of Houston, Houston, Texas, USA.

Sarah Murray, Department of Mental Health, Johns Hopkins Bloomberg School of Public Health, Baltimore, Maryland, USA.

Natasha Prosperi, Julia's Counseling & Play Therapy Group, Houston, Texas, USA.

Kholisa Rani, Centre for Development Support, University of the Free State, Bloemfontein, South Africa.

Ravit Rozenfeld Kraft, School of Education, Bar-Ilan University, Israel.

Ora Segal-Drori, Faculty of Education and Early Childhood Department, Levinsky College of Education, Israel.

Motsaathebe Serekoane, Department of Anthropology, University of the Free State, Bloemfontein, South Africa.

Carla Sharp, Department of Psychology, University of Houston; Centre for Development Support, University of the Free State, Bloemfontein, South Africa.

Cilly Shohet, I.B. Harris Program, Bar Ilan University, Israel.

Amanda Venta, Department of Psychology, University of Houston, Houston, Texas, USA.

Kiana Wall, Department of Psychology, University of Houston, Houston, Texas, USA.

Quenette Walton, University of Houston Graduate College of Social Work, Houston, Texas, USA.

1 The Mediational Intervention for Sensitizing Caregivers

A Pathway to Resilience

Carla Sharp and Lochner Marais

1.1 Introduction

The United Nations' Global Strategy for Women's, Children's and Adolescents' Health (2016–2030) outlines a threefold agenda to ensure that children and adolescents reach their full developmental potential. These include Survive (end preventable deaths), Thrive (ensure health and wellbeing), and Transform (expand enabling environments). Ending preventable deaths, enhancing health and wellbeing, and expanding enabling environments are worthy goals, but their feasibility and sustainability in the low-to-middle-income (LMIC) countries are challenged by significant adverse childhood experiences (ACEs). These forms of adversity include war, poverty, malnutrition, discrimination, and the effects of HIV/AIDS and other chronic illnesses, among other forms of adversity. For instance, the United States Government Action Plan on Children in Adversity reports that 200 million children under 5 (more than 30% of the world's children) fail to reach their developmental potential in LMIC; 6.9 million children die before their fifth birthday of largely preventable causes; an estimated 300,000 children are associated with armed forces or groups; 70 million children are affected by natural disaster; 3.3 million children under 15 are living with HIV and AIDS, and 17.3 million children under 18 have lost one or both parents to it; and 1.8 million children are victims of sex trafficking or pornography. These adversities seldom occur in isolation and tend to co-occur with cascading and accumulating downstream effects for children across multiple domains of function across the lifespan, increasing the risk for premature death (see Figure 1.1).

While ACEs appear at a higher frequency and among larger proportions of the population in LMIC, they are common in high-income countries like the United States for populations who are negatively affected by the social determinants of health (SDOH). SDOH are defined by the Centers for Disease Control and Prevention (CDC, 2018) as the "conditions in the places where people live, learn, work and play that affect a wide range of health risks and outcomes". SDOH include gender, social and economic opportunity, food security, social interactions and relationships, and quality

DOI: 10.4324/9781003145899-1

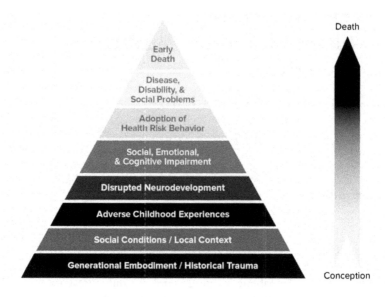

Figure 1.1 Mechanisms by which childhood experiences influence health and wellbeing throughout the lifespan

of education. When exposed to ACEs and other negative SDOH, a child's stress response system is activated, which, if prolonged and excessive, can derail healthy development; this is called toxic stress (Fuller-Rowell, Curtis, Chae, & Ryff, 2018).

For populations affected by SDOH, as for the populations in LMIC, surviving, thriving, and transforming cannot be taken for granted. Special resilience is needed to overcome adversity and stay on track to meet socio-emotional and cognitive developmental milestones. Yet, it is important to recognize that many children and adolescents with multiple ACEs thrive in adulthood. In these cases, ACEs were balanced out by protective or resiliency factors that mitigated the negative effects of ACEs (Garner et al., 2012). Put differently, toxic stress can be buffered and returned to baseline if certain protective factors are in place. Both the United Nations' Global Strategy for Women's, Children's and Adolescents' Health (2016–2030) and the United States Government Action Plan on Children in Adversity, as well as decades of developmental research, agree that arguably the most potent protective factor for children growing up in adversity is an environment of supportive and responsive relationships. The United Nations' Global Strategy for Women's, Children's and Adolescents' Health (2016–2030) identified responsive and sensitive caregiving as the central mechanism for transforming and expanding enabling environments that may enhance surviving and thriving of children.

The question then becomes what sort of intervention frameworks are best suited for transforming and expanding enabling environments. Considering intervention frameworks that may be fit for purpose, it is worth recognizing that thriving is an ongoing and unfolding process. Therefore, it requires an intervention framework that can offer ongoing interventions at different time points throughout development while flexibly adapting to the unique characteristics of each developmental epoch. Second, thriving requires an intervention framework that can be adapted cross-culturally, across caregiving contexts and low-resource settings. These are the settings where caregiving capacity is most likely to be disrupted. Third, because thriving has multiple dimensions that cut across physical growth, cognitive and socio-emotional learning, and the development of healthy interpersonal relationships, creativity, empathy, and the capacity for moral reasoning, it requires a holistic intervention framework that approaches the child as more than the sum of its parts. Put differently, an intervention framework is needed that can simultaneously address both cognitive and socio-emotional developmental needs. Finally, an intervention framework is needed that has the flexibility to serve in a one-on-one context and group settings and, critically, which can be learnt and taught by laypersons or professionals from multiple backgrounds, without which scalability would be severely limited. In short, what is needed is an agile intervention that can be easily adapted across cultures, settings, and developmental stages and does not require an undergraduate or graduate degree.

Informed by a life-course developmental framework of early childhood and development, this volume discusses an approach to child development intervention that meets the previously given criteria. This intervention was designed to allow children to thrive by enhancing a responsive and sensitive caregiving environment. It is universally accepted that sensitive and responsive caregiving leads to positive cognitive and socio-emotional outcomes for children. Therefore, several intervention approaches exist, each with its advantages and disadvantages. The current volume brings together the rationale and current evidence base for the Mediational Intervention for Sensitizing Caregivers (MISC). The MISC is a culturally and developmentally transportable intervention framework to improve caregiver-child interactions in populations who have experienced ACEs. The standard structure of MISC is a year-long video-feedback intervention. It is typically implemented by trained lay persons (MISC "trainers") without an advanced degree. Caregivers can include parents, teachers, or other caregivers (e.g. foster parents, after-school carers). Grounded in both attachment theory and theories of learning, the MISC trainer "sensitizes" the caregiver to the child's needs by using emotional (attachment-oriented) and cognitive (mediational/learning-oriented) components of adult behavior to build trust, mental flexibility, a capacity for learning, and resilience in the child. Because MISC uses everyday situations and interactions in children's lives (making a sandwich together, doing homework, playing, reading, etc.), it is highly scalable. It does not require any special workbooks, tools, or equipment.

Consistent with the primary rationale behind MISC, various global health institutions are investing in a range of parenting and educational programs to promote the development of children. Like MISC, these programs assume that investing in children do have social and economic benefits in adulthood. However, MISC differs from other programs in that it integrates aspects of socio-emotional health and cognitive development simultaneously. MISC is not instructional either but targets the "serve-and-return" between caregiver and child in real time through non-instructional means. This feature of MISC makes it less culturally intrusive than other approaches, which are developed based on Westernized ideas of caregiving. Finally, MISC is a strengths-based program complementing existing practices and cultures in caregiving rather than promoting "best practice" as if one culture or approach has privilege over another.

MISC was developed by Dr. Pina Klein in Israel. The first MISC volume was published in 1996 (Klein, 1996), which, up until the current volume was produced, constituted the most authoritative, comprehensive description of MISC. While the 1996 volume laid out the underlying theory and application of MISC, it did not necessarily include the research conducted over the last two decades in empirically evaluating MISC and/or adapting MISC to new and different contexts. In addition, while several individual peer-reviewed papers and chapters have been published on MISC, the current volume is the first compilation of MISC projects beyond the group that initially developed and evaluated the intervention. We are excited to bring together, for the first time, in one volume the theory, intervention, and training model and the most recent research evidence from the last decade supporting the MISC approach across different countries and settings. In the following, we summarize the contributions of various research and clinical applications of MISC as they are presented in the chapters that follow; and we complete the chapter with a brief discussion of future directions for MISC research and practice.

1.2 Chapter Summaries and Overview

Readers' MISC journey will begin with Chapters 2 and 3 by co-developers of the MISC, Cilly Shohet and Deborah Givon. For many years, these authors, who have worked alongside Pnina Klein, introduce the MISC interventional model (Chapter 2) and the MISC training Program (MISC-TP; Chapter 3). These two chapters lay the foundation for the chapters to follow. Therefore, it is critical that readers first read these chapters before perusing the application of the MISC model in different settings and populations. Chapter 2 introduces the basic MISC model. It explains that the acronym MISC stands for both the process and the objective of the intervention. The intervention's objective is to help children become **M**ore **I**ntelligent and **S**ocially **C**ompetent individuals. And the process through which this is achieved is through the **M**ediational **I**ntervention for **S**ensitizing **C**aregivers.

Shohet and Givon highlight that the MISC is based on the idea that specific components in an adult's behavior within adult-child interaction affect the flexibility of mind in young children, which affects a child's need and desire for learning. These components in adults' behavior include broadly two types: emotional components and cognitive components. Each chapter that follows Chapter 2 will reference these components, as they form the basic structure of the MISC intervention, as depicted in the MISC tree (see Chapter 2, Figure 2.1). Emotional components, which form the roots of the MISC tree, include eye contact, smiles, vocalization, touch, physical closeness, turn-taking, sharing of joy, expression of positive affect, synchrony, length of communication chains, and excitement expressed towards things, people, and experiences in the environment. The basic messages communicated through these emotional components are "I love you," "I'm with you," and "It's worthwhile to act" in addition to "I have time for you," "I enjoy being with you," and "I am proud of you." In the MISC model, the emotional components are necessary but not sufficient for learning ("love/attachment is not enough"), and therefore form the foundation on which the cognitive (mediational) components (the tree trunk of the MISC tree) are built. These include focusing, affecting (providing meaning), expanding, regulating, and rewarding (see Chapter 2 for a full definition and description of these components). The mediational components provide caregivers with the step-by-step know-how of how to interact with their child to slow down the interaction and mediate a child's subjective experience so that both cognitive and socio-emotional learning occurs. As conveyed in Chapter 2, what is special about MISC is that it focuses on cultural re-sensitization and the adult's capacity to elicit quality interactions as prerequisites for social-emotional and cognitive development. Put differently, MISC fosters cultural learning to take place—it allows information and knowledge to be passed on from caregiver to child in a way that it can effectively be received and trusted by the child as being in their best interest—a process captured well by the concept of epistemic trust. The concept of epistemic trust was developed by developmental psychologists (Sperber et al., 2010) and refers to an individual's willingness to consider communication conveying the knowledge from someone as trustworthy, generalizable and relevant to the self. Epistemic trust catalyzes learning (Fonagy & Allison, 2014; Sharp et al., 2021). It is a biological signal that conveys that knowledge about to be passed on is reliable since it came from a trusted source. In an attachment context of background security, an individual will be more likely to learn from their caregiver (Harris & Corriveau, 2011). Epistemic trust contributes to resilience in a child, enabling adaptation to change environments and protecting the child from developing psychopathology as he/she matures (Sharp et al., 2021).

In Chapter 3, Shohet and Givon elaborate the basic model introduced in Chapter 2 by guiding the actual training process that caregivers undergo as they become effective mediators for children in their care. Critical to understand is that the same emotional and cognitive (mediational) components are used by the MISC trainer in her caregiver training, as the caregiver uses with the child in her care. It is also the same components that a MISC supervisor uses to oversee the work of a MISC trainer. As such, the emotional and cognitive (mediational) components of MISC (the roots and the trunk of the tree) provide the glue that binds together all levels of the MISC intervention: child-to-caregiver; caregiver-to-MISC-trainer; and MISC trainer-to-MISC-supervisor. Put differently, the MISC training process refers to two parallel levels of relationships: adult–child interactions and trainer–trainee interactions. In both levels of relationships, based on the MISC interventional model, quality interactions have the same "building blocks" (emotional and cognitive components) that will result in an internalized mental change in the child, as well as in the adult (the parent, the educator, or the MISC trainer herself). This feature of MISC provides coherence and a shared language for changing the way we think about human interactions. It also has practical value. When the same components to intervene in caregiver-child interactions as are used in training and supervision are employed, consolidation of learning across levels of the MISC intervention occurs.

Chapter 4 is the first chapter in this volume to offer an example of a practical application of MISC. This chapter, written by Ravit Rozenfeld Kraft, was chosen to immediately follow from Chapters 2 and 3 because it describes the original implementation of MISC as intended by Dr. Pnina Klein and her collaborators, Cilly Shohet and Deborah Givon, in early childhood education settings in Israel in children ages birth to 3. Like Chapters 2 and 3, this chapter is somewhat foundational to all the other chapters that follow. It addresses the challenges facing the implementation of the MISC-TP principles as a training model in childcare settings. Similar challenges are faced by many other childcare settings and include challenges related to child characteristics and structural and process challenges. Challenges include, for instance, the implementation of MISC in group settings, managing individual differences in temperament and development between children, group size, level of professional training and staff qualifications, characteristics of the physical environment, working conditions, and program structure. While the program described in this chapter has never been evaluated in a randomized controlled trial, it has undergone multiple internal audits by it being delivered in Israel since the 1990s in various settings (daycare settings for infants and toddlers, pre-k, kindergarten), within various populations and various places (urban, rural). This early childhood intervention program in Israel has received financial support from both governmental and private foundations. It continues to be evaluated qualitatively as part of a report to funding bodies. As will become clear in the chapters that follow, assessing the quality of the interaction is a built-in component of the MISC intervention program. It serves as a tool for evaluating the training process and its outcomes. MISC program evaluation, therefore, occurs naturally as part of the tracking of improvement in quality caregiving. Chapter 4 provides a rich first case example of the MISC application in a real-life educational setting focused on developmental learning outcomes of children.

Chapter 5, by Ora Segal-Drori and Ofra Korat, continues on the theme of early developmental learning outcomes in children and describes how the MISC model has been applied to facilitate emergent literacy through book-reading activities with preschool children in Israel. The chapter describes a study in which 94 kindergarteners (equally divided into middle and low SES families) and their mothers participated in a mother-child book-reading interaction program. Results showed that the MISC cognitive (mediational) components correlated with children's emergent literacy in mother-child dyads from middle socio-economic groups but not low socio-economic groups. Apart from exciting comments on the effects of socio-economic status on MISC mechanisms and outcomes, this chapter illustrates the benefits of taking an everyday situation, such as reading to one's child, and turning it into a learning experience that stands to promote cognitive and socio-emotional development. Mediational actions taken by mothers during reading—including naming details and objects in the illustrations; relating the text to the illustrations; naming details in the illustrations that were not mentioned in the text; paraphrasing the text; interpreting words; discussing personal experiences; making connections beyond the text; and discussing the written language—were found to be essential components in advancing literacy in children.

Staying with the theme of enhancing early neurocognitive development in preschoolers but shifting geographical location to Africa, Chapter 6 by Monica K. Gentchev, Michael Boivin, and Sarah Murray discuss the impressive MISC research program implemented over the last decade in Uganda. The chapter describes a first pilot randomized control trial for mothers with HIV/AIDS and their preschoolers, who were HIV-infected or -affected (i.e. caregiver with HIV/AIDS or orphaned), followed by a larger cluster randomized control trial with the same population. Both studies were funded by the National Institutes of Health and therefore represented the most mature application of MISC in terms of US-based federal funding. The chapter helpfully outlines a critical battery of outcome measures that can be used to evaluate cognitive developmental outcomes in African countries, including cutting-edge eye-tracking technology. The chapter also highlights potential adaptations of MISC that mitigate the financial costs and human resources associated with the classic one-to-one delivery method of MISC and describe a skills-focused parenting program for group delivery supported with SMS technology that can efficiently and synergistically improve related maternal and infant health outcomes. The chapter also usefully describes potential future directions for MISC dissemination and implementation research, which will be essential for future scale-up efforts of MISC.

Michael J. Boivin's research group is also in the beginning phases of a MISC application to prevent konzo disease in the Democratic Republic of

Congo. Chapter 7, by Monica Gentchev, Michael Boivin, and Esperance Kashala-Abnotnes, outlines the effects of konzo on the neurodevelopment of children and discusses the implementation of the current hybrid model for community intervention utilizing the MISC to prevent konzo—a study currently underway and funded by the National Institute of Health. Of particular interest in this chapter is the innovation associated with combining a method that removes toxins from the Casava plant (the Wetting Method; WTM) with MISC. WTM has the potential to reduce the burden of konzo. However, it is labour-intensive for caregivers preparing food, so consistent and long-term adherence to the WTM may be problematic. Furthermore, it may detract from other essential daily caregiving activities for children in the home, placing them at risk neurodevelopmentally in other ways. Finally, the WTM, while effective in minimizing nutritional risk for konzo when consistently implemented, does not address other risk factors for impaired neurodevelopment of children in impoverished konzo-affected areas. The basic premise of combining WTM and MISC is that the latter will improve mothers' sensitivity to the development of their children and their emotional wellbeing and functionality, which will result in better adherence to WTM. Gentchev and colleagues helpfully lay out the rationale, implementation, and outcome assessment for implementing a hybrid WTM and MISC and illustrate the agility of MISC to be combined with existing health interventions.

In Chapter 8, we turn to a new geographic location for MISC, in addition to switching outcomes more explicitly to socio-emotional or mental health outcomes in 7–11-year-old orphan and vulnerable children (OVC). In this chapter, Carla Sharp, Madeleine Allman, Jan Cloete, and Lochner Marais describe their study, funded by the National Institute of Health, and conducted in collaboration with Michael Boivin, in which MISC was adapted and evaluated for mental health outcomes in a quasi-experimental trial. An additional innovation in this work was that the strategic point of intervention shifted from educational childcare settings (e.g. Chapter 3) and parent-child households (Chapters 4–7) to community-based organizations (CBOs). In many LMIC, CBOs offer an essential solution to the lack of a mental health workforce to address significant mental health problems associated with the impact of HIV/ AIDS on children. In this chapter, Sharp and colleagues describe how MISC was adapted for the CBO environment with mental health outcomes in mind and explicitly link the MISC model with social-cognitive function (mentalizing) due to attachment disruption associated with orphanhood.

Continuing with the theme of mental health outcomes, Chapter 9 by Nurit Jaegermann and Ornit Freudenstein, discusses the use of MISC for toddlers with sensory processing and self-regulation disorder (MISC-Sensory Processing; MISC-SP). Building on an early efficacy trial in which the effects of the MISC-SP intervention were compared to those of another intervention designed to enhance children's sensory functioning and to a control group receiving no intervention, the authors describe how MISC has been tailored specifically to address the unique challenges of children with sensory processing difficulties. The chapter elaborates how problems in arousal, attention, affect, and action can be ameliorated by more sensitive maternal behavior and supporting toddlers' communication and better regulating their behavior through the application of MISC components.

The self-regulatory functions of MISC also form the basis of the MISC adaptation discussed in Chapter 10, by Kiana Wall, Sophie Kerr, and Carla Sharp. In this chapter, the rationale and method of an ongoing study, funded by the National Institute of Mental Health, for mothers with Borderline Personality Disorder (BPD) are presented. BPD is a complex psychiatric disorder most often diagnosed in women, many of whom are mothers. Research has demonstrated that the offspring of mothers with BPD have a greater risk of poor mental health outcomes than the children of mothers without BPD, and mothers with BPD often experience more stress and lower levels of satisfaction and competency than mothers without BPD. Therefore, supportive caregiver interventions that focus on enhancing the caregiver-child relationship are important for reducing suffering for mothers with BPD, improving outcomes for their offspring, and breaking the intergenerational transmission of non–optimal caregiver-child interactions. The chapter helpfully introduces a framework for intervention adaptation, called the ADAPT-ITT model, and discusses the steps underway to adapt MISC for this population. As such, the chapter provides a helpful example of how MISC can be adapted to new settings and populations.

Chapter 11, by Itziar Familiar, describes the application of MISC in another group of vulnerable mothers and children, namely mothers who suffer from depression. While the project for borderline mothers described in Chapter 10 takes place in the United States, Familiar describes a program of research planned for maternal depression in LMIC, who may face additional and unique challenges compared to mothers in Western countries. She reviews the rich literature on the effects of maternal depression on child development and brain outcomes and mothers' own sense of self-efficacy as mothers. She builds a compelling case for adapting MISC for this context.

Chapter 12, by Venta and colleagues, transports us back to the United States and grapples with the devastating impact of the separation of caregivers and children due to migration. The authors point out that approximately 85% of the 200,000 Mexican and Central American youth who traveled to the US between 2013 and 2018 have experienced long-term separation from their parents. Once they reunify with their parents in the US, youth often undergo significant attachment distress and behavioral disturbances. Yet, there are no interventions that target the quality of the parent-child relationship during the reunification process. Their chapter discussed a study funded by an internal seed grant from their institution to use the ADAPT-ITT framework to adapt MISC for mothers and children undergoing reunification after separation and assess acceptability. Results of interviews with mothers and offspring revealed that parents are exposed to significant adversity before reunification (e.g., domestic violence) and continue to struggle with grief about having been separated from their children and stress associated with getting to know one another again. Youth also faced adversity before reunification (e.g., trauma exposure, economic instability) and reported struggling with school adaptation, continued grief associated with maternal migration in their earlier childhood, and adjustment difficulties, including missing extended family and struggling to accept rules and norms in the US. The formative work summarized in this chapter suggests that MISC is acceptable and feasible for delivery in this setting. Further adaptation may offer a behavioral approach to re-establish relational patterns that may positively affect reunification.

Chapter 13 by Brashear and colleagues describe another formative study underway to adapt MISC for yet another setting in which attachment disruption may derail the capacity to learn and thrive. Intimate Partner Violence (IPV; or domestic violence) is a highly prevalent form of trauma with devastating effects on children's educational and socio-emotional outcomes. This chapter discusses the intersectional implications of IPV for Black women, the intergenerational patterns that put IPV-exposed children at risk for later IPV perpetration and victimization, and the impacts that IPV exposure has on mothers, children, and the relationships between them. It highlights the current gaps in intervention research for mothers and children exposed to IPV and builds the rationale for MISC as an intervention that can innovatively combine the shelter work for women that typically focus on the mother's wellbeing, with the focus of Child Protective Services on child wellbeing. Current work adapting this intervention to this context is discussed, and preliminary findings from caseworkers and mothers who have experienced IPV are presented.

In Chapter 14, we change gears to consider MISC as an example of asset-based community development. In this chapter, Lochner Marais, Kholisa Rani, and Molefi Lenka describe a recent shift in community development from a needs-based approach to asset-based community development. This has occurred because a focus on needs could disempower communities and increase the need for welfare services. It can create the impression that government, business, or society can fix societal problems. In contrast, asset-based community development starts from the premise that communities can use community assets as a springboard for development. Against this background, the authors compare their experiences of implementing MISC in South African Community Based Organizations (described in Chapter 8 by Sharp and colleagues; MISC-CBO) and argue that there are substantial similarities between MISC and asset-based community development (ABCD) that required further development. They advance the argument that the overall approach to MISC allows for linking MISC and community development. They develop a framework for such integration. As such, Chapter 14 offers a blueprint for the hybrid application of MISC alongside other community development projects, similar to how and Gentchev and colleagues described a hybrid integration of MISC with existing health interventions in Chapter 7.

The volume concludes with a unique perspective provided by Motsaathebe Serekoane in Chapter 15. Serekoane is an anthropologist who served as a cultural consultant in the MISC application in South African OVC described in Chapter 7. His chapter emphasizes that even though MISC is considered a culturally transportable intervention, child-rearing and caregiving practices are embedded within local cultural structures, beliefs, and practices, despite the emergence of 20th-century idealism of global culture. Consistent with the community participatory research framework, Serekoane emphasizes the need for a negotiated and situated conceptual practice model that is responsive to contextual nuances to enhance acceptability and sustainable use. Drawing from the South African MISC project, this chapter presents valuable discernment emerging from the consideration of "culture" and "context", aided by forging a partnership with a community advisory board, with specific comment on how culture and context may influence MISC components.

1.3 Conclusion

We are excited to welcome readers to join us on the MISC journey we have collectively enjoyed over the last several decades. We hope that this volume will stimulate further research evaluating additional adaptations of the MISC approach. And we also hope that this volume will provide an important foundation for those wishing to implement MISC in their clinical, educational, or community-based settings. As such, this volume is appropriate for those working in educational and/or clinical settings where individuals are tasked with intervening or developing policy to ensure optimal child developmental outcomes. Therefore, the volume is appropriate for professionals from a wide variety of disciplines, including clinical, counselling and educational psychology, psychiatry, paediatrics, nursing, social work, education, and public health. The volume is also appropriate for researchers working in these disciplines as the following chapters reflect the ongoing or completed federally and foundation-funded MISC research projects. Beyond the interest in the MISC intervention specifically, we also believe that this volume will be of interest to anyone who wishes to advocate for a paradigm shift in early child development, which, in our view, has come to rely too heavily on instructional, quick-fix options based on psychoeducation, with uncertain long-term impact. This volume will invite readers to reconsider an alternative approach to these mainstream approaches by bringing together the evidence across multiple settings to support such a paradigm shift. Consistent with the MISC ethos, we believe that changing the basic caregiving environment takes time and energy and should be prioritized. In the same way that we invest millions of dollars in math and reading literacy, we advocate for similar, if not more investment, in the literacy of interaction—the serve-and-return between caregiver and child. The sky is the limit.

References

Centers for Disease Control (CDC). (2018). *Social determinants of health*. Retrieved June 19, 2018, from www.cdc.gov/socialdeterminants/index.htm. Published February 15, 2018.

Fonagy, P., & Allison, E. (2014). The role of mentalizing and epistemic trust in the therapeutic relationship. *Psychotherapy, 51*, 372–380.

Fuller-Rowell, T. E., Curtis, D. S., Chae, D. H., & Ryff, C. D. (2018). Longitudinal health consequences of socioeconomic disadvantage: Examining perceived discrimination as a mediator. *Health Psychology, 37*(5), 491–500.

Garner, A. S., Shonkoff, J. P. et al. (2012). Early childhood adversity, toxic stress, and the role of the pediatrician: Translating developmental science into lifelong health. *Pediatrics, 129*(1), e224–e231.

Harris, P. L., & Corriveau, K. H. (2011). Young children's selective trust in informants. *Philosophical Transactions of the Royal Society of London. Series B, Biological Sciences, 366*, 1179–1187.

Klein, P. S. (1996). *Early intervention: Cross-cultural experiences with a mediational approach*. Oxford: Routledge.

Sharp, C., Kulesz, P., Marais, L., Shohet, C., Rani, K., Lenka, M., . . . Boivin, M. (2021). Mediational Intervention for Sensitizing Caregivers to improve mental health outcomes in orphaned and vulnerable children. *Journal of Clinical Child and Adolescent Psychology, 49*(4), 545–557.

Sharp, C., Shohet, C., Givon, D., Penner, F., Marais, L., & Fonagy, P. (2021). Learning to mentalize: A mediational approach for caregivers and therapists. *Clinical Psychology: Science and Practice, 27*(3), 1–17.

Sperber, D., Clement, F., Heintz, C., Mascaro, O., Mercier, H., Origgi, G., & Wilson, D. (2010). Epistemic vigilance. *Mind and Language, 25*, 359–393.

2 An Introduction to the MISC Interventional Model

Cilly Shohet and Deborah Givon

2.1 Background and Rationale for the MISC

The future of any society depends on its ability to foster the next generation's health and well-being. Today's children will become tomorrow's citizens, workers, and parents. When we fail to provide children with what they need to build a strong foundation for healthy and productive lives, we put our future prosperity and security at risk (National Scientific Council on the Developing Child, 2007). Young children's growth and development are profoundly shaped by the opportunities for learning, education, economic resources, and interactions provided by adults—whether they encounter these adults in home, out-of-homecare, or community contexts (Thematic Group on Early Childhood Development, Education, and Transition to Work, 2014).

The development of children is a highly complex process that is influenced by the interplay of genetic and environmental factors. Accumulating evidence reveals that the relationship between heredity and environment is not a one-way path from genes to environment to behavior. Instead, it is bidirectional: genes affect children's behavior and experiences; experiences and behavior affect gene expression (Gottlieb, 2000). These processes are expressed in the brain architecture, composed of highly integrated sets of neural circuits. These circuits are hard-wired under the continuous and mutual influences of genetics and environment. Genes determine when specific brain circuits are formed and individual experiences then shape how that information unfolds (National Scientific Council on the Developing Child, 2007).

Early experiences create the foundations for life-long learning, behavior, and both physical and mental health. A strong foundation in the early years increases the probability of positive outcomes, and a weak foundation increases the odds of later difficulty (National Scientific Council on the Developing Child, 2007).

There is a consensus supporting the idea that early intervention can change and have lasting and valuable effects on young children's development and well-being. This is especially true during the *sensitive period* of rapid brain development and learning, and the formation of caregiver-child attachment that characterizes children under three years. However, since the

DOI: 10.4324/9781003145899-2

capacity to be modified due to new learning is a characteristic of human beings throughout their entire lifecycle, even adults or older people change following life experiences (Klein, 1996; Lifshitz & Klein, 2011; Lifshitz, 2020). Although it is possible to affect children's behavior even at a later age, it is probably more rewarding, easier, and more economical in terms of time and effort to begin early in infancy, to prevent difficulties, rather than engage in correcting them (Black et al., 2017; Heckman, Moon, Pinto, Savelyev, & Yavitz, 2010; Klein, Shohet, & Givon, 2018).

Despite general agreement regarding the need and importance of early interventions for at-risk young children, there is no consensus regarding criteria for quality early intervention programs. The MISC interventional model provides a clear framework for identifying and quantifying the emotional and cognitive processes that young children experience within their human environment vis-à-vis what they need for optimal development in a rapidly changing world. The MISC interventional model is based on the knowledge that the environment has an immense effect on children's development. One of the environmental factors that seems to have a dominant role in the developmental interplay between heredity and environment is the quality of human relationships and care experienced by children (Ainsworth, Blehar, Waters, & Wall, 1978; Phillips & Shonkoff, 2000). Children's early development requires nurturing care, defined as health, nutrition, security and safety, responsive caregiving, and early learning—provided by parents and family interactions and supported by an environment that enables these interactions (Black et al., 2017).

Parents and caregivers around the globe share a common interest: to enhance the well-being and the emotional, social, cognitive, and physical development of children who are under their care. Development is a process that includes growth, maturation, and learning. There is an unresolved professional debate among theoreticians, researchers, and professionals, of what is the relationship between learning and development in children. The Vygotskian position is one in which learning and development are neither separate nor identical processes. Instead, they combine in a complex, interrelated fashion (Berk & Winsler, 2002). Following Vygotsky's theory (1978), according to Feuerstein's theory of cognitive modifiability (1979), learning is a process in which an individual is modified through interaction with his environment. It is a basic process of adjustment and socialization in all societies and cultures.

An individual can be modified through interaction with his environment in two basic ways: the first occurs due to direct exposure to stimuli; the second occurs with the assistance and guidance of an "expert". Children learn through both ways, and both are important for their development. An adult can assist a child's learning process in different modes. Questions that might arise about the adult's teaching modes are: *What would be an optimal mode of a teaching-learning process? Do all adult-child interactions are equally contributive to differential cognitive development?* The MISC represents an educational approach, the MLE (Mediated Learning Experience) (Feuerstein, 1979,

1980) grounded in the theoretical framework of Cognitive Modifiability, and defines intelligence as the capacity of an organism to use previous experiences for future learning. According to the MLE approach, an optimal learning process occurs when the adult serves as a *mediator* between the environment and the child, preparing and reinterpreting stimuli from the environment to become meaningful and relevant for the child. The mediator takes an active role in making components of the environment compatible with the child's needs, interests, and capacities (Feuerstein & Feuerstein, 1991; Klein, 2000; Vigotsky, 1978). The MLE approach and the MISC model are based on the understanding that child development (both social-emotional and cognitive) is deeply influenced by the caregiver, and by the *quality of interactions* between him/her and the developing child. Through the suggested model, parents, caregivers, and teachers are helped to recognize and understand how they affect the child's development. They learn to identify a set of components that characterizes the adult's behavior during an adult-child interaction, which may turn the interaction into an enriching learning experience for the child. Since these components may be identified within any existing child-rearing practices, the MISC model is suitable for cross-cultural adaptation. As this book will attest, research suggests that mediated learning experiences affect *flexibility* of children's minds and consequently promote their mental and emotional development. According to the MISC model, flexibility of mind serves as a disposition for learning from new experiences that children may encounter within their traditional cultural setting or confront in the constant changing world.

2.2 The MISC Model

"MISC" stands for both the objective and the process of the intervention. The objective is More Intelligent and Sensitive (socially competent) Children. This is what most parents and educators want for young children to develop properly and to adjust to life. "MISC" also stands for the process of the intervention: Mediational Intervention for Sensitizing Caregivers. Through the process of sensitizing, parents, caregivers, and teachers become more aware and sensitive to their behavioral components in their interactions with children and the effects of the quality of their interactions on children's development. The MISC model consists of three basic "building blocks" that lay the ground for understanding and assessing adult-child interactions: cultural-environmental, emotional, and cognitive. Each of these consists of specific components affecting adult-child interaction.

2.2.1 Culture and Environment

Environmental factors make up the physical, social, and attitudinal environment in which people live and conduct their lives. They can act as facilitator or barrier to child development (de Kleijn-de Vrankrijker & Ten Napel,

2017). In infancy and early childhood, children are most susceptible to environmental effects. One significant factor that defines children's environment is *culture*. All cultures include specified traditions, customs and attitudes, beliefs, goals, and values. Culture has a strong effect on parents' and educators' values, assumptions, educational philosophy, and perception of the child and their role in children's lives (Klein, 2000).

There are cross-cultural differences in parental philosophy of child-rearing or perception of their child's development (Keller et al., 2004). However, the most dramatic differences appear in parents' view of the "ideal child", and consequently their objectives for the child (Klein, 1996). In addition to the socio-cultural effects on parents' view of their child, parents' perceptions of themselves as effective agents in child development, their styles of coping with their life stresses, their support systems, and their life experiences must be taken into serious consideration in an attempt to understand and affect parental mediation to the child. It should be noted that the factor of cultural impact on parental behavior is especially dramatic in populations of children at risk for environmental causes and genetic or other physiological risk factors.

Based on their cultural perceptions and educational philosophy, parents typically carry *short-term* and *long-term objectives* for the children they care for; both are important in the educational process. Short-term objectives refer to specific skills or knowledge, which the adult aims to provide the child with, in the present. Long-term objectives are associated with plans or educational objectives of child-rearing; either caregivers are aware of it, or not (Klein, 1996). One of the major challenges in applying research and practical knowledge on upbringing practices and child development, in different cultures, is related to the major differences in culturally based orientations to child development and socialization. Socialization is the critical process in the upbringing of children, a process through which the child internalizes and adjusts behavior to norms, values, and ways of living in the family, society, and culture. The orientations to the upbringing of children, to cultural values and traditions, are central to this model.

The MISC interventional model fits in with the family's cultural background and does not depend upon importing external methods, ideas, and tools, since it operates inside the existing child-rearing practices. It is built on collaboration with caregivers, and relates to the caregivers' functioning and resources, within the social and cultural context. Its approach is not instructive, but rather a support for the caregiver to discover his or her own resources or potentials for enhancing the child's development in a better way through improved experiences in daily life. This collaboration "from within" allows parents and caregivers to preserve their values and beliefs regarding child-rearing, while becoming aware of their qualitative behavioral components during their interaction with the child, through a process of conceptualization of those components. A careful assessment of cultural and psychological variables should constitute a major prerequisite of any early intervention, especially in cross-cultural intervention programs, because of the dramatic effects of these variables on the quality and style of parental interaction with their children.

2.2.2 Emotional Components in Adult–Child Interaction

The emotional and cognitive development of young children is closely related and interdependent. In theory and practice, the two areas of development must be addressed concurrently. Experts in child development emphasize the importance of making children aware that they are accepted and loved, and the importance of positive affect on learning. In the MISC model, the intricate interplay between the emotional and cognitive aspects of learning is addressed and recognized.

Emotions, positive and negative, have an enormous effect on the development of young children. The effect is not limited to the behavior occurring during an actual interaction with an adult. Its effect may be accumulative and make a real impact on brain development through secreting chemicals and hormones (Panksepp, 2003; Schore, 2001). To ensure children's healthy intellectual development—i.e., satisfy their curiosity, urge to explore their environment, and relate to others—children need to have a warm, stable, and secure relationship, with a least one other person. Numerous studies have highlighted the importance of close physical contact and expressions of love, sensitivity, and responsiveness, leading to secure attachment (Ainsworth et al., 1978; Cassidy, 2000; Hazan, Campa, & Gur-Yaish, 2013; Rosenblum & Muzik, 2018). According to the MISC interventional model, positive emotions expressed by the adult lay the basis for quality adult-child interactions and serve as a bridge to learning and intellectual development.

Features of the MISC model can be represented using the metaphor of a **tree** (see Figure 2.1). The roots of the tree represent the basic elements constituting expressions of love and positive affect towards the child. These are regarded as the "ABC of love". Affect variables relate to the type and intensity of emotional expressions, manifested in the interaction: positive and negative emotions of different intensity. Positive affect can be expressed in various behaviors, each impacting the child's emotional state and well-being.

Smiles: A smile is a human signal expressing positive affect, which arouses social interaction from the very beginning of child development.

Eye Contact: A basic component of any human interaction that involves at least two people communicating and is regarded as a meaningful nonverbal way of communication.

Turn-taking: A fundamental innate component in any human interaction. Since the brain is a social organ, even newborns express the ability to maintain short back-and-forth facial signals, an ability that develops through social interactions with their environment. The ability to maintain turn-taking within an interaction requires being sensitive and responsive to the other's initiatives.

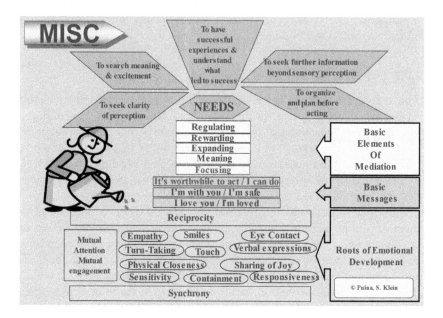

Figure 2.1 The MISC tree

Sensitivity: The ability to "read" (or to be alert to) the other's signals, gestures, or verbal expressions.

Responsiveness: Acting upon the signals, gestures, or verbal expressions of another person. Sensitivity and responsiveness are basic requirements for human relationships and interactions.

Physical closeness and **touch**: Two physical behaviors that reflect positive emotional affect and create an atmosphere of emotional closeness.

Verbal expressions: Human interaction consists of verbal and non-verbal communication. Children develop language and communication skills through experiences with their social environment. Communicating with children verbally and non-verbally and having a conversation with them affects their emotional and cognitive development and sense of self.

Empathy: The ability to understand and share the feelings of another.

Containment: A state in which another person takes the emotional experience of the child, modulates it in him/herself, and conveys to the child an understanding of these emotions in a "digested" form. Then, contained emotions are no longer so difficult to bear; one can say they are "detoxified" and need not be overwhelming.

Synchrony: An optimal timing of the adult's behaviors in the process of interaction with the child. It occurs when the adult is conscious and able to "read" the child's behavior, facial expressions, or body language and respond and match, moment to moment, their own behavior to that of the child.

The existence of positive, warm, responsive, and reciprocal behaviors paves the road for mutual attention and mutual engagement and enables two-way communication between the partners in the interaction. Initiating and maintaining communication exchanges with the child is a goal of itself and a ground for continued mediational interaction. During the developmental process, children experience a wide range of positive and negative feelings. However, quality interactions with young children are usually characterized by positive affect, which, as opposed to a stressful interaction, may create openness for learning and social interactions.

In the tree metaphor of the MISC interventional model (see Figure 2.1), the "soil", in which the tree grows, represents the partners' cultural background in an interaction. The roots of the tree are nourished by values, beliefs, and rules of the culture, and by basic conceptions of child-rearing, the image of the "ideal parent or caregiver", the "ideal child", and long-term educational objectives for the child's development and well-being.

As part of the attempts to enhance the roots of the mediational process, according to the MISC model, the adult has to ensure that each child receives three basic messages during the interaction with the child: 1. "I love you," conveying to the child that he or she is important and loved (rather than worthless); 2. "I am with you," conveying the message that he or she is secure and supported, and can initiate new explorations in the environment (as opposed to insecurity and fear to act); 3. "It is worthwhile to act," conveying the message that the environment responds to the child's actions and that good or interesting things may happen (as opposed to learning to be passive and acquire "learned helplessness"). Love is very important for adequate psychological development. However, having loving, caring, affectionate, positive, and containing caregiving does not guarantee a child's intellectual development. Love opens the gate for learning and mental development, but does not in itself determine what will pass through the gate.

2.2.3 Cognitive (Mediational) Components in Adult-Child Interaction

In today's rapidly changing world, one can hardly predict the situations that a child will be required to cope with in the future. Under such conditions, preparing a young person for future development must include provisions for developing flexibility of mind, which is a predisposition for learning from new experiences.

Flexibility of mind cannot be defined merely by the quantity or variety of content areas acquired by the child, but rather by the action patterns, needs, or "appetites" the child acquires for modes of perception, elaboration, and expression. These will enable him/her to learn from new experiences and become a more intelligent, sensitive, and socially adjusted person.

Several basic characteristics of adults' behavior, necessary to create positive mediated learning experiences for children, were identified and described by Feuerstein (Feuerstein, 1979, 1980; Feuerstein, Rand, & Rynders, 1988). Klein (1988, 1991, 1996; Klein & Alony, 1993) empirically defined five basic adult behavioral components that can turn any adult-child inter-action into an enriching learning (mediational) experience for the child. The identified behaviors were found to be significantly related to children's learning processes in their early years, and consequently to their cognitive and social-emotional behavior (Klein & Alony, 1993; Klein & Rye, 2004; Nir-Gal & Klein, 2004, Schiff & Rosenthal, 2005; Tzuriel, 1999; Tzuriel & Caspi, 2017).

As distinct from direct learning, mediational learning occurs when the environment is interpreted for the child by another person. It is an *inten-tional*, *reciprocal*, and *active* process—a process in which the adult develops consciousness of his/her actions during the interaction with the child. The conscious and sensitive adult will ask himself: "What are the behaviors in my interaction with the child that will enhance the child's emotional and cog-nitive development and increase flexibility of mind and the ability to learn effectively from new experiences?" Mediational learning is a dynamic pro-cess of *matching*, moment to moment, to the child's behaviors and character-istics. Being familiar with the child's personal characteristics (i.e., the child's temperament, her sensory sensitivity, her age and developmental stage, her attention span, etc.), and being mindful to the child's behaviors and cues (i.e., the child's physical and emotional state, her interest and engagement in the activity, her alertness, etc.), all are a prerequisite for obtaining a quality mediational interaction.

In addition to the ABC of love, and the basic messages, the tree metaphor includes five essential cognitive components that characterize any mediational teaching behavior, depicted as the trunk of the MISC tree (see Figure 2.1).

Focusing. Any adult's act or sequence of acts that appears to be directed towards focusing a child's attention and achieving a change in the child's perception, or response (e.g., selecting, exaggerating, grouping, sequencing, or pacing stimuli).

Focusing may be expressed verbally, non-verbally, or in a combined manner.

Providing meaning (affecting). Any adult's behavior expressing mean-ing, excitement, appreciation, or affect, verbally or non-verbally, in relation to people, objects, animals, or concepts and values.

Expanding. Any adult's behavior directed towards the broadening of a child's cognitive awareness, beyond the immediate experience (e.g., explain-ing, relating to past and future, relating to cause and effect, reasoning, com-paring, making analogies, rules, WH questions).

Rewarding (mediated feelings of competence). Any adult's verbal or non-verbal behavior expressing satisfaction with a child's behavior, intend-ing to encourage the child. A more effective rewarding is expressed verbally with the adult's identification of specific components of the child's behavior, which the adult considers as successful. In addition, breaking a task into smaller components or making it easier for the child allows the child to experience success, and be rewarded by the adult.

Regulation of behavior. Any adult's behavior that models, demonstrates, and/or verbally suggests to the child how to do things better in relation to the specific requirements of a task, or to any other cognitive process required prior or during an overt action (e.g., modelling, sequencing, planning, matching speed and intensity to the task).

It is important to note that for the adult's behaviors in the interaction to be considered mediational, there must be a clear indication of the adult's intentionality to engage the child, and a child's clear behavior that indicates responsiveness. However, sometimes interactions are initiated by children. In this case, the child shows an attempt to draw the adults' attention, and the adult must be sensitive and responsive to these attempts.

Many differences between children in their capacity to benefit from new experiences are linked to the type of interaction they had with adults who cared for them. These differences are apparent in the way these children approach new experiences, in the way they express themselves, in the way they explore their environment, how much they are interested in what they see, hear, smell, in the way they are enthusiastic or involved in what is going on around them (Klein, Shohet, & Givon, 2017; Tzuriel & Shomron, 2018).

One of the basic differences between the MISC and other early intervention programs is related to its objectives. While many programs aim primarily to affect social-emotional or cognitive skills and processes, the prime objective of the MISC is to affect a child's *need system*, to create new, more differentiated needs that will promote his or her future capacity for learning. Merely bringing a child into contact with new experiences will not help him or her develop a differentiated "taste" or need for them. Through human mediation, an infant or a young child learns to need and seek deeper understandings and achieve skills, which will lead him/her to a better adaptation to the constantly changing world.

In the MISC tree metaphor (see Figure 2.1), the branches represent a set of needs and dispositions for learning that a mediator aims to reach through on-going quality mediational interactions.

The following are the basic cognitive and social-emotional needs fostered by quality mediation:

- The need to seek clarity of perception;
- The need to search for meaning and excitement;
- The need to seek further information beyond sensory perception;
- The need to have successful experiences and understand what led to success; and
- The need to organize and plan before acting

In Table 2.1, we summarize the contribution of each cognitive (mediational) component to the child's need system.

Table 2.1 MISC program: cognitive and social-emotional needs in relation to mediation

Cognitive (Mediational) Components	Examples	Cognitive Needs	Social-Emotional Needs
1. Focusing Any adult's act or sequence of acts that appears to be directed towards focusing a child's attention and achieving a change in the child's perception or response.	"Look!" "See that!" "Let's see it." "Listen," "Feel it," "Touch it." Pointing, moving objects closer to the child, changing the volume of sounds, clearing the environment from stimuli that may distract the child's attention, exaggerating the size, or intensity of something.	Need for precision in perception (vs. scanning exploration). Need for precision in expression.	Need to focus on and decode facial and body expressions of emotion. Need to modify one's own behavior or the environment in order to mediate to others (to make the other person see or understand).
2. Providing Meaning (Affecting) Any adult's behavior expressing meaning, excitement, appreciation, or affect, verbally or non-verbally, in relation to people, objects, animals, or concepts and values	"This is a serious storm." "I see that you are happy . . ." "I see that you are digging a big hole . . ." "You are a good friend . . ." Wow! OH! Mmmm . . . Shsh. . . . Facial expressions of delight, anger, sadness, or gestures like touching, caressing, smiling, shedding tears.	Need to search for meaningful new experiences. Need to respond in a way that conveys meaning and excitement. Need to invest energy in meaningful activities.	Need to think about one's own feelings and the feeling of others.
3. Expanding Any adult's behavior directed towards the broadening of a child's cognitive awareness, beyond the immediate experience	"The beans must be soaked in water for a few hours to get soft enough for cooking." "This flower blooms in the spring only." "How do we solve this problem?" "What do you think about it?" "You are feeling sad because your friend insulted you in front of the whole group. "Yesterday when we came to the community center it didn't rain heavily like today."	Need to go beyond what meets the senses. Seek out further information through exploration. Request information from other people and from other sources. Need to seek generalizations. Need to link, to associate, to recall past information and anticipate future experiences.	Need to understand cause and effect sequences in social interaction. Need to associate between experiences, to recall past information and anticipate future experiences.

Component	Example		
4. Rewarding Any adult's verbal or non-verbal behavior expressing satisfaction with a child's behavior, intending to encourage the child. Identification of specific components of the child's behavior that the adult considers as successful. Breaking a task into smaller components to allow success	"Good", "Great", "Fine", "O.K.". Clapping hands, smiling. "Very good, you were a great helper in arranging the classroom". "I am proud of you! You were generous to your friend and helped him solve the problem."	Need to seek more success in experiences. Need to summarize one's own activities and determine what led to success	Need to please others and gain more mediated feelings of competence. Need to identify what pleases different people. Need to provide others with mediated feelings of competence.
5. Regulation of Behavior Any adult's behavior that models, demonstrates, and/or verbally suggests to the child how to do things better in relation to the specific requirements of a task, or to any other cognitive process required prior or during an overt action	"Look at me. I'll show you how to do it . . ." "This is the base; we'll start with it, so that the building that we are building will be stable." "Try to be careful and not press too hard, because the paper is thin and it might tear."	Need to plan before acting, to consider possible solutions prior to responding. Clarifying goals, meeting subgoals. Need to pace one's activities. Need to regulate the level of energy invested in any given task.	Need to control one's impulses in social situations. Need to adopt acceptable ways of expressing one's emotions

The MISC model is grounded in recognition of the powerful effect of adult-child interactions on children's development. The model presents a broad conception of adult-child interactions: social-emotional, communicational, cognitive, environmental, and developmental aspects. A human interaction is an event where two or more people communicate with or react to each other. From a communicational point of view, according to the MISC model, quality interactions include well-synchronized communication chains; i.e., both partners initiate or respond in accordance with the other partner in good timing. Quality interactions characteristically include long chains of communication, i.e., longer back-and-forth responses of one partner to the other's behavior, in an atmosphere of *positive affect* (as opposed to a stressful interaction) that sets the stage for continued mediation. The two partners in a quality interaction—the adult and the child—are equal partners in the interaction. However, the adult is the one who is responsible for matching his initiations and responses to the child's, and for keeping a sequence of communication exchanges throughout the mediational interaction with the child.

The model's structure represented in this chapter enables experts to evaluate and assess the "mental diet" that the child receives throughout any interaction. "Mental diet" refers to the emotional and cognitive "ingredients" that the child is provided with throughout the interaction, just like caring for the nutritious balance of the alimentation provided to the child. In the long run, a balanced and rich "mental diet" enhances the child's cognitive and socio-emotional development, and prepares him or her to benefit from future learning. To assess emotional and cognitive components systematically, researchers and trainers may use the observational measure developed for the MISC intervention called the Observing Mediational Interaction (OMI; Klein, 2014). The OMI makes use of real-life video recordings of the caregiver-child interactions that are the focus of the intervention, and codes blow-by-blow events and utterances as they occur, thereby allowing a profile of positive, sensitive, and responsive interactions, as well as negative and unresponsive interactions, to be summarized quantitatively and visually through graphs. The original validation study of the OMI was conducted by Klein, Wieder, and Greenspan (1987) in a sample of mother-child dyads across varying age ranges. It demonstrated good interrater reliability and criterion validity through cross-sectional and prospective relations with child outcomes. In addition, caregiver behavior rated using the MISC components was relatively stable over a four-year follow-up.

2.3 Conclusion: The Sky Is the Limit

The essence of the MISC interventional model is sensitization and awareness-raising of adults (parents, caregivers, and teachers) regarding the characteristics of their interactions with the children they care for. In practice, it requires adults caring for children to develop sensitivity and a practical understanding of each child's needs, abilities, and behavior, vis-à-vis their own behavior in the interaction. The process that parents, caregivers, and teachers go through during the intervention empowers and enables them to be more efficient, sensitive, and responsive, and provide children with an appropriate enriching "mental diet".

Since the MISC interventional model is focused on the quality of interaction between the caregiver and the child, and not on the content or the material used in the interaction, it is not a "program" in the traditional sense. It is more a framework, a model or method for sensitizing parents or caregivers to the positive aspects of their existing daily interactions with the children, within their child-rearing objectives and practices.

The intervention has been implemented with various groups of children, in various contexts where interaction takes place, from home, nursery, and preschool to large-scale community-based projects, involving local resource persons who are trained to implement the intervention with caregivers (Boivin et al., 2013a, 2013b; Penner et al., 2020; Klein, 2001; Sharp et at., 2021). In addition, it has been used cross-culturally with different groups of children, including very poor children in six cultures (Klein, 1996), children with sensory processing and regulatory disorders (Jaegermann & Klein, 2010), children with Down Syndrome (Klein, Japha, & Rosenthal, 2010), as well as gifted children (Klein & Tannenbaum, 1992), HIV-exposed children, and children with human immunodeficiency virus (Boivin et al., 2013a, 2013b; Penner et al., 2020).

Despite these differences in target groups, the MISC interventional model includes a structured aspect of implementation, common to all target groups. This aspect relates to the procedure of the intervention's implementation process, carried out by the MISC trainers. In addition, the model includes an unstructured aspect that allows cultural interpretations of the model's objectives within various contexts, in which the MISC components are implemented. The intervention is carried out through regular training sessions based on video guidance of adult-child interactions. Chapter 3 will expand on the training model designated for parents, caregivers, and educators, in light of the MISC's basic objectives, and elaborate on its possible implementation modes.

In the chapters that follow, the contributing authors to this volume will show the impact that MISC has had across settings, cultures, developmental epochs, and various adverse childhood experiences that challenge the capacity for resilience. The MISC's objective is based on an optimistic approach to human development and human modifiability. Therefore, the unfolded message to the adults who care for children is that "*the sky is the limit*": every child can do more with an adult's appropriate support.

References

Ainsworth, M. D. S., Blehar, M. C., Waters, E., & Wall, S. (1978). *Patterns of attachment.* Hillsdale, NJ: Erlbaum.

Berk, E., & Winsler, A. (2002). *Scaffolding children's learning. Vygotsky and early childhood education.* Washington, DC: National Association for the Education of Young Children.

Black, M. M., Walker, S. P., Fernald, L., Andersen, C. T., DiGirolamo, A. M., Lu, C., . . . Lancet Early Childhood Development Series Steering Committee (2017). Early childhood development coming of age: Science through the life course. *Lancet, 389*(10064), 77–90.

Boivin, M. J., Bangirana, P., Nakasujja, N., Page, C. F., Shohet, C., Givon, D., Bass, J. K., Popka, R. O., & Klein, P. (2013b). A year-long caregiver training program improves cognition in preschool Ugandan children with human immunodeficiency virus. *The Journal of Pediatrics, 163*(5), 1409–1416.

Boivin, M. J., Bangirana, P., Page, C. F., Shohet, C., Givon, D., Bass, J. K., Opoka, R. O., Nakasujja, N., & Klein, P. S. (2013a). A year-long caregiver training program to improve neurocognition in preschool ugandan HIV-exposed children. *Journal of Behavioral & Developmental Pediatrics, 34,* 269–278.

Cassidy, J. (2000). The complexity of the caregiving system: A perspective from attachment theory. *Psychological Inquiry, 11*(2), 86–91.

de Kleijn-de Vrankrijker, M. W., & Ten Napel, H. (2017). *Environmental factors: Classification and measurement expert meeting.* WHO Collaborating Centre FIC in the Netherlands. https://unstats.un.org/unsd/demographic-social/meetings/2017/new-york-disability-egm/Session%206/UNSD.pdf

Feuerstein, R. (1979). *The dynamic assessment of retarded performers.* New York: University Park Press.

Feuerstein, R. (1980). *Instrumental enrichment: Redevelopment of cognitive functions of retarded performers.* New York: University Park Press.

Feuerstein, R., & Feuerstein, S. (1991). Mediated learning experience. In R. Feuerstein, P. Klein, & A. Tannenabaum (Eds.), *Mediated learning experience: Theoretical, psychosocial, and social implications* (pp. 3–52). Tel Aviv: Freund Publishing House.

Feuerstein, R., Rand, Y., & Rynders, J. E. (1988). Mediated learning experience. In *Don't accept me as I am* (pp. 59–93). Boston, MA: Springer.

Gottlieb, G. (2000). Environmental and behavioral influences on gene activity. *Current Directions in Psychological Science, 9,* 93–97.

Hazan, C., Campa, M., & Gur-Yaish, N. (2013). Attachment across the lifespan. In P. Noller & J. A. Feeney (Eds.), *Close relationships: Functions, forms and processes* (pp. 189–209). Hove: Psychology Press.

Heckman, J. J., Moon, S. H., Pinto, R., Savelyev, P. A., & Yavitz, A. (2010). The rate of return to the HighScope perry preschool program. *Journal of Public Economics, 94*(1–2), 114–128.

Jaegermann, N., & Klein, P. S. (2010). Enhancing mothers' interactions with toddlers who have sensory-processing disorders. *Infant Mental Health Journal, 31*(3), 291–311.

Keller, H., Lohaus, A., Kuensemueller, P., Abels, M., Yovsi, R., Voelker, S., . . . Mohite, P. (2004). The bio culture of parenting: Evidence from five cultural communities. *Parenting Science and Practice, 4,* 1.

Klein, P. S. (1988). Stability and change in interaction of Israeli mothers and infants. *Infant Behavior and Development, 11*(1), 55–70.

Klein, P. S. (1991). Improving the quality of parental interaction with very low birth weight children: A longitudinal study using a mediated learning experience model. *Infant Mental Health Journal, 12*(4), 321–337.

Klein, P. S. (1996). *Early intervention: Cross cultural experiences with a mediational approach.* New York: Garland Publications.

Klein, P. S. (2000). A developmental mediation approach to early intervention: Mediational intervention for sensitizing caregivers (MISC). *Educational and Child Psychology*, *17*(3), 19–31.

Klein, P. S. (Ed.). (2001). *Seeds of hope: Twelve years of early intervention in Africa*. Oslo: Unipub forlag.

Klein, P. S. (2014). *OMI—observing mediational interaction Manual*. Unpublished manuscript.

Klein, P. S., Adi Japha, E., & Rosenthal, V. (2010). Maternal teaching behavior and pre-verbal development of children with Down syndrome and typical developing children. *Down Syndrome Research and Practice*. doi:10.3104/reports.2105.

Klein, P. S., & Alony, S. (1993). Immediate and sustained effects of maternal mediation behaviors in infancy. *Journal of Early Intervention*, *71*(2), 177–193.

Klein, P. S., & Rye, H. (2004). Interaction-oriented early intervention in Ethiopia: The MISC approach. *Infants & Young Children*, *17*(4), 340–354.

Klein, P. S., Shohet, C., & Givon, D. (2017). A mediational intervention for sensitizing caregivers (MISC): A cross-cultural early intervention. In A. Abubakar, & F. Van de Vijver (Eds.). *Handbook of applied developmental Science in sub-saharan Africa* (pp. 291–312). New York: Springer.

Klein, P. S., & Tannenbaum, A. J. (1992). *To be young and gifted*. Norwood: Ablex Publishing Corp.

Klein, P. S., Wieder, S., & Greenspan, S. I. (1987). A theoretical overview and empirical study of mediated learning experience: Prediction of preschool performance from mother-infant interaction patterns. *Infant Mental Health Journal*, *8*(2), 110–129.

Lifshitz, H. (2020). *Growth and development in adulthood in persons with intellectual disability: New frontiers in theory, research, and intervention*. Cham, Switzerland: Springer Nature.

Lifshitz, H., & Klein, P. (2011). Mediation between staff and elderly persons with intellectual disability with Alzheimer Disease as a means of enhancing their daily functioning. *Education and Training in Autism and Developmental Disabilities*, *46*(1), 106–115.

National Scientific Council on the Developing Child. (2007). *The science of early childhood development: Closing the gap between what we know and what we do*. Retrieved from www.developingchild.harvard.edu.

Nir-Gal, O., & Klein, P. S. (2004). Computers for cognitive development in early child-hood—the teacher's role in the computer learning environment. *Information Technology in Childhood Education Annual*, *2004*(1), 97–119.

Panksepp, J. (2003). At the interface of the affective, behavioral, and cognitive neuro-sciences: Decoding the emotional feelings of the brain. *Brain and Cognition*, *52*(1), 4–14.

Penner, F., Sharp, C., Marais, L., Shohet, C., Givon, D., & Boivin, M. (2020). Community based caregiver and family interventions to support the mental health of orphans and vulnerable children: Review and future directions. In M. Tan (Ed.), HIV and Childhood: Growing up Affected by HIV. *New Directions for Child and Adolescent Development*, *2020*(171), 77–105.

Phillips, D. A., & Shonkoff, J. P. (Eds.). (2000). *From neurons to neighborhoods: The science of early childhood development*. Washington, DC: National Academies Press.

Rosenblum, K. L., & Muzik, M. (2018). Infant social-emotional development. Emerging competence in a relational context. In C. H. Zeanah (Ed.), *Handbook of infant mental health* (pp. 103–125). Milton Keynes: Guilford Publications.

Schiff, R., & Rosenthal, V. (2005). *A first-grade reading intervention program: The effects of teacher-pupil interactions and meta-cognitive strategies on reading achievement*. Paper presented at the International Association for Cognitive Education and Psychology (IACEP) Conference, Durham University, Durham.

Schore, A. N. (2001). Effects of a secure attachment relationship on right brain development, affect regulation, and infant mental health. *Infant Mental Health Journal, 22*(1–2), 7–66.

Sharp, C., Kulesz, P., Marais, L., Shohet, C., Rani, K., Lenka, M., . . . Boivin, M. (2021). Mediational Intervention for Sensitizing Caregivers to improve mental health outcomes in orphaned and vulnerable children. *Journal of Clinical Child and Adolescent Psychology, 49*(4), 545–557.

Thematic Group on Early Childhood Development, Education, and Transition to Work. (2014). *(Rep.). Sustainable development solutions network.* Retrieved January 18, 2021, from www.jstor.org/stable/resrep16105

Tzuriel, D. (1999). Parent-child mediated learning interactions as determinants of cognitive modifiability: Recent research and future directions. *Genetic, Social, and General Psychology Monographs, 125*(2), 109.

Tzuriel, D., & Caspi, R. (2017). Intervention for peer mediation and mother-child interaction: The effects on children's mediated learning strategies and cognitive modifiability. *Contemporary Educational Psychology, 49*, 302–323.

Tzuriel, D., & Shomron, V. (2018). The effects of mother-child mediated learning strategies on psychological resilience and cognitive modifiability of boys with learning disability. *British Journal of Educational Psychology, 88*(2), 236–260.

Vigotsky, L. (1978). *Mind in society: The development of higher mental functions.* Boston, MA: Harvard University Press.

3 MISC Training Program (MISC-TP)

Cilly Shohet and Deborah Givon

3.1 Introduction

To survive and thrive, children need adults who can provide them with good care and meet their physical, emotional, and learning needs. Good care means keeping children safe from harm and giving them love, attention, and many opportunities to learn. Infants are "hardwired" to relate to their social environment (Music, 2016). From birth, they build ties to special adults with whom they develop relationships. Consistent relationships with caring adults are essential for healthy development (National Scientific Council on the Developing Child, 2004) therefore, relationships matter critically from birth. What children learn from these relationships helps to prepare them for life. To ensure children's healthy intellectual and socio-emotional development (i.e., satisfy their curiosity, their urge to explore their environment, and relate to others), children need to have a warm, stable, and secure relationship, with at least one other person (a parent, or an educator) (Klein, 2001). The relationship "dance" between the adult and the child delivers essential elements for successful development. Through the pleasure and emotional sharing of a warm, loving, reciprocal exchange with an emotionally available adult, a child learns about people and the world and grows cognitively, socially, and emotionally in manageable steps (Edwards & Raikes, 2002). Numerous studies have highlighted the importance of close physical contact and expressions of love, sensitivity, and responsiveness, leading to secure attachment and serving as a springboard for leaning (Ainsworth, Blehar, Waters, & Wall, 1978; Black et al., 2017; Cassidy, 2000; Hazan, Campa, & Gur-Yaish, 2013; Music, 2016; Rosenblum, Dayton, & Muzik, 2018). All learning takes place in the context of relationships and is critically affected by the quality of those relationships (Norman-Murch, 1996).

Recognizing that children grow and develop in the context of their ongoing relationships with their parents, their families, and their other caregivers or educators, the best way to support young children is to support their relationships with the adults who care for them. In this chapter, we use the word "parent" to also include other caregivers who care for children at home, and "educator" to denote any adult working with children in out-of-home

DOI: 10.4324/9781003145899-3

settings. According to the National Research Council (2000), the ultimate impact of an intervention to enhance the quality of adult-child interactions is dependent not only on the expertise of professional practitioners who train and mentor the parents or the educators but also on the quality and continuity of the personal relationship established between them and the family that is being served. Researchers and professionals have recorded similar understandings regarding the impact of interventions in educational settings (Eggbeer, Shahmoon-Shanok, & Clark, 2010; Tal, 2019).

The MISC interventional model is *relationship-based*—acknowledging the significant impact of adult-child relationships on children's development. The model's long-term objective is **M**ore **I**ntelligent and **S**ensitive (socially competent) **C**hildren. This objective is achieved through a process of **M**ediational **I**ntervention for **S**ensitizing **C**aregivers, focusing on the relationships between the caregiver and the child within their daily interactions (Klein, Shohet, & Givon, 2018).

3.1.1 What Do We Mean by Mediation?

As distinct from direct learning, mediation is a process of learning that occurs when another person serves as a *mediator* between the child and the environment (Feuerstein, Rand, & Rynders, 1988; Klein, 1996, 2001). Mediated learning experiences take place in the context of relationships and are critically affected by the quality of those relationships. An optimal learning process occurs when the adult, who serves as a mediator, prepares and reinterprets stimuli from the environment to become meaningful and relevant for the child. The mediator takes an active role in making components of the environment compatible with the child's needs, interests, and capacities (Feuerstein & Feuerstein, 1991; Klein, 2000; Vigotsky, 1978). Mediational interaction enables the individual to benefit from the experience; it prepares the individual to learn and be modified (Klein, 2001). Mediational experiences are *learning-teaching* processes. The mediator acts in an *intentional* and *reciprocal* teaching mode while developing consciousness to his or her actions during the interaction with the child.

3.1.2 What Do We Mean by "Sensitization"?

Sensitization means trying to enhance the adult's awareness of the positive aspects of her interaction with the child and the inner beliefs that underlie her behavior. This process provides the adult with "new glasses", a new way of understanding and conceptualizing the characteristics of her interpersonal interaction with the child and recognizing the connection between her actions with the child's best interests in mind. The "new glasses" enable the adult to view things in the interaction from the child's perspective and communicate that their needs and interests are being recognized (Sharp et al., 2020). As a result of the sensitization process, the adult realizes what is important in what he or she may be doing while interacting with children and doing it even better. It enhances the awareness of people who are interacting face to face with children to their power to change and affect children's learning experiences.

As part of sensitization, the mediator has to acknowledge that both partners in an interaction affect each other based on their personal characteristics and on the "what" and "how" that is occurring between them. This fact is supported by the basic idea of the transactional model (Sameroff & Chandler, 1975), that children affect their environments while their environments affect them. The process of sensitization requires time and constant personal development and change. The MISC interventional model adheres to the notion that sustained change is likely when the adult implicitly discovers needed change through a *reflective process* (Sharp et al., 2020). As opposed to more instructional skills-based approaches, implicit change involves facilitating the development of a reflective (or mentalizing) capacity so that the adult may reach insights and discover solutions or answers regarding the future, independently (Schön, 1988; Shulman, 1993). The sensitized adult has the tools and the power to positively affect children's development and learning skills, leading to a more optimal adjustment to a constantly changing world.

According to the MISC interventional model, sensitization is a long and deep process that requires the training and supervision of a professional trainer. The concept of "supervision" brings up two meanings. In respect to inspection and control, the trainer acts as an inspector of the trainee's work and behavior. Second, in respect to "supervision", the trainer, as an observer, can view things from a broader angle. In the field of children's development and education, supervision relates to *marking* the route by the trainer and to the journey that both the trainer and the trainee march together, side by side, a journey in which both go through a process of change and development (Kadushin & Harkness, 2014).

3.2 The Structure, Content, and Goals of the MISC Training Program (MISC-TP)

As with other relationship-based early interventions, the MISC interventional model is concerned with fostering the learning and growth of children, parents, educators, and their trainers, based on the quality of the relationships they form throughout their interactions (Kelly, 1999). The MISC-TP has a hierarchical structure: parents and educators receive training from professional MISC trainers who have been trained and supervised by MISC qualified *mentors* (supervisors). All adults participating in the program receive training to become mediators.

A trainer's experience in supervision delivered by her mentor directly affects her interactions with her trainee (Shamoon-Shanok, Gilkerson, Eggbeer, & Fenichel,1995). Interactions are foundational to forming interpersonal relationships. The structure of the MISC-TP provides support to trainers in their relationship-based work and provides a model of the kinds of interpersonal interactions that characterize all levels of the relationships in the hierarchy. According to the MISC-TP, quality interaction has the same components, be it an adult–child or trainer–trainee interaction.

As part of the MISC interventional model, the MISC training program aims to enhance the quality of interactions that occur in various levels of personal relationships and thus the *flexibility of mind* of all participants in the web of connections. In all levels of the hierarchy mentioned earlier, the training program reflects the concept of "parallel processes" (Campbell, 2013; Tracey, Bludworth, & Glidden-Tracey, 2012) occurring during adult–child interactions as well as trainer–trainee interactions. Thus, the same objectives for training parents and educators to be successful mediators apply to the MISC trainers who are trained by their mentors. This process creates a common professional language: a "MISC language".

Professional literature acknowledges that the web of relationships, created through interactions among the various connected partners, is crucial to the effective delivery of support that will produce learning, growth, and wellbeing to children, their families, and those who support them (Weston, Ivins, Heffron, & Sweet, 1997; Wilcox & Weber, 2001; Pilkington & Malinowski, 2002; Gilkerson & Taylor Ritzler, 2005). By recognizing and nurturing the many interrelated relationships associated with early intervention, programs can achieve a high level of service delivery in which children participate, learn, and develop in the context of their everyday routines, activities, places, and relationships.

The main content of the MISC-TP is the *interaction* between two partners: adult–child (or children) and trainer–trainee (or trainees). The program's main objective is to sensitize the mediator to the emotional and cognitive-behavioral components of her interaction with her partner (the child or the trainee) to the MISC model's objectives and her own educational beliefs. When the mediator (the parent, the educator, or the trainer) is sensitized, there is a higher probability that the interaction will follow the needs of the partner. Such an interaction may be defined as a quality interaction, providing an enriching learning experience for the child or the trainee.

In the following, we summarize the training program's goals for the trainee (parent, educator) to enhance the learning and development of children:

1. To provide knowledge regarding the MISC model, its structure, its components, and the educational approach that the model represents.
2. To enhance the adult's (parent, or educator) awareness of the emotional and cognitive characteristics of their interaction with the child (or children) in relation to the MISC model.
3. To enhance the adult's (parent or educator) awareness of the relationship between their educational philosophy, their values and beliefs, and the characteristics of their interactions with the child (children).
4. To enhance child-oriented interactions between adults and children.

5. To enhance understanding of specific situations and concepts related to children (i.e. milestones in child development, temperament characteristics, educational approach).
6. To learn how to *match* the adult's behavior to the characteristics and needs of the child (children) in the interaction, in the context they occur.
7. To enhance the adult's trust in her competencies, autonomy of thought, and mind flexibility.

3.3 The Theoretical Background of the MISC-TP

Like the MISC model itself, the definition of quality interaction and learning in the MISC-TP is also based on Vygotsky's contextual theory (1978) and Feuerstein's cognitive modifiability theory (1979, 1980). According to these theories, learning is considered a mediated learning experience (MLE), in which a constant process of change of the learner's cognitive structures takes place. This process eventually leads to flexibility of mind and further development.

Mediated learning experiences take place in the context of relationships and are critically affected by the quality of those relationships. These learning experiences are the outcome of adults' actions to make the physical and social world more accessible, reinterpreted, based on verbal and non-verbal communication, and the arrangement of the physical environment with, and for, children. The perception of mediated learning experiences is based on the socio-constructivist assumption (Vigotsky, 1978; Feuerstein & Feuerstein, 1991) that an individual's ability to learn is critically affected by interactions with more capable individuals (parents, educators, siblings, peers). Bronfenbrenner and Morris (2006) claim that direct, intensive, bidirectional interactions between children and their social and physical worlds constitute "proximal processes", the primary mechanism that explains human development. According to Feuerstein and Feuerstein (1991), the ability to learn is modified by social and physical stimuli and phenomena. Thus, Vigotsky (1978) and Feuerstein and Feuerstein (1991) claim that cognitive modifiability and the child's knowledge depend on the quality of the interaction between the person and the environment.

Klein (1988, 1991) empirically defined five interaction components that lead to cognitive modifiability in an MLE: *focusing, providing meaning (affecting), expanding, rewarding, regulating behavior* (see Chapter 2). Klein found that interactions based on these components predicted a child's later cognitive development.

One of the important contributions of the criteria defining mediated learning experiences, suggested by Klein's MISC model (Sobelman-Rosenthal & Klein, 2010), is the inclusion of social-emotional components and the reference to the cultural-environmental characteristics of the adult into the model of adult-child interaction, explaining cognitive modifiability (see Chapter 2).

The MLE approach and the MISC model are based on the understanding that child development is deeply influenced by the caregiver and the *quality of interactions* between him/her and the developing child. The suggested program (MISC-TP) helps parents and educators to recognize and understand how they may affect the child's development. They learn to identify a set of components that characterizes the adult's behavior during an adult-child interaction, which may turn the interaction into an enriching learning experience for the child and eventually affect her flexibility of mind. According to the MISC model, flexibility of mind serves as a disposition for learning from new experiences that children may encounter within their traditional cultural setting or confront in the constantly changing world.

3.4 The MISC "Building Blocks" in Practice

The MISC-TP, as part of the MISC interventional program, focuses on the interaction occurring between the MISC trainer and her trainee (parent, educator). Its quality is measured by the same characteristics that define a quality interaction between an adult and a child (as mentioned earlier), leading to flexibility of mind. The MISC trainer uses MISC components in the interaction to create an MLE for her trainee (parent, educator), just as the trainee (parent, educator) uses MISC components in the interaction to create MLEs for the child. This basic concept of the training process represents the idea of parallel processes that take place in both types of interaction: adult-child interaction and trainer-trainee interaction. Therefore, each interaction should relate to the same three "building blocks" mentioned in Chapter 2: cultural-environmental, emotional, and cognitive.

Every MISC trainer must have a deep understanding of these building blocks of the interaction to be able to reflect on her interaction characteristics with her trainee (parent, educator), thus helping her trainee understand and reflect on her own interaction with the child in relation to those central building blocks.

It is impossible to expect long-term sustainable effects of any intervention if the trainer does not cooperate and work within the cultural norms of the trainee. Therefore, the trainer must be acquainted with her trainee's cultural-environmental and socioeconomic reality and the trainee's beliefs and values regarding child-rearing. The MISC trainer should be capable of forming a warm, empathic, respectful, and trusting relationship with her trainee and function in a supportive, caring, and non-authoritative manner. Establishing a positive expressive interaction is a necessary condition for mediation in adult-child interaction and the trainer-trainee interaction.

The following are examples of each of the five cognitive mediational components in both types of interactions (adult-child, trainer-trainee):

Focusing: Any mediator's act or sequence of acts that appear to be directed towards focusing the partner's attention and achieving a change in his or her perception or response (e.g., selecting, exaggerating, grouping, sequencing, or pacing stimuli). Focusing may be expressed verbally, non-verbally, or in a combined manner. At times the child, or the trainee, may initiate the act of focusing.

Examples of focusing in adult-child interaction:

- A mother points out to a cat sitting on a garbage-tin saying to her infant: "Look at the cat."
- A teacher claps her hands at the beginning of a lesson to attract the children's attention.
- A child turns to his teacher and says, "Look what I have built."

Examples of focusing in trainer-trainee interaction:

- The trainer points to a child while observing a group of children with the trainee.
- The trainer presents a new issue to discuss on.
- The trainee brings up a new challenge and asks for help, despite the trainer's plan for that meeting.

Providing meaning (Affecting): Any mediator's behavior expressing meaning, excitement, appreciation, or affect, verbally or non-verbally, concerning people, objects, animals, or concepts and values. At times, the child, or the trainee, may initiate the act of providing or asking for meaning.

Examples of providing meaning (affecting) in adult-child interaction:

- The teacher presents to the children a flower and names it and its parts: "This is a rose, this is the stem, and these are stamens."
- The mother asks the child: "Describe what you see in the picture."
- While walking in the garden, the mother points to a colorful bird and says with excitement: "Oh, what a beautiful bird!"
- The child asks the mother: "What is it?"

Examples of providing meaning (affecting) in trainer-trainee interaction:

- The trainer points out specific child behavior and asks the trainee: "To your understanding, what does this behavior mean?"
- The trainer asks the trainee: "How did you feel during this activity with the children?"
- The trainer moves her chair closer to the trainee, looks at her and smiles.
- The trainee turns to the trainer and says: "I don't understand the meaning of this mediational component."

Expanding: Any mediator's behavior directed towards broadening a partner's cognitive awareness, beyond the immediate experience (e.g., explaining, relating to past and future, relating to cause and effect, reasoning, comparing, making analogies rules, questions). At times, the child, or the trainee, may initiate the act of expanding or asking for it.

Examples of expanding in adult-child interaction:

- The teacher explains: "These plants that I've brought you are part of our environmental components. They are living organisms, just like animals . . ."
- The teacher asks the children in her group: "What is common to all the objects you see on the table? Can we sort them into groups? According to what?"
- A mother explains to her child, as they are looking together at a picture-book: "This is a cow, and next to her is the calf. A calf is the baby of the cow, just as you are my baby . . . see how big the cow is and how small the calf is . . ."
- A child asks his father: "How come that nothing happens to a bird who stands on an electric pole?"

Examples of providing expanding in trainer-trainee interaction:

- The trainer points to a child's behavior that seems "aggressive". She explains that this behavior may be an expression of the child's temperament and/or her developmental stage.
- The trainer asks her trainee: "Does the interaction that you have experienced with this child characterize other interactions that you have with him? . . . How do you feel about it?"
- The trainer asks the trainee to reflect on her progress with implementing the new knowledge she acquired on enhancing the quality of her interaction with her child.
- The trainee asks the trainer: "How do you differentiate between 'providing meaning' and 'expanding'? Sometimes they seem almost alike, especially when it comes to interactions with very young children."

Rewarding (mediated feelings of competence): Any mediator's verbal or non-verbal behavior expressing satisfaction with a partner's behavior, intending to encourage the partner. A more effective reward is expressed verbally with the mediator's identification of specific components of the partner's behavior, which the mediator considers successful. In addition, breaking a task into smaller components or making it easier for the partner allows the partner to experience success and be rewarded by the mediator. At times, the child, or the trainee, may initiate the act of rewarding or ask for it.

Examples of rewarding in adult-child interaction:

- A mother and her young child are assembling a puzzle. The mother says to her child: "Good for you! You have succeeded in placing the right piece so that now we can see the lion's face!"
- The teacher observes a toddler who shares a toy with another toddler. The teacher says: "It is so nice of you to share the doll with Miriam! Now both of you can play together and take turns."
- The teacher asks: "What does a worm eat?" A child responds: "Lettuce." The teacher approves and says: "Right" (with no explanation).
- A toddler is struggling to string beads with no success. The caregiver says: "Let's find beads with a bigger hole so that it will be easier for you to string them."
- A child has solved a math exercise. He asks her father: "Did I do it right?"

Examples of rewarding in trainer-trainee interaction:

- The trainer praises the trainee on her progress since the beginning of the year.
- The trainer says to the trainee: "You paid attention to the child's initiation and responded to it verbally. Your response elicited a big smile on his face. By doing so, you have transmitted a very important message to the child: It is worthwhile to act!"
- Following a movement activity of the caregiver with a group of children, the trainer praises her and explains: "This was a successful activity. It was well planned, matched to the children, you have related to each child personally, and the children were very engaged in the activity. Good job!"
- The trainee says to her trainer: "I'm not sure I did it right . . . what do you think?"

Regulation of Behavior: Any mediator's behavior that models, demonstrates, and/or verbally suggests to the partner how to do things better concerning the specific requirements of a task or to any other cognitive process required before or during an overt action (e.g., modelling, sequencing, planning, precision matching speed, and intensity to the task). It should be noted that at times the child, or the trainee, may initiate the act of regulation of behavior or ask for it.

Examples of regulation of behavior in adult-child interaction:

- The teacher suggests the child build a wide base for the Lego-tower he intends to build.
- While getting dressed, the father says to his young girl: "When putting our shoes on, what do we do first?"

- Before leaving home for a walk in the park, the mother says to her child: "Let's see what we need to take with us . . ."
- While trying to assemble the puzzle pieces, the child says to his mother: "I don't know how to start . . ." The mother responds: "Before starting, let's look at the picture on the box and think: what will be the easiest way to start? I suggest starting from the frame . . ."

Examples of regulation of behavior in trainer-trainee interaction:

- The trainer asks the caregiver to observe the children before planning the next activity.
- The trainer sets up "rules" for a regular set of her meetings with the trainee. She asks the trainee to keep the "rules" precisely and explains the importance of the regularity, continuity, and persistence of the training process.
- The trainee asks the trainer for advice in planning effective ways of coping with challenging behaviors of a child in her group. The trainer says: "First, tell me about the child. Where do you feel challenged? Try to think what can help you . . ."

3.5 Interaction Profiles

According to Klein (Sobelman-Rosenthal & Klein, 2010), interactions among people and interactions between adults and children may be described and categorized in personal and unique profiles. The interaction profile reflects the interaction's quality: its components and the nature of the relationship between the two partners.

Tal, Bachar, Sandroviz, Wisebrod, and Shemer (2001) have developed a categorization method for characterizing different teaching–learning interaction profiles. According to them, the frequency of each mediational component in the interaction, and the combinations among them, reflect the integration between the biological and cultural characteristics of each partner in the interaction, as well as personal philosophy and beliefs:

1. <u>An interaction profile focused on the learner (the child or the trainee) versus an interaction profile focused on the mediator</u> who is responsible for the interaction (the parent, educator, or trainer): When the interaction is focused on the learner, one will observe a higher frequency of initiations by the learner (child or trainee), which provides him or her the opportunity to develop his or her own ideas. Whereas, when the interaction is characterized by a higher frequency of the mediator's initiations, the learner is less active in the interaction.

   An interaction profile might be balanced when the frequency of the mediator's and the learner's initiations are even.

2. An emotional interaction profile versus a cognitive interaction profile: An emotional profile is characterized by higher frequencies of positive or negative affect expressed towards the learner (child or trainee). Mediators, whose interaction profile is mainly cognitive, tend to use higher frequencies of cognitive mediational components (providing meaning and expanding) and tend to ignore the learner's emotional expressions. A balanced interaction profile combines emotional and cognitive components in the interaction.

3. An interaction profile that encourages autonomy versus an interaction profile that reflects control: A mediator whose profile reflects encouragement of autonomy will convey feelings of competence to the learner regarding her ability to think, solve problems, and develop ideas of her own and express higher frequencies of expansion. Whereas a mediator with a tendency to control the interaction will express higher frequencies of regulation of behavior and rewarding with no explanation. This interaction profile is defined as "adult-centered" ("trainer-centered"), characterized by a high frequency of the mediator's initiations and less acceptance of ideas that are not her own.

3.5.1 How to Build an Interaction Profile Based on Video-Recorded Interactions

The MISC-TP consists of implementing a method using video recordings of interactions. This method (i.e. Video Interaction Guidance: VIG) is a means to promote the objective of enhancing quality interaction competencies in all dyads by analysis of its profile components and providing feedback and supervision by the trainer. The process of identifying the profile components allows the quantification of the quality of the interaction and Klein considers it as the "literacy of interaction" (Shohet & Jaegermann, 2012). The VIG method has been used in numerous intervention and research projects as a primary method to promote quality of interactions among various populations (Jilink, Fukkink, & Huijbregts, 2018; Kennedy, Landor, & Todd, 2011). It is often part of a broader professional development program that also includes additional methods and processes. Pianta, Mashburn, Downer, Hamre, and Justice (2008) found that teachers that received feedback targeting videotapes of their interactions and online consultation showed significantly greater increases in the quality of interactions than did teachers that only received access to a website with video clips.

Using the VIG method allows for analysis, providing feedback, discussion, demonstration, and reflection on reinforcing, enriching, and developing mediational learning experiences through reciprocal communication chains occurring between adults (parents, educators) and children and between trainers and their trainees. According to the MISC-TP, the value that guides the VIG method is creating partnerships with families

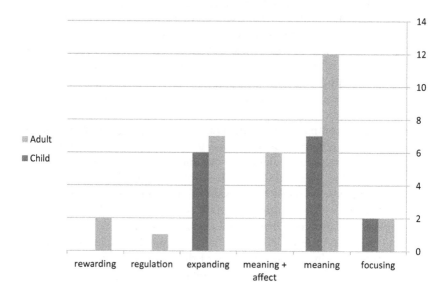

Figure 3.1 Frequencies of mediational behaviors in an adult–child interaction

and educators. Training and supervision sessions occur in a home context or educational settings context, respecting cultural diversity, attitudes, and beliefs. The MISC-TP is "client-oriented" and is focused on relationships, based on strengths, on an ecological and reflective approach and the VIG method, as part of the means for achieving the program's objectives.

The following are the steps in building an interaction profile of the mediator:

1. Video recording of an interaction
2. Observation of the video-recorded interaction
3. Encoding the interaction according to the MISC components
4. Summary of frequencies of the MISC components
5. Graphical presentation of the frequencies
6. Conclusions regarding the interaction profile

Figure 3.1 is an example of a graphical representation of an observation on an adult–child interaction focused on a dialogue between a teacher and a 10-year-old child. The graph indicates that the child was interested, active, and involved in the dialogue and that the adult's mediational behaviors in the interaction were balanced.

Based on the previous, the trainer plans the training process for his or her trainee (parent, educator). The process comprises several training meetings that include a reference to the trainee's cultural-environmental characteristics and the interaction's emotional and cognitive components.

In the following, we summarize the steps of a training meeting between the MISC trainer and the trainee (parent, educator), based on a video-recorded interaction:

1. Presenting the objectives of the training meeting.
2. Joint observation of the videotaped interaction.
3. Allowing the trainee to share and reflect on her feelings and thoughts regarding the observed interaction.
4. Pointing out the positive aspects of the trainee's interaction using the MISC's terminology (emotional and cognitive components).
5. Joint focus on various parts of the interaction that represent MISC components or issues that require the trainee's change of behavior or attitude and reflection on possible ways of realizing the change.
6. Summing up the meeting and planning the implementation of the new knowledge that has been acquired throughout the meeting.

3.5.2 Professionalizing the New MISC Trainer

As mentioned earlier, MISC-TP has a hierarchical structure in which trainers are trained and supervised by experienced professional and acknowledged MISC mentors. The professionalizing process of new MISC trainers is carried out by MISC mentors (supervisors) and consists of similar procedures described earlier: 1. Video recording of training sessions between the MISC trainer and her trainee (parent, educator). 2. Forming a profile of the trainer's interaction with her trainee. 3. Establishing an ongoing training session process that each follows the steps mentioned earlier.

The training process of the new MISC trainer aims to promote the development of competencies of identification and analysis of the interaction profile and communicational behaviors with their trainees. Alongside the training program's structural characteristics, reflective processes take place as an inseparable part of the program, leading to high levels of competencies (i.e. self-awareness, meta-cognition, autonomy).

Becoming a sensitized mediator, in all types of interaction (adult-child, trainer-trainee), is a long process that requires an investment of time, thought, and practical experiences, escorted by a professional expert capable of handling important issues related to interaction and communication, child development, children's and adults' learning processes, and their appropriate practice in everyday life. MISC-TP is the process through which the MISC intervention's long-term objective—More Intelligent and Sensitive (socially competent) Children—is achieved.

3.6 A Bird's Eye View on the Training Process

The MISC-TP focuses on two main groups of trainees: caregivers and educators. Each training process is initiated with a stage of *acquaintance* with the caregiver or the educator, which includes a semi-structured interview with the trainee, aiming to acquire a deep understanding of the trainee's cultural and socioeconomic reality. This stage of the training program reflects one of the basic concepts of the MISC model: the need to be matched to the trainee's characteristics and needs throughout the interaction. This concept of matching to the partner in the interaction depicts the whole training process and supports the establishment of trust between the trainer and the trainee.

Following the stage of acquaintance between the trainer and her trainee (caregiver, educator), a 10-minute video of a regular daily interaction (e.g. a meal, a joint play activity, storytelling) with a child or a small group of children is recorded. A trainee's interaction profile is formed (see steps for building a profile earlier) and analyzed by the MISC trainer, based on the video recording. The video provides the content of the training process that, along the way, will result in learning and sensitization and eventually will turn the mediator to be a competent mediator.

Three basic modes of training are implemented according to the characteristics and needs of each group of trainees:

Training through individual video guidance (based on the trainee's videotaped interactions with a child or a small group of children). Each meeting focuses on the trainee's two or three behaviors, which the trainer conceptualizes in terms of the MISC components to which they relate. During the meetings, the trainer and the trainee reflect on the thoughts and feelings that the trainee experienced during the interaction, on the extent of matching of the trainee's behavior to the child's (or children's) and ways of generalization and transfer of the new knowledge acquired, in other situations.

Training through individual "in-service" training (training the trainees during their interaction with the children). The training takes place during everyday interactions between the trainee and the child (or children). The MISC trainer, who is present during the interaction, identifies *teachable moments* where the trainer can help the trainee by providing meaning, expanding, and/or modeling, to implement in the "here-and-now" MISC concepts and ideas that were discussed during video guidance.

Training through group meetings, where discussion, elaboration, sharing of issues raised in the individual training sessions occur. This mode enables establishing a learning group of parents or educators. In the group meetings they have the opportunity to share and elaborate on issues related to their personal experiences with a child (or a group of children), especially on the MISC concepts and components. Sharing experiences, thoughts, and feelings in a group of peers, with the trainer's guidance, enables the participants to be exposed to various attitudes and individual differences among adults and children related to daily interactions. This shared process allows individual participants to learn from others' experiences with the support of the trainer's mediation.

All three training modes may be implemented with parents and with educators. All three are complementary. However, it is possible to carry out the first and third training modes independently.

All training processes in any kind of training mode are characterized by empathic relationships between the trainer and the trainee (or the trainees) and being supportive, caring, and non-judgmental. MISC trainers are trained to listen carefully, demonstrate concern and empathy, promote reflection, observe, respond thoughtfully, encourage autonomy of thought, and convey enthusiasm and hope regarding the role of the parent or the educator in promoting the chances of child development and learning. By emphasizing solid relationships with parents and educators, trainers attend to *what* they do and *how* they do it. They can most effectively share their knowledge, perspective, and resources with their trainees in the context of a trusting relationship that will eventually be delivered to the trainee's relationships with the child or children.

3.7 Conclusion

The basic idea behind the MISC intervention, carried out by the MISC-TP, is not to teach parents and educators specific behaviors, but rather to help them through the process of MISC-TP identify behaviors that exist within their own repertoire and explain why behaviors of this nature may help the children learn and develop. The intervention's objective is to overcome generalization and transfer, which plague many educational programs (Klein et al., 2018).

When supported by trained professionals, the trainees, who learn to meditate, may develop communication and responsiveness competencies to meet the children's needs better. These changes will be visible through a higher ability to identify the needs and resources necessary to ensure the wellbeing, functioning, and better opportunities for learning and development for the children.

References

Ainsworth, M. D. S., Blehar, M. C., Waters, E., & Wall, S. (1978). *Patterns of attachment.* Hillsdale, NJ: Erlbaum.

Black, M. M., Walker, S. P., Fernald, L., Andersen, C. T., DiGirolamo, A. M., Lu, C., . . . Lancet Early Childhood Development Series Steering Committee. (2017). Early childhood development coming of age: Science through the life course. *Lancet, 389*(10064), 77–90.

Bronfenbrenner, U., & Morris, P. A. (2006). The bioecological model of human development. In W. Damon & R. M. Lerner (Series Eds.) & R. M. Lerner (Vol. Ed.), *Handbook of child psychology: Vol. 1. Theoretical models of human development* (6th ed., pp. 793–828). New York: Wiley.

Campbell, J. (2013). *Becoming an effective supervisor: A workbook for counselors and psychotherapists.* London: Routledge.

Cassidy, J. (2000). The complexity of the caregiving system: A perspective from attachment theory. *Psychological Inquiry, 11*(2), 86–91.

Edwards, C. P., & Raikes, H. (2002). Extending the dance: Relationship-based approaches to infant/toddler care and education. *Faculty Publications, Department of Child, Youth, and Family Studies, 16.*

Eggbeer, L., Shahmoon-Shanok, R., & Clark, R. (2010). Reaching toward an evidence base for reflective supervision. *Zero to Three (J)*, *31*(2), 39–45.

Feuerstein, R. (1979). *The dynamic assessment of retarded performers*. New York: University Park Press.

Feuerstein, R. (1980). *Instrumental enrichment: Redevelopment of cognitive functions of retarded performers*. New York: University Park Press.

Feuerstein, R., & Feuerstein, S. (1991). Mediated learning experience. In R. Feuerstein, P. Klein, & A. Tannenabaum (Eds.), *Mediated learning experience: Theoretical, psychosocial, and social implications* (pp. 3–52). Tel Aviv: Freund Publishing House.

Feuerstein, R., Rand, Y., & Rynders, J. E. (1988). Mediated learning experience. In *Don't accept me as I am* (pp. 59–93). Boston, MA: Springer.

Gilkerson, L., & Ritzler, T. T. (2005). The role of reflective process in infusing relationship-based practice into an early intervention system. In K. Finello (Ed.), *The handbook of training and practice in infant and preschool mental health* (pp. 427–452). Singapore: Wiley.

Hazan, C., Campa, M., & Gur-Yaish, N. (2013). Attachment across the lifespan. In P. Noller & J. A. Feeney (Eds.), *Close relationships: Functions, forms and processes* (pp. 189–209). Hove: Psychology Press.

Jilink, L., Fukkink, R., & Huijbregts, S. (2018). Effects of early childhood education training and video interaction guidance on teachers' interactive skills. *Journal of Early Childhood Teacher Education*, *39*(4), 278–292.

Kadushin, A., & Harkness, D. (2014). *Supervision in social work*. New York: Columbia University Press.

Kelly, J. F. (1999, Fall). Parent education within a relationship-focused model. *Topics in Early Childhood Education*, *19*(3), 151–157.

Kennedy, H., Landor, M., & Todd, L. (2011). *Video interaction guidance*. London: Jessica Kingsley.

Klein, P. S. (1988). Stability and change in interaction of Israeli mothers and infants. *Infant Behavior and Development*, *11*(1), 55–70.

Klein, P. S. (1991). Improving the quality of parental interaction with very low birth weight children: A longitudinal study using a mediated learning experience model. *Infant Mental Health Journal*, *12*(4), 321–337.

Klein, P. S. (1996). *Early intervention: Cross -cultural experiences with a mediational approach*. New York: Garland Publications.

Klein, P. S. (2000). A developmental mediation approach to early intervention: Mediational intervention for sensitizing caregivers (MISC). *Educational and Child Psychology*, *17*(3), 19–31.

Klein, P. S. (Ed.). (2001). *Seeds of hope: Twelve years of early intervention in Africa*. Oslo: Unipub forlag.

Klein, P. S., Shohet, C., & Givon, D. (2018). A mediational intervention for sensitizing caregivers (MISC): A cross-cultural early intervention. In A. Abubakar & F. Van de Vijver (Eds.), *Handbook of applied developmental Science in Sub-Saharan Africa* (pp. 291–312). New York: Springer.

Music, G. (2016). *Nurturing natures: Attachment and children's emotional, sociocultural and brain development*. Hove: Psychology Press.

National Research Council. (2000). *From neurons to neighborhoods: The science of early childhood development*. The science of early childhood development. Committee on Integrating the Science of Early Childhood Development. Washington, DC: National Academy Press.

National Scientific Council on the Developing Child. (2004). *What science is telling us: How neurobiology and developmental psychology are changing the way policymakers and communities should think about the developing child.* Waltham, MA: Heller School for Social Policy and Management at Brandeis University.

Norman-Murch, T. (1996, October–November). Reflective supervision as a vehicle for individual and organizational development. *Zero To Three, 20*(1), 16–20.

Pianta, R. C., Mashburn, A. J., Downer, J. T., Hamre, B. K., & Justice, L. M. (2008). Effects of web-mediated professional development resources on teacher-child interactions in pre-kindergarten classrooms. *Early Childhood Research Quarterly, 23*, 431–451.

Pilkington, K. O., & Malinowski, M. (2002). The natural environment II: Uncovering deeper responsibilities within relationship-based services. *Infants & Young Children, 15*(2), 78–84.

Rosenblum, K. L., Dayton, C. J., & Muzik, M. (2018). Infant social and emotional development: Emerging competence in a relational context. In C. H. Zeanah (Ed.), *Handbook of infant mental health* (pp. 103–125). New York: Guilford Publications.

Sameroff, A. J., & Chandler, M. J. (1975). Reproductive risk and the continuum of caretaking casualty. *Review of Child Development Research, 4*, 187–244.

Schön, D. A. (1988). Coaching reflective teaching. In P. Grimmet & G. L. Erickson (Eds.), *Reflection in teacher education* (pp. 19–29). New York: Teacher College Press.

Shamoon-Shanok, R., Gilkerson, L., Eggbeer, L., & Fenichel, E. (1995). *Reflective supervision: A relationship for learning, a discussion guide.* Washington, DC: Zero to Three.

Sharp, C., Shohet, C., Givon, D., Penner, F., Marais, L., & Fonagy, P. (2020). Learning to mentalize: A mediational approach for caregivers and therapists. *Clinical Psychology: Science and Practice, 27*(3), e12334.

Shohet, C., & Jaegermann, N. (2012). Integrating infant mental health into primary health care and early childhood education settings in Israel: "The mediational intervention for sensitizing caregivers" Approach. *Zero to Three (J), 33*(2), 55–58.

Shulman, L. (1993). *Interactional supervision.* Washington, DC: NASW Press.

Sobelman-Rosenthal, V., & Klein, P. S. (2010). *Together and alone. Inclusion of children with special needs in regular early childhood educational settings.* Israel: Hebrew.

Tal, C. (2019). Core practices and competencies in teaching and teacher education: Definitions, implementation, challenges and implications. In P McDemott (Ed.), *Teacher training: Perspectives, implementation and challenges* (pp. 1–74). New York: Nova Science.

Tal, C., Bachar, E., Sandroviz, R., Wisebrod, D., & Shemer, O. (2001). *Mediational training towards autonomy* (in Hebrew). Tel-Aviv: Moffet.

Tracey, T. J., Bludworth, J., & Glidden-Tracey, C. E. (2012). Are there parallel processes in psychotherapy supervision? An empirical examination. *Psychotherapy, 49*(3), 330.

Vygotsky, L. (1978). *Mind in society: The development of higher mental functions.* Boston, MA: Harvard University Press.

Weston, D., Ivins, B., Heffron, M., & Sweet, N. (1997). Formulating the centrality of relationships in early intervention: An organizational perspective. *Infants and Young Children, 9*(3), 1–12.

Wilcox, M. J., & Weber, C. A. (2001). *Relationship-based practice in early intervention.* Poster presented at NAEYC's National Institute for Early Childhood Professional Development, Washington, DC.

4 Considerations for Implementing MISC in Early Childhood Education Care Settings

Ravit Rozenfeld Kraft

4.1 The Early Childcare Environment

Early childhood education and care (ECEC) settings are characterized by group setting care. In practice, a caregiver or kindergarten teacher is responsible for a group of infants or toddlers, and therefore most of the interactions take place with a group of children. From an attachment theory perspective (Bowlby,1969), a relationship characterized by closeness, warmth, and responsiveness allows infants and toddlers to develop a safe base. They can explore the environment and develop independence and autonomy (OECD, 2012). Interactions with educators are an essential quality factor of ECEC, affording a positive influence on children's developmental and learning outcomes and social competence (Brock & Curby, 2014; Mashburn et al., 2008; Hamre, Hatfield, Pianta, & Jamil, 2014; Jamison, Cabell, LoCasale-Crouch, Hamre, & Pianta, 2014). The relationships between infants and toddlers and their caregivers in ECEC settings is one of the main components that define the quality of the educational setting (Slot, Leseman, Verhagen, & Mulder, 2015; OECD, 2012; Ruzek, Burchinal, Farkas, & Duncan, 2014).

Assessment tools designed to measure the quality of ECEC settings, such as the Classroom Assessment Scoring System (CLASS-Toddlers; La Paro, Hamre, & Pianta, 2009), and Infants Toddlers Environment Rating Scale—third edition (ITERS-3; Harms, Cryer, Clifford, & Yazejian, 2017) include extensive reference to the quality of interaction between caregivers, infants, and toddlers in these settings. The CLASS, for example, includes components for estimating the quality of interaction such as "the degree to which the caregiver responds to children's signals concerning their needs" or "the degree to which the caregiver recognizes the children's emotions and accepts them". The ITERS-3 also include several components aimed to evaluate the quality of interaction between infants and toddlers such as: "Talking with children", "Encouraging children to communicate", "staff-child interaction", "Providing Physical Warmth/touch", etc. (Harms et al., 2017).

DOI: 10.4324/9781003145899-4

4.2 The Challenge of Working With a Group of Infants and Toddlers

The caregiver establishes an attachment relationship with the infants and toddlers under her responsibility and gradually acquaints herself with them so that she/he can provide them with the most appropriate response to their needs. The process of getting to know the group of infants or toddlers includes getting acquainted with various features like the age when entering the setting, family characteristics, the infant or toddler's developmental features from birth to entering the setting, sleeping and eating habits, and more. The caregiver establishes a relationship with each infant or toddler in the group, allowing them to feel safe while learning and exploring the environment. Establishing sensitive and responsive relationships and interactions with a group of infants or toddlers and providing support beneficial to a child's development can also pose a complex implementation challenge for the caregiver. The MISC intervention model (see Chapter 2) aims to match between an adult and one child. This matching considers the child's cues to create as long communication chains as possible between adult and child. This goal can be difficult to implement when it comes to a group of infants or toddlers who are interacting simultaneously with one caregiver. There are several difficulties or challenges in educational work with a group of infants and toddlers. There are temperamental and other individual differences that make it difficult for the caregiver to adapt the most appropriate response to a group of infants or toddlers who are different from each other. The differences between the infants or toddlers also exist regarding their physical needs, like different sleep times during the day, different feeding times from each other, and different developmental needs. Therefore, the goal of applying the MISC-TP in group settings is to increase the sensitivity and responsiveness of the educators to the group of infants or toddlers or young children under their responsibility. This is done while the educator is aware of the limitations that exist in her work as long as she is in charge of a group of infants or toddlers.

4.2.1 The Challenge of Temperamental Differences Between Children

Infants and toddlers are born with unique temperamental characteristics related to a congenital biological structure, which refers to their behavioral and emotional style. The temperament primarily expresses the personality of the child (Rothbart & Ahadi, 1994). Temperament is based on individual differences in responsiveness and self-regulation and includes attentional reactivity, emotionality, and motor activity (Rothbart & Bates, 2006). To support the optimal development of infants and toddlers in ECEC settings, caregivers should identify different temperamental and biological characteristics and adjust their interaction with the toddlers according to their needs (Harkoma, Sajaniemi, Suhonen, & Saha, 2021). In practice, when there is a group activity with infants or toddlers in the setting, the caregiver needs to adapt herself and the characteristics of her interaction to different temperamental characteristics of each infant or toddler in the group. This adaption might be a complex challenge. Young children with low self-regulating abilities are at risk of experiencing insensitive interactions, such as negative and controlling discipline from caregivers, which may cause vulnerability to stress (Tarullo & Gunnar, 2006).

4.2.2 *The Challenge of Individual Developmental Differences Between Children*

The ECEC setting for infants and toddlers (birth and up to 3) contains different age groups. Typically, infants include children aged 3 months to 1 year, young toddlers include children of 1–2 years of age, and older toddlers include children of 2–3 years of age. The grouping together of children of different developmental ages and stages poses additional challenges for the caregiver. The caregiver must adapt at any given moment to the different needs of all the infants or toddlers in the group. For example, a caregiver may have to respond to the fatigue of a 15-month-old toddler while having a music and movement activity with a group of 1 to 2 years old. The caregiver must decide how to respond to the toddler's need to sleep while she/ he is in the middle of the activity with the rest of the group.

4.2.3 *Structural and Process Challenges*

The quality of an educational setting for infants and toddlers includes structural and process features. Structural features include government or regional policy and entail components such as the number of children in the classrooms, the number of educational staff in the classroom, the level of education of the staff, the level of training and supervision, and physical data of the setting's space and the quality of the equipment. The process features refer to the quality of the care and educational processes that occur during the day in the setting and include the characteristics of the caregiver's relationship with children, the quality of activities, and the educational program.

In Israel, ECEC settings for ages birth to 3 are under the supervision of the Ministry of Labor and Social Affairs. The Ministry of Education supervises ECEC for ages 3 to 6 years. Studies show that structural features such as a smaller group size and a better staff-to-child ratio are related to a better quality of the process features within the setting, including the quality of interaction between educators and children (OECD, 2012). High quality of interaction between educators and children is related to the promotion of development and wellbeing and constitutes one of the process variables in educational settings (Van Schaik, Leseman, & de Haan, 2018; Williams, Mastergeorge, & Ontai, 2010). Studies show that the recommended group size for infants is six to eight infants, and the recommended ratio is one adult

Table 4.1 Current adult-to-child ratio and group size in ECEC settings in Israel in comparison to the recommended standards

Age	*Current Group Size in Israel*	*Current Staff-to-Child Ratio—in Israel*	*Recommended* Group Size*	*Recommended Staff-to-Child* Ratio*
3–15 months	18 infants	1:6	6–8 infants	1:3
16–24 months	27 toddlers	1:9	8–10 toddlers	1:5
25–36 months	33 toddlers	1:11	10–12 toddlers	1:6

* Ministry of Industry, Commerce, and Employment. Standards for operating educational settings for toddlers. Rosenthal's advisory committee report. 2009

to three infants. For toddlers, the recommendation is a maximum of 12 toddlers or young children in the group and a ratio of 1:4 (Campbell, Pungello, Miller-Johnson, Burchinal, & Ramey, 2001; De Schipper, Marianne Riksen- Walraven, & Geurts, 2006).

In Israel, the standard public day-care center is characterized by relatively large groups of infants and toddlers, and the staff-to-child ratio is lower than the recommended standard. For example, the infants age group (6 months to 1 year of age) can reach 18 infants, with three caregivers, according to the ratio of 1:6. Toddlers have a maximum group size in Israel of 33 children, and an adult-to-child ratio is 1:11. In other words, the challenges involved in group work with infants and toddlers are intensified in Israel because the groups are much larger than the recommended standard. Table 4.1 (following) summarizes the current adult-to-child ratio and group size in ECEC settings in Israel compared to the recommended standards.

4.3 Professional Training in ECEC

Training programs aimed at promoting the professional development of ECEC caregivers are associated with a higher quality of education and care (Burchinal, Peisner-Feinberg, Pianta, & Howes, 2002; Cassidy, Buell, Pugh-Hoese, & Russell, 1995; Hamre et al., 2012). The importance of professional "in-service training" in ECEC has been studied and identified as an important and significant factor related to the quality of care and education provided to infants and toddlers in the ECEC (Eurofound, 2015; Oberhuemer, Schreyer, & Neuman, 2010; Oecd, 2012; Urban, Vandenbroeck, Van Laere, Lazzari, & Peeters, 2012). Studies have found that a continuous, frequent, reflective training model delivered by professional trainers improves the quality of interaction with children (Howes, James, & Ritchi, 2003). Recent studies show the advantage of training and training programs, such as Video Interaction Guidance (VIG), including personal training for professionals (Fukkink & Tavecchio, 2010; Werner, Linting, Vermeer, & Van IJzendoorn, 2016). The MISC-TP is, therefore, a unique and focused training model for the guidance of educators in early childhood education and care.

4.4 Characteristics of the MISC -TP in ECEC Settings

The MISC Training Program for ECEC has two *long-term objectives*: (1) to support the optimal development of children and prepare them to adapt to a changing world that requires new dimensions and possibilities to create and initiate; and (2) to prevent delays or impairment in emotional, cognitive, and motor development due to a lack of awareness or neglect of parents or caregivers. Another *short-term objective* is to improve the quality of interaction between caregivers and the infants or toddlers in their care by increasing their sensitivity to the characteristics of their interaction with the children (see Chapter 2), thereby contributing to improving the quality of education and care provided to children. Quality interaction in the context of a group setting is defined as the caregiver's ability to create an emotionally positive and supportive atmosphere using emotional components such as warm tone, positive affect, physical closeness, responsiveness, and sensitivity when interacting with the group of children. During the interaction, the caregiver can take into account the children's perspectives, and as a result, give them autonomy alongside being sensitive to their needs and feelings (Goble, Sandilos, & Pianta, 2019; Klein, 1996).

A training program implemented in the ECEC—based on the MISC model intervention (MISC-TP)—includes elements of content and process. The training content is based on the interaction between the caregiver and the infants or toddlers within the daily activities during the ECEC program schedule (e.g., meals, creative activity, group play activities, free play, etc.). The training process is based on observations and video recordings of the interaction between the caregiver and the infants or toddlers. By this method (i.e., Video Interaction Guidance: VIG—see Chapter 3), the caregiver has the opportunity to observe her interaction with the infants or toddlers. The VIG allows both the trainer and the caregiver to examine the interaction together, thereby enhancing the awareness of quality interaction components. The issues that typically arise in this type of training include recognizing individual differences between the infants or toddlers in the group; identifying infant and toddler cues and their meaning; the use of the mediation components during the activity with the children; and identifying the degree of infant or toddler initiatives and involvement in the activity. The training process includes stages and a dialogue between the trainer and caregiver, designed to allow a reflective process through an online consultation (see Chapter 3).

The focus of the training session is the interaction with the infants/toddlers group, and therefore pedagogical issues arise in the training session vis-à-vis the features of the group activity, including the degree to which developmentally appropriate practices are implemented in the activity, as well as examining the caregiver's decision-making process at a given time pertaining to the infants and toddlers signals and behaviors (Copple & Bredekamp, 2009).

The experience in implementing the model in Israel and abroad shows that using the MISC model as a training model in ECEC settings raises the caregiver's awareness of quality interaction components and raises sensitivity when working with a group of infants or toddlers. However, in our experience in training staff in ECEC settings, we know that such training—which focuses on components of interaction between caregiver and the infants or toddlers in care—is not suitable for all settings. We found that settings must include certain conditions, or specific quality components, or "basic infrastructures", which form a necessary basis for the staff to learn and implement the principles of the model. These "basic infrastructures" are related to several components that define the quality of the settings for infants and toddlers and include a tailored physical environment, a certain level of staff qualification and training, adequate working conditions and wellbeing of staff, a developmentally appropriate educational program structure, and the existence of certain pedagogical principles that promote quality interaction in the group. In the following, each of these is elaborated on in more detail.

4.4.1 The Physical Environment in the Setting

The physical environment in the ECEC includes variables such as the size of the indoor space, the presence of suitable furniture adapted for care and play, the room arrangement in a way that provides various stimuli according to the needs of the infants and toddlers, and the display in the room space. An adapted physical environment is a necessary infrastructure for the caregiver to have a quality interaction with a group of toddlers. For example, the room space divided into distinct and defined activity centers that offer a variety of play and relaxation areas allows toddlers to choose a preferred activity. It, therefore, also allows the caregiver to recognize a toddler's initiatives and have quality interaction around play or activity in a way that expands and enriches them. In contrast, a poorly adapted play environment or lack of basic furniture (cushions and carpeting that allow relaxation or dramatic play accessories for imaginative games) deprives children of play options necessary to promote development, making it difficult for caregivers to have meaningful play activities with children.

4.4.2 Staff Qualification and Training

A training program's effectiveness depends on the starting level of the professional qualification (Kalliala, 2011; OECD, 2012). An ECEC staff member who lacked academic, professional education in early childhood education and care, or did not participate in professional courses, will find it difficult to derive meaningful learning from the MISC training program. The lack of basic professional training makes it difficult to maintain the efficiency of the learning process. For example, a basic familiarity with the stages of infant and toddler development fosters an understanding of children's behaviors.

In addition, knowledge of developmentally appropriate practice serves as the basis for planning a suitable educational program. Therefore, appropriate qualification constitutes a basis for a quality setting and enables the staff to be available for continued learning and professional development while working.

4.4.3 Working Conditions and Wellbeing of Staff

The working conditions of the professional staff in ECEC settings, such as the salaries and general wellbeing, influence the quality of adult-child interaction (OECD, 2012). For instance, recent studies have found a link between professional wellbeing and process components (Cassidy et al., 2017). Variables such as autonomy of caregivers in decision-making, caregivers' feelings about their work, and the degree to which they think their salary is fair are all related to process variables. The more the caregivers perceived the pay as unfair, this will reduce the process quality characteristics (OECD, 2012). The wellbeing of the staff also includes characteristics of an organizational climate.

4.4.4 The Structure of the Educational Program in the Day-Care Center

The structure of a developmentally appropriate daily educational program is essential to addressing infants and toddlers' unique educational needs. A high-quality program includes free playtime, along with group play activities, as well as well-planned transition times so that infants and toddlers will not have to wait for the next activity. A low-quality educational program may adversely affect the quality of caregiver/child interactions. For example, in an educational program in which toddlers must participate in a group activity, and no alternative activity is allowed for toddlers who do not wish to participate, there may be adverse interactions with the toddlers who are forced to participate involuntarily, contrary to developmentally appropriate practice.

4.4.5 Implementation of Pedagogical Principles That Promote Quality Group Interaction

Working with caregivers and with ECEC managers, we found that the more the setting uses pedagogical principles that promote quality group interaction, the greater the chance of the caregivers to be open to learning the principles of quality interaction. These principles include:

- **Small group activity.** Activity in a small group enables the educator to identify and respond individually to the personality, needs, and initiatives of each infant and toddler. Responsiveness to the needs of infants and toddlers enables quality interaction and support the development of physical, language, and social-emotional skills.

- **Primary caregiver for each infant or toddler.** A primary educator is an attachment figure for the infant or toddler, knows his temperament and preferences well, and is in constant contact with his parents.
- **Maintaining adapted expectations from infants and toddlers.** This pedagogical principle is to use the educator's familiarity with the specific developmental characteristics of the age group in their care and the personal characteristics of each infant or toddler in their group. For example, when working with crayons, the toddlers will often turn their personal basket of crayons into a senso-motor exploration. Recognizing this developmental feature helps the caregiver to accept and contain behavior, despite being "contrary" to the purpose of drawing activity.
- **Identifying and connecting to the initiatives of infants and toddlers.** Infants and toddlers by nature are curious and active. They initiate interaction with caregivers through internal motivation and experiences to explore and learn of the environment. The caregiver's ability to observe infants and toddlers, and to identify interest and initiatives for play and inquiry, enables her to respond to initiatives, thus providing a meaningful basis for learning and development.

4.5 Implementation of the MISC-TP Training Program in Early Childhood Educational Settings

One of the first steps in training the ECEC staff includes a video recording of the interaction of the activity with an infant or toddler or a group of infants or toddlers. The video recording is conducted after an introductory period with the caregiver. The video-taking takes place after the trainer held some introductory sessions with the caregivers and observed several times during the activity in the various classes in the setting. The video recording that handles the activity is used to assess the quality of the caregiver's interaction with one infant or toddler or with a group and as an initial basis for the beginning of the training process. Usually, the video recording is planned before the training process. The trainer can also capture group activities spontaneously from the ongoing activities in the setting, with prior agreement with caregivers. This spontaneous video recording also forms the basis for training sessions with staff in the setting.

4.6 Adult-Infant or -Toddler Quality Interaction in a Group Setting: Global Assessment Description

Group activity video recording of infants or toddlers allows the MISC trainer to evaluate the profile of the caregiver's interaction globally with the entire group (see Chapter 3). As described, this allows the assessment of the quality of the caregiver's interaction with a group of infants or toddlers according to the MISC components (see Chapters 2 and 3) by forming a profile of the caregiver interaction with the group of infants or toddlers. For example, the trainer estimates to what extent, on a scale between 1 and 10, the caregiver expresses encouragement and conveys a feeling of competence (Rewarding). In this way, a global profile picture of the caregiver is obtained, expressing the style of her interaction with the group of infants or toddlers. The trainer uses the caregiver's profile (during an individual training meeting) to raise the caregiver's awareness of her group interaction characteristics (see Chapter 3). For example, following the interaction analysis, the trainer may convey to the caregiver her tendency to re-focus the children on stimuli such as characters that appear in the book and that she uses a tone of voice characterized by a positive emotion. Equally, the trainer may convey that the caregiver rarely expands around the stimuli and does not stimulate the child to think about expansions in the context of the stimulus. This discovery can lead to a discussion with the caregiver about the term "Expanding", which is one of the cognitive components (see Chapters 2 and 3) and its contribution to children's learning and flexibility of mind (see Chapter 3).

4.7 The Training Content Deriving From the MISC-TP

4.7.1 Identifying Individual Differences in the Group and Caregiver Reflection

One of the advantages of VIG is the ability of both the trainer and the caregiver to observe the caregiver's interaction jointly. The caregiver sees herself and is slowly exposed to her behavior and the characteristics of her interaction with the infants or toddlers in the group. When watching together, the caregiver can discover the reactions and behaviors of infants and toddlers. In this way, the meaning of the individual differences between the infants or toddlers is revealed. For example, the VIG sessions may reveal that there are very active motorized toddlers, characterized by a high level of activity, which often attracts the caregiver's attention at the expense of other toddlers characterized by a lower level of activity and therefore tend to be neglected.

The VIG also allows the construction of individual profiles that reflect its interaction with each child in the group individually. The trainer can count the frequency of the MISC components that the caregiver expresses in front of each child, and each receives a unique individual profile. It is also possible to examine the differences in the profile of the interaction among the infants or toddlers in the group and study the possible reasons.

4.7.2 Identifying Infant's or Toddler's Initiatives as an Opportunity for Learning

While watching the video, during the MISC TP, the caregiver becomes aware of how she allows infants or toddlers to take the initiative and develop ideas of their own within the interaction. As a learning approach, the MISC model sees value in an interaction characterized by both the adult's and the child's initiatives. Very often, the caregiver comes up with her/his own "plan", for example, to encourage building blocks with a group of toddlers; in contrast, the toddler may want to tap the blocks into each other, enjoying producing sounds. The caregiver can see herself re-focusing the toddlers on placing one block on top of another through the training sessions, ignoring the tapping initiative. The training session can facilitate a discussion about the importance of connecting with the toddler's initiative while maintaining appropriate communication chains to encourage learning (see Chapters 2 and 3). Why is it important to give meaning to a child's initiative to tap with blocks and produce a sound? Making the connection to the child's initiative instils in him a need to continue exploring the environment, and therefore encourages learning. At the same time, responding to children's initiatives does not contradict or eliminate the importance of the caregiver's plan to teach how to build a tower from blocks. There are a place and importance for both.

4.7.3 Social Mediation and Learning of Socio-Emotional Skills

Analyses of a video recording of a group activity allow examining the reactions and behaviors of infants and toddlers directed at each other. For example, suppose a toddler expresses distress and cries because one of the toddlers accidently stepped on another toddler's finger while looking for a place to sit on the carpet. In that case, the caregiver seems to try to calm him down and comfort him. While watching the video, it becomes apparent that several toddlers had stopped their activities and turned their attention to the crying toddler. The caregiver did not notice this until the moment she watched the video with the trainer. The trainer can then raise the possibility of using the toddlers' focus on the distress and addressing them in the future while giving meaning to the occurrence and encouraging empathy: "Dina cries because Joey accidentally stepped on her finger, she cries because it hurts her a lot. . . . Soon she will overcome," etc. Even in everyday situations such as conflicts over objects, which are very common at the ages of 2 to 3, the joint viewing of the conflict raises questions about the caregiver's mediational role in teaching social skills. For example: encouraging a toddler to ask for an object from a friend, or during an emotional storm, the caregiver provides meaning to the turbulent emotion that arises at the moment: "I understand that you are very angry about Mona, because she does not want to give you the doll . . ."

4.7.4 Learning Mediation Skills for the Entire Group

As mentioned earlier (see Chapters 2 and 3), the MISC intervention model was originally developed for a parent or educator and one child (Klein, 1996). One of the main challenges of the caregiver working with a group of toddlers or young children is the adult's ability to adapt to the different needs, characteristics, and temperaments of the infants or toddlers all at the same time. Using VIG enables the caregiver to learn more effective mediational strategies for the entire group. One of the key strategies is focusing the entire group on a particular child's needs when the caregiver is required to respond specifically to a particular toddler's distress or need. For example, while there is an activity with books, one toddler points to a high shelf and points at a particular book that he is interested in. The caregiver often feels that by answering the child's need, she may neglect the rest of the group. The caregiver can give meaning to what is happening in the "here and now" for the whole group. For example, the caregiver will give meaning to what she does while addressing the whole group: "What is Danny pointing to? Do you want the book, Danny? Kids . . . what book does Danny want?" The training sessions enable the trainer to discuss the possibilities of response with the entire group with the caregiver, thereby studying the important strategy aimed at responding to the need of an individual child in the group while continuing to "hold" the entire group.

4.8 Challenges Associated With Implementing the MISC-TP

Along with the benefits of training staff working in group settings, there are also difficulties implementing the training program. Sometimes, the caregiver's awareness of the importance of her sensitivity and responsiveness to all children's signals and needs may frustrate her due to the challenges involved in adapting herself to all the children in the group. Another pitfall relates to the training resources needed to implement the MISC-PT with the staff of ECEC settings. Time resources are needed, and therefore, a budget that allows for several hours of training is needed. Such a training program also requires electronic equipment and devices such as a projector, screen, and computer for the VIG sessions and a separate room where training sessions can be held individually, without interruptions.

4.9 Ways of Implementing the MISC-TP in ECEC

MISC-TP is implemented in several ways: as an in-service training in public and private day-care centers (birth to 3); as part of courses and workshops for kindergarten teachers of children ages 3–6; and as part of the training program for early childhood educational counselors.

- **In-service training in public and private day-care settings for birth-to-3 infants and toddlers.**
  - A trainer who attends a staff of day-care centers through in-service training arrives approximately every two weeks and operates in the following modes of training:
    - Observation and training in the classroom
    - Personal training sessions with caregivers with or without video (VIG)
    - Group training sessions with or without video (VIG)

- **Training workshops for kindergarten teachers (ages 3–6).** As part of these training sessions, educators participate in a group meeting with the trainer for a series of sessions (between four and seven sessions, depending on the length of the course). The program structure includes two content sessions and exposure to the nature of the MISC intervention model (see Chapter 2) and practice sessions in identifying the MISC components based on video recording of themselves with children.
- **Training program for ECEC counselors and trainers.** As part of a counselor training program that aims to train the participants as counselors and trainers in ECEC settings, the students are exposed to the MISC intervention model (see Chapter 2). The students are also trained as a "MISC trainers" through the experience of training a caregiver in a setting as a part of the practicum in the program. This qualification includes practicing video training with a caregiver (VIG) while receiving professional supervision throughout the process.

According to the concept of "parallel process" (see Chapter 3), the interaction between the trainer and the caregiver is defined with the same MISC interventional model components concerning adult-child interaction. The trainer acts intentionally while he/she is aware of the meaning and quality of interactions that appear in all kinds of relationships in the setting. The MISC trainer must also express expertise in various issues related to the ECEC settings: child development, assessment of the quality of the day-care center, pedagogical issues, and developmentally appropriate practices. When caregivers receive professional training to connect to their professional needs within a sensitive and supportive relationship, they may promote quality interactions with infants or toddlers and foster optimal development and learning.

4.10 Conclusion

The importance of the quality of the interaction between educators and children in their care is the focus of the MISC training program. This chapter described the modes of implementation of MISC-TP in early childhood settings, along with the many challenges underlying these applications. One of the critical ideas brought here is the understanding that adults, serving as caregivers, need appropriate conditions to learn and maintain quality interactions with infants and toddlers during all kinds of play/learning and daily routine activities. Commitment to improving the quality of education and care in out-of-home settings requires policymakers to consider existing disparities regarding the quality characteristics of early childhood setting. This involves making responsible decisions, including prioritizing the quality educational infrastructure that is important for enhancing the wellbeing and healthy development of infants and toddlers in early childhood settings.

References

Bowlby, J. (1969). *Attachment and loss: Vol. 1. Attachment.* New York: Basic.

Brock, L. L., & Curby, T. W. (2014). Emotional support consistency and teacher—child relationships forecast social competence and problem behaviors in prekindergarten and kindergarten. *Early Education and Development, 25*(5), 661–680.

Burchinal, M. R., Peisner-Feinberg, E., Pianta, R., & Howes, C. (2002). Development of academic skills from preschool through second grade: Family and classroom predictors of developmental trajectories. *Journal of School Psychology, 40*(5), 415–436.

Campbell, F. A., Pungello, E. P., Miller-Johnson, S., Burchinal, M., & Ramey, C. T. (2001). The development of cognitive and academic abilities: Growth curves from an early childhood educational experiment. *Developmental Psychology, 37*(2), 231.

Cassidy, D. I., Buell, M. I., Pugh-Hoese, S., & Russell, S. (1995). The effect of education on child care teachers' beliefs and classroom quality: Year one evaluation of the TEACH early childhood associate degree scholarship program. *Early Childhood Research Quarterly, 10*(2), 171–183.

Cassidy, D. et al. (2017). Teacher work environments are toddler learning environments: Teacher professional wellbeing, classroom emotional support, and toddlers' emotional expressions and behaviours. *Early Child Development and Care, 187*(1), 1666–1678.

Copple, C., & Bredekamp, S. (2009). *Developmentally appropriate practice in early childhood programs serving children from birth through age 8* (Vol. 1313, pp. 22205–4101). Washington, DC: National Association for the Education of Young Children.

De Schipper, E. J., Marianne Riksen-Walraven, J., & Geurts, S. A. (2006). Effects of child—caregiver ratio on the interactions between caregivers and children in childcare centers: An experimental study. *Child Development, 77*(4), 861–874.

Eurofound. (2015). *Working conditions, training of early childhood care workers and quality of services—A systematic review.* Luxembourg City, Luxembourg: Publications Office of the European Union. doi:10.2806/69399

Fukkink, R. G., & Tavecchio, L. W. C. (2010). Effects of video interaction guidance on early childhood teachers. *Teaching and Teacher Education, 26*, 1652–1659.

Goble, P., Sandilos, L. E., & Pianta, R. C. (2019). Gains in teacher-child interaction quality and children's school readiness skills: Does it matter where teachers start? *Journal of School Psychology, 73*, 101–113.

Hamre, B. K., Hatfield, B., Pianta, R., & Jamil, F. (2014). Evidence for general and domain-specific elements of teacher-child interactions: Associations with preschool children's development. *Child Development, 85*(3), 1257–1274.

Hamre, B. K., Pianta, R. C., Burchinal, M., Field, S., LoCasale-Crouch, J., Downer, J. T., . . . Scott-Little, C. (2012). A course on effective teacher-child interactions: Effects on teacher beliefs, knowledge, and observed practice. *American Educational Research Journal, 49*(1), 88–123.

Harkoma, S. M., Sajaniemi, N. K., Suhonen, E., & Saha, M. (2021). Impact of pedagogical intervention on early childhood professionals' emotional availability to children with different temperament characteristics. *European Early Childhood Education Research Journal, 29*(2), 183–205.

Harms, T., Cryer, D., Clifford, R. M., & Yazejian, N. (2017). *Infant or toddler environment rating scale (ITERS-3).* New York, NY: Teachers College Press, 1234 and Amsterdam Avenue, 10027.

Howes, C., James, J., & Ritchie, S. (2003). Pathways to effective teaching. *Early Childhood Research Quarterly, 18*(1), 104–120.

Jamison, K. R., Cabell, S. Q., LoCasale-Crouch, J., Hamre, B. K., & Pianta, R. C. (2014). CLASS—Infant: An observational measure for assessing teacher—infant interactions in center-based child care. *Early Education and Development, 25*(4), 553–572.

Kalliala, M. (2011). Look at me! Does the adult truly see and respond to the child in finnish day-care centres? *European Early Childhood Education Research Journal, 19*(2), 237–253.

Klein, P. S., & Hundeide, K. (1996). *Early intervention: Cross-cultural experiences with a mediational approach* (Vol. 887). London: Routledge.

La Paro, K. M., Hamre, B. C., & Pianta, R. C. (2009). *The classroom assessment scoring system, toddler version.* Charlottesville, VA: Teachstone.

Mashburn, A. J., Pianta, R. C., Hamre, B. K., Downer, J. T., Barbarin, O. A., Bryant, D., . . . Howes, C. (2008). Measures of classroom quality in prekindergarten and children's development of academic, language, and social skills. *Child Development, 79*(3), 732–749.

Oberhuemer, P., Schreyer, I., & Neuman, M. J. (2010). *Professionals in early childhood education and care systems. European profiles and perspectives.* Opladen, Germany: Barbara Budrich Publishers.

OECD. (2012). *Starting strong III—a quality toolbox for early childhood education and care.* Paris, France: Author.

Rothbart, M. K., & Ahadi, S. A. (1994). Temperament and the development of personality. *Journal of Abnormal Psychology, 103*(1), 55.

Rothbart, M. K., & Bates, E. (2006). Temperament. In N. Eisenberg, W. Damon, R. Lerner (Eds.), *Handbook of child psychology: Social, emotional, and personality development* (pp. 99–166). Hoboken, NJ: John Wiley & Sons Inc.

Ruzek, E., Burchinal, M., Farkas, G., & Duncan, G. J. (2014). The quality of toddler child care and cognitive skills at 24 months: Propensity score analysis results from the ECLS-B. *Early Childhood Research Quarterly, 29*(1), 12–21.

Slot, P. L., Leseman, P. P., Verhagen, J., & Mulder, H. (2015). Associations between structural quality aspects and process quality in Dutch early childhood education and care settings. *Early Childhood Research Quarterly, 33*, 64–76.

Tarullo, A. R., & Gunnar, M. R. (2006). Child maltreatment and the developing HPA axis. *Hormones and Behavior, 50*(4), 632–639.

Urban, M., Vandenbroeck, M., Van Laere, K., Lazzari, A., & Peeters, J. (2012). Towards competent systems in early childhood education and care; Implications for policy and practice. *European Journal of Education, 47*(4), 508–526.

van Schaik, S. D., Leseman, P. P., & de Haan, M. (2018). Using a group-centered approach to observe interactions in early childhood education. *Child Development, 89*(3), 897–913.

Werner, C. D., Linting, M., Vermeer, H. J., & Van IJzendoorn, M. H. (2016). Do intervention programs in child care promote the quality of teacher-child interactions? A meta-analysis of randomized controlled trials. *Prevention Science, 17*, 259–273.

Williams, S. T., Mastergeorge, A. M., & Ontai, L. L. (2010). Caregiver involvement in infant peer interactions: Scaffolding in a social context. *Early Childhood Research Quarterly, 25*(2), 251–266.

5 Mothers' Mediation in Book-Reading Activities Through the Lens of the MISC Model

Relation to SES and Children's Early Literacy

Ora Segal-Drori and Ofra Korat

5.1 Introduction

Shared storybook reading is a cultural and familial activity, which often occurs between parents and young children, and is one of the major activities that affect children's development. Research in the field has been tracking the nature of this activity for nearly 50 years and examines its impact on children's language and literacy achievements (Dickenson & Morse, 2019).

5.1.1 Book Reading and Early Literacy

Early literacy (EL) knowledge (e.g., letter naming, word reading, word writing, concepts about print) before formal schooling is known to be an important factor for reading and writing acquisition and for general academic achievement throughout the school years (Whitehurst & Lonigan, 2001). Several researchers on adult-child storybook reading indicated the contribution of book-reading activities to children's spoken language, while only a few studies reported the contribution of this activity to children's EL knowledge (Han, 2015). Some researchers stated that shared book reading is an important predictor of literacy achievement, even though the stability and reliability of the connections found between reading books to children and measures of literacy were relatively low (Mol, Bus, de Jong, & Smeets, 2008; Noble et al., 2019). The considerably low effects of book reading on children's EL can be explained by the fact that young children are not engaged with print during their everyday or natural activity (without special intervention) and that parents and teachers rarely discuss the written text when reading a book to children (Justice, Pullen, & Pence, 2008). Although this behavior is rare, there is some evidence that when parents discuss the written text with kindergarten-age children during joint book reading, this predicts high literacy achievement in school. Results showed an improvement in parents' discussion of the written text during the reading activity and children's progress in print awareness and word reading (Justice & Ezell, 2000). Piasta, Justice, McGinty, and Kaderavek (2012) conducted a

DOI: 10.4324/9781003145899-5

longitudinal study in which preschoolers participated in a 30-week shared reading program implemented by their teachers, who related to print verbally and nonverbally (talking about or pointing to print within the text). The longitudinal results showed that the use of print references made a significant impact on children's EL skills (reading, spelling, story comprehension) for two years post-intervention. The controversy over the contribution of adult-child printed book reading to EL shows that different ways of adults' reading and mediation may impact children's literacy in different ways.

5.1.2 Parents' Reading Mediation Behavior

Researchers investigating joint parent-child reading emphasize the importance of parents' mediation during book reading to young children. Two main models are known for analyzing parent-child book reading activities: "distancing" (Sigel, 1982) and the "dialogic reading" model (Whitehurst et al., 1988). Sigel's (1982) model is grounded in a discourse-oriented theoretical framework suggesting that there are different aspects of parental talk while interacting with young children during book-reading activities, referred to as "distancing". More specifically, some parents describe and elaborate on the book's pictures and focus more on specifics and less on general knowledge. Some parents discuss issues that relate to general knowledge about the world and the child's own experiences. In contrast, others may discuss issues with the child beyond the text's information (inferences, predictions, etc.). Some researchers emphasize the importance of decontextualized language when reading a book with the young child, such as talking about future and past events, inferencing meanings, understanding definitions, and linking abstract concepts to everyday experiences. This language enables young children to infer non-immediate meanings from words and promotes comprehension and elaboration from the narrative language (Seven, Ferron, & Goldstein, 2020).

Whitehurst et al.'s (1988) model of "dialogic reading" focuses on teaching children to become storytellers and active partners instead of passively listening to the story. Adults ask questions during the process of dialogic reading, add information, and prompt the children to increase the sophistication of their descriptions of the material in the book. For example, Lever and Sénéchal (2011) tested whether an eight-week shared-reading intervention will enhance the fictional narrative skills of 40 kindergarten children. Dialogic reading was used to engage children in oral interaction during reading and to emphasize elements of story knowledge. The results indicated that the children improved their narrative construction knowledge and vocabulary.

The models previously presented emphasize mainly cognitive aspects during the adult-child joint reading. To the best of our knowledge, this is the first study to analyze the joint book reading event using the MISC model (Klein, 2000), which is more comprehensive and incorporates instructional, cognitive, emotional, and cultural aspects. Based on the MISC model, Korat and Klein (2004) developed the OLMI (Observing Literacy Mediational Interaction) tool, which focuses on the literacy interaction between the adult and the child in general book-reading interaction in particular. This tool relates to various aspects of the interaction, analyzing general characteristics such as the adults' and children's participation in the discourse, their initiations and their style as providing (information) and demanding (asking questions), as well as the adults' cognitive and emotional mediation to the children.

5.1.3 SES and Book Reading

The relationship between parent-child shared book-reading activities and the family's socioeconomic status (SES) was at the focus of many pieces of research in the last few decades (e.g., Arafat, Korat, Aram, & Saiegh-Haddad, 2017; Mol & Neuman, 2014). The importance of investigating how low-SES parents behave toward their children in the shared reading event stems from the compelling evidence that such children are at greater risk for school failure as a result of the literacy practices in their homes, compared to children from middle-SES families (Phillips & Lonigan, 2009). These studies found that middle-SES parents used higher levels of mediation during a book-reading activity than did lower-SES parents (Barnes & Puccioni, 2017; Chang & Huang, 2016; De la Rie, van Steensel, van Gelderen, & Severiens, 2020). De la Rie et al. (2020), for example, found that middle-SES parents produced higher distancing talk (such as inferencing) during book reading with children than did low-SES parents, who produced more low distancing talk (such as labeling).

Very few studies examined parents' emotional mediation and its relation to SES. For example, Baker and colleagues (2001) found that middle-SES mothers were more positive than low-SES mothers during shared storybook reading with their children and exhibited more emotional support. There is literature on parents' mediation during storybook reading with young children on socio-emotional themes raised in the story (such as mental terms, mental causality, the characters' intentions, relationships, and emotions) regarding SES (Aram, Deitcher, Shoshan, & Ziv, 2017). However, these studies did not research the emotional atmosphere during the reading interaction and the parents' emotional mediation to the children.

Another aspect that was researched regarding book reading and SES was parents' beliefs about reading a book to their child (see Goodnow & Collins, 1990; Miller, 1988). The literacy activities in which parents engage with their children are influenced by their beliefs relating to these activities, including reading a book with their children (Gonzalez et al., 2017; Weigel, Martin, & Bennett, 2006). For example, Bingham (2007) examined the association between the quality of mother-child interactions around reading practices, such as visiting the library and the frequency of joint reading, and mothers' affect during joint reading practice. The results showed that mothers' beliefs about the importance of reading significantly predicted the quality of literacy activities in the home, even after taking the mothers' education level into account.

Some studies showed differences in parents' literacy beliefs (e.g., belief that they should play an active role in promoting the child's literacy or regarding ways for promoting it) between parents from different SES groups (Fitzgerald, Spiegel, & Cunningham,1991; Meehan, 1998). However, some researchers did not find these differences between parents from different SES groups, but found differences in the mediation level of those parents during the literacy activities (Korat & Haglili, 2007; Korat & Levin, 2001). For example, Korat and Haglili (2007) did not find differences regarding literacy beliefs on children's emergent literacy level between mothers from low and middle SES. Still, they did find differences in their mediation level while reading a book to the child in favor of the middle-SES mothers.

In this chapter, we present an example of a study (based on Korat, Klein, & Segal-Drori, 2007) that investigated mothers' mediation in a book-reading activity through the lens of the MISC model, aiming to expand and deepen our understanding of the nature of this activity in families from different SES groups. A few studies found connections between adults' mediation to young children during book reading and children's EL achievements, and there is no information about these connections within different SES groups. Our research aims were to (1) research whether mothers' reading mediation behavior using the MISC model relates to children's early literacy level; (2) investigate whether these relationships are different or similar in low- versus middle-SES families.

5.2 Methods

The participants included 94 children aged 5–6 years, of whom 54 are girls (low SES n=26, middle SES n=28) and 40 are boys (low SES n=21, middle SES n=19), and their mothers. They were recruited from 41 kindergarten classes located in urban neighborhoods in the greater Tel-Aviv area. Twenty-two of the 41 kindergarten classes were located in middle-SES neighborhoods, and 19 were located in low-SES neighborhoods. Between two to four children from each of the 41 kindergartens participated in the study.

A seven-factor index was used to calculate the families' SES level. This index took the educational level, the profession and occupation of the father and mother, and the family's income level into account. A "z" score was used to calculate the mean for the SES variable (range 1–5; a=0.90). All families that had a score above the median were categorized as middle SES (n=47). Families scoring below the median were categorized as low SES (n=47).

Data were collected in three sessions. In the first session, the children's EL was assessed individually within their kindergarten setting. In the second session, mother-child dyads were involved in a joint storybook-reading activity in their homes. In the third and final session, demographic information was gathered from the mothers. Three to four days after testing the children individually in their kindergartens, the researcher visited the children's home. She gave the mother a book and asked whether it was familiar to her or the child. No child or mother in the study answered this question affirmatively. The mother was asked to read the book to the child as she usually would any other book.

We decided on a non-familiar, rather than a familiar, book for two reasons: (1) to avoid the possibility of different levels of previous exposure to the book, and (2) the expectation that a new book might present more of a challenge to the mother to elaborate on the book's content (De Temple & Snow, 1996; Haden, Reese, & Fivush, 1996; van Kleeck, Gillam, Hamilton, & McGrath, 1997). The book was *Frog and a Very Special Day* by Velthuijs (2000). The book has 30 pages, and each page has a big colored drawing and three to five written sentences (of about 30 words). The story is about a frog that one day discovers that all his friends suddenly seem to be avoiding his company. This makes him very sad, and he is very offended. But, at the end of the book, when he discovers that all of them had disappeared to prepare a birthday party for him, he feels loved by his friends and becomes very cheerful. The story has all the traditional characteristics of a "written" story: a full story scheme and inferential passages, and the language in it is typical of that found in such books. It includes illustrations and written text in pointed Hebrew, which employs the diacritical marks or points (nekudot) that are usually used in texts intended for young children to more easily relate to the text. A VHS camcorder on a tripod, placed at the far end of the room, videotaped the session. The researcher left the room while the mother and the child completed the task.

The mother-child book-reading interaction occurred in the participants' chosen place at home (the living room, the child's room, or the kitchen) and lasted, on average, for about 15 minutes (M=15 min; range=10–25 min). Videotapes of the dyadic interactions were transcribed verbatim, and the transcripts were used to code the interactions. In several cases, when coding was difficult to decide, videotapes were examined together with the transcripts. Mother-child interactions were analyzed according to the OLMI tool (Korat & Klein, 2004). The interaction was segmented into verbal units. Verbal units constitute the smallest unit of meaning and are usually comprised of sentences. Single or multiple verbal units may be found within a speaking turn. Inter-rater reliabilities for segmenting the interaction into units were computed based on a random selection of 10% of the dyads. Reliability measured by Cohen's j=0.80, p < 0.001. Each unit was coded in three ways: (1) who is speaking (the mother or the child); (2) the function of the unit (a new unit or a continuation); and (3) the subject or topic of the unit (e.g., naming details in illustrations or discussing the written system). The content was coded only when a new subject was added to the previous discourse. A repetition of content or comments was not coded as new content.

The verbal units were classified into the following aspects:

- General characteristics of the reading interaction according to the number of statements said by the child and the mother, the number of new initiatives of the child, and the number of giving or demanding of the mother.
- The mother's mediating behaviors in the interaction according to focusing, excitement, expansion, encouragement, and behavioral regulation.
- The level of cognitive mediation of the mother to the child coded and based on the types of expansions the mother made while reading, according to eight levels, from low to high: (1) naming details and objects in the illustrations; (2) relating the text to the illustrations; (3) naming details in the illustrations that were not mentioned in the text; (4) paraphrasing the text; (5) interpreting words; (6) discussing personal experiences; (7) making connections beyond the text; (8) discussing the written language.
- The mother's level of emotional support was measured by tone, closeness, supportive physical contact, and lack of cooperation. The score of the tone component was determined according to a scale of five, from the lowest to the highest. The score in the closeness component was determined according to a scale of four, from the lowest to the highest. The score in the components of supportive physical contact and lack of cooperation was determined by the number of times this component appeared in the interaction.
- Mother's text reading level: accuracy, fluency, and intonation.
- Children's EL skills were assessed before the interaction: concepts about print, the ability to read a familiar book, word recognition, phonological awareness, and naming letters.

5.3 Results

Comparisons between the two SES groups regarding the mothers' mediating level while reading a book to their young children showed no differences in the general characteristics between the groups. Expansion was the most common mediating behavior, beyond SES groups and within each SES group. Furthermore, a difference between the groups was found only in the mediating behavior of expansion: middle-SES mothers made more expansions than low-SES mothers.

Low-SES mothers related to details in the illustrations and made more text paraphrasing (low level) than did middle-SES mothers. In contradistinction, middle-SES mothers discussed the written language (high level) more than the low-SES mothers did.

Middle SES mothers were more emotionally supportive of their children in all the emotional characteristics. Additional results show that the mothers' level of text reading (accuracy and fluency) was higher in the middle than in the low-SES group and that low-SES children exhibited lower levels of EL skills than did middle-SES children.

Correlations were found between middle-SES mothers' cognitive mediation and children's EL measures (concepts about print, phonological awareness, and the child's general reading level). No such correlations were found in the low-SES group. No correlations were found between mothers' emotional mediation and children's early literacy level, except for phonological awareness in the low-SES group. Regression operations were performed beyond the SES and within each SES group to explore the contribution of the study's variables to the children's general EL level and each of the individual EL task levels. The dependent variables included the children's EL level (general score) and the five reading measures: concepts about print, the ability to read a familiar book, word recognition, phonological awareness, and naming letters. The independent variables included the SES group, the mothers' cognitive mediation level, the mothers' emotional mediation level, and the mothers' reading level.

The data show that family SES contributed to children's emergent literacy (this variable explains 20% of the differences). Mothers' cognitive mediation contributed to children's emergent literacy in the middle-SES group (this variable explains 13% of the differences). Mothers' emotional mediation contributed to children's phonological awareness in the low-SES group (this variable explains 14% of the differences). No other mediation was found.

Several important results emerged in the current study. First, the findings show that low-SES mothers' cognitive and emotional mediation levels are lower than those of middle-SES mothers. The findings regarding cognitive mediation are consistent with the literature (Barnes & Puccioni, 2017; Chang & Huang, 2016; De la Rie et al., 2020). The findings regarding emotional mediation are also consistent with the limited studies available on this aspect. For example, Baker, Mackler, Sonnenschein, and Serpell (2001) found that in reading a book to children, mothers' emotional support in the middle-SES group was more positive than that of low-SES mothers. The current findings also support research that suggests differences in emotional aspects between SES groups during other literacy activity interactions, such as co-writing. Korat (1998) examined differences in the tone of mothers from two different SES groups in Israel in joint writing activities with their children. She found that low-SES mothers used a less positive tone than middle-SES mothers. These results could be explained by environmental stress (Perkins, Finegood, & Swain, 2013). The pressure stems from family demographics, including the family's income, living conditions, and parents' education. It seems that these factors directly affect mothers' behavior (Weinfield, Egeland, & Ogawa, 1998).

The findings of the current study also show that the general EL level of the middle-SES children is higher than that of the low-SES children. This finding is consistent with the available literature (Strang & Piasta, 2016). These results are significant since early literacy skills at kindergarten age are considered reliable predictors for school-age literacy achievements (Dickenson & Morse, 2019).

Our results also show a correlation between the mothers' cognitive mediation and the children's EL. The higher the mothers' cognitive mediation, the higher the children's EL level. It should be stressed that this was found only in the middle-SES group.

The findings regarding the middle-SES group are consistent with the literature, which shows a correlation between non-immediate discourse that occurs when a parent reads letter names to a young child and the child's EL abilities, such as concept about print (De Temple, 1994) and recognition of letter names (Dickinson & Tabors, 2001; Haden et al., 1996; Hockenberger, Goldstein, & Sirianni Haas, 1999). Such a correlation was also found between discussion of the written language in the book-reading activity and the children's own ability "to read" from a book (pretend reading) and recognition of letter names (Bus & van IJzendoorn, 1988).

Regarding the low-SES group, only a few studies found a correlation between non-immediate parent-child dialogue in the book-reading activity and children's EL (De Temple, 1994), while other studies did not find such a correlation (Korat, Aram, & Hassunha-Arafat, 2014; Sparks & Reese, 2013). The lack of correlation might be due to the low level of mothers' cognitive mediation in the reading activity, including discussing the written text, which could support children's EL level. The literature presents conflicting results regarding the impact of intervention programs that included coaching parents from different SES groups in cognitive mediation while reading a book to their child (e.g., dialogic reading) on their child's literacy and language. Regarding the parent's cognitive mediation level, some meta-analyses found no differences between parents from different SES groups after these interventions (Noble et al., 2020), while others found differences between parents from low and middle-high SES in favor of parents from the middle-high SES (Manz, Hughes, Barnabas, Bracaliello, & Ginsburg-Block, 2010; Mol et al., 2008). Regarding the influence of these interventions on children's literacy and language abilities, some meta-analyses found no differences between children from different SES groups in their emergent literacy (Noble et al., 2020) and vocabulary (Dowdall et al., 2020), while others found differences between children from low SES and middle-high SES in their emergent literacy (Manz et al., 2010) and vocabulary (Mol et al., 2008), in favor of children from the middle-high SES. Possible explanations that the researchers gave for these results were that it is difficult to distinguish between the parent's reading mediation (or style) in reading the book to the child, which was learned by the intervention. In addition, it might be easier for parents whose reading mediation is naturally more interactive to adopt new reading styles. It may also be related to the parents' attitudes and beliefs about reading books to children and their purposes like enjoyment, religious goals, or social goals, and this may make it harder for some parents to adopt one specific reading approach (e.g., interactive reading) that they need to learn over other approaches (Noble et al., 2020).

These findings point to the importance of exploring parents' natural cognitive mediation style as the OLMI tool allows but raises the need to expand the tool to another important aspect in the MISC model: the cultural aspect. It is essential that follow-up studies also examine parents' attitudes and beliefs about mediation in reading a book to a child. Examining these aspects will enable better targeting of the parents' training and intervention programs of mediation when reading a book to the child.

As for the mothers' emotional mediation found in the current study, only one correlation with EL was found in the low SES group with phonological awareness. This finding is consistent with the limited literature in this context (Aram, 1998; Sonnenschein & Munsterman, 2002). For example, Aram's (1998) study examined interactions of co-writing between low-SES mothers and their preschool children. She found no correlation between the emotional aspects of the joint writing interaction and children's emergent writing. The lack of this correlation could be explained by the notion that parents perceive joint book reading as an opportunity to support cognitive abilities rather than emotional ones. It is also recommended to investigate parents' beliefs on this issue to test our assumptions in future studies. Reading books to young children in a positive and supportive atmosphere seems important for all children, especially for low-SES children who might benefit from it by expanding their motivation for repeated reading and advancing their language and literacy skills.

5.4 Conclusion

In conclusion, we used the MISC model and the OLMI tool as a framework to provide a comprehensive picture of adult-child reading activities and learn about their nature in different SES groups and their relations to children's skills. These findings can serve as a good foundation for educators and policymakers to propose suitable programs for parents that incorporate cognitive and emotional principles in parent-child interactions as a better start for literacy learning, especially for low-SES children.

References

Arafat, S. H., Korat, O., Aram, D., & Saiegh-Haddad, E. (2017). Continuity in literacy achievements from kindergarten to first grade: A longitudinal study of Arabic-speaking children. *Reading and Writing*, *30*(5), 989–1007. doi:10.1007/s11145-016-9709-x

Aram, D. (1998). *How mothers help their children to cope with writing tasks* (Unpublished doctoral dissertation). Tel Aviv University, Tel-Aviv. [Hebrew]

Aram, D., Deitcher, D. B., Shoshan, T. S., & Ziv, M. (2017). Shared book reading interactions within families from low socioeconomic backgrounds and children's social understanding and prosocial behavior. *Journal of Cognitive Education and Psychology*, *16*(2), 157–177. doi:10.1891/1945-8959.16.2.157

Baker, L., Mackler, k., Sonnenschein, S., & Serpell, R. (2001). Parent's interactions with their first-grade children during storybook reading and relations with subsequent home reading activity and reading achievement. *Journal of School Psychology, 39*(5), 415–438. doi:10.1016/S0022-4405(01)00082-6

Barnes, E., & Puccioni, J. (2017). Shared book reading and preschool children's academic achievement: Evidence from the early childhood longitudinal study-birth cohort. *Infant and Child Development, 26*(6), e2035. doi:10.1002/icd.2035

Bingham, G. E. (2007). Maternal literacy beliefs and the quality of mother-child book-reading interactions: Associations with children's early literacy development. *Early Education and Development, 18*(1), 23–49. doi:10.1080/10409280701274428

Bus, A. G., & van IJzendoorn, M. H. (1988). Mother-child interactions, attachment, and emergent literacy: A cross-sectional study. *Child Development, 59,* 1262–1272. doi:10.2307/1130489

Chang, C. J., & Huang, C. C. (2016). Mother-child talk during joint book reading in two social classes in Taiwan: Interaction strategies and information types. *Applied Psycholinguistics, 37*(2), 387.

De la Rie, S., van Steensel, R. C., van Gelderen, A. J., & Severiens, S. (2020). Level of abstraction in parent-child interactions: The role of activity type and socioeconomic status. *Journal of Research in Reading, 43*(1), 140–159. doi:10.1111/1467-9817.12294

De Temple, J. M. (1994). *Book reading styles of low-income mothers with preschoolers and children's later literacy skills* (Unpublished doctoral dissertation). Harvard Graduate School of Education, Cambridge, MA.

De Temple, J. M., & Snow, C. (1996). Styles of parent-child book reading as related to mothers' view of literacy and children's literacy outcomes. In J. Shimron (Ed.), *Literacy and education: Essays in memory of Dina Feitelson* (pp. 49–68). Cresskill, NJ: Hampton Press.

Dickenson, D. K., & Morse, A. B. (2019). *Connecting through talk: Instructing children's development with language.* Baltimore: Brookes.

Dickinson, D. K., & Tabors, P. O. (2001). *Beginning literacy with language.* Baltimore: Brookes.

Dowdall, N., Melendez-Torres, G. J., Murray, L., Gardner, F., Hartford, L., & Cooper, P. J. (2020). Shared picture book reading interventions for child language development: A systematic review and meta-analysis. *Child Development, 91*(2), e383–e399. doi:10.1111/cdev.13225

Fitzgerald, J., Spiegel, D. L., & Cunningham, J. W. (1991). The relationship between parental literacy level and perceptions of emergent literacy. *Journal of Reading Behavior, 23*(2), 191–213. doi:10.1080/10862969109547736

Gonzalez, J. E., Acosta, S., Davis, H., Pollard-Durodola, S., Saenz, L., Soares, D., . . . Zhu, L. (2017). Latino maternal literacy beliefs and practices mediating socioeconomic status and maternal education effects in predicting child receptive vocabulary. *Early Education and Development, 28*(1), 78–95. doi:10.1080/10409289.2016.1185885

Goodnow, J. G., & Collins, W. A. (1990). *Development according to parents: The nature of the sources and consequences of parents' ideas.* Hillsdale, NJ: Lawrence Erlbaum.

Haden, C. A., Reese, E., & Fivush, R. (1996). Mothers' extratextual comments during storybook reading: Stylistic differences over time and across texts. *Discourse Processes, 21,* 135–169. doi:10.1080/01638539609544953

Han, J., & Neuharth-Pritchett, S. (2015). Meaning-related and print-related interactions between preschoolers and parents during shared book reading and their associations with emergent literacy skills. *Journal of Research in Childhood Education, 29*(4), 528–550. doi:10.1080/02568543.2015.1073819

Hockenberger, E. H., Goldstein, H., & Sirianni Haas, L. (1999). Effects of commenting during joint book reading by mothers with low SES. *Topics in Early Childhood Special Education, 19*(1), 15–27. doi:10.1177/027112149901900102

Justice, L. M., & Ezell, H. K. (2000). Enhancing children's print and word awareness through home-based parent intervention. *American Journal of Speech-Language Pathology, 9*(3), 257–269. doi:10.1044/1058-0360.0903.257

Justice, L. M., Pullen, P. C., & Pence, K. (2008). Influence of verbal and nonverbal references to print on preschoolers' visual attention to print during storybook reading. *Developmental Psychology, 44*(3), 855–866. doi:10.1037/0012-1649.44.3.855

Klein, P. S. (2000). A developmental mediation approach to early intervention: Mediational intervention for sensitizing caregivers (MISC). *Educational and Child Psychology, 17*(3), 19–31.

Korat, O. (1998). *Mother-child interactions, mother's beliefs and the development of children's writing texts: Comparison between two SES* (Unpublished doctoral dissertation). Bar-Ilan University, Ramat Gan. [Hebrew]

Korat, O., Aram, D., & Hassunha-Arafat, S. (2014). Mother-child literacy activities and early literacy in the Israeli Arab family. In E. Saiegh-Haddad & M. Joshi (Eds.), *Handbook of Arabic literacy* (pp. 323–350). New York: Springer.

Korat, O., & Haglili, S. (2007). Maternal evaluations of children's emergent literacy level, maternal mediation in book reading, and children's emergent literacy level: A comparison between SES groups. *Journal of Literacy Research, 39*(2), 249–276. doi:10.1080/10862960701331993

Korat, O., & Klein, P. S. (2004). *OLMI: Observing literacy mediational interaction.* Israel: Bar Ilan University.

Korat, O., Klein, P. S., & Segal-Drori, O. (2007). Maternal mediation in book reading, home literacy environment, and children's emergent literacy: A comparison between two social groups. *Reading and Writing, 20*(4), 361–398. doi:10.1007/s11145-006-9034-x

Korat, O., & Levin, I. (2001). Maternal beliefs, mother-child interaction, and child's literacy: Comparison of independent and collaborative text writing between two social groups. *Journal of Applied Developmental Psychology, 22*(4), 397–420. doi:10.1016/S0193-3973(01)00080-6

Lever, R., & Sénéchal, M. (2011). Discussing stories: On how a dialogic reading intervention improves kindergartners' oral narrative construction. *Journal of Experimental Child Psychology, 108*(1), 1–24. doi:10.1016/j.jecp.2010.07.002

Manz, P. H., Hughes, C., Barnabas, E., Bracaliello, C., & Ginsburg-Block, M. (2010). A descriptive review and meta-analysis of family-based emergent literacy interventions: To what extent is the research applicable to low-income, ethnic-minority or linguistically-diverse young children? *Early Childhood Research Quarterly, 25*(4), 409–431. doi:10.1016/j.ecresq.2010.03.002

Meehan, E. (1998). *Parents' knowledge of emergent literacy.* Partial fulfillment of the requirement of the master degree, Kean University, Newark, New Jersey

Miller, S. A. (1988). Parents' beliefs about children's cognitive development. *Child Development, 59*, 259–285. doi:10.2307/1130311

Mol, S. E., Bus, A. G., de Jong, M. T., & Smeets, D. J. H. (2008). Added value of dialogic parent-child book readings: A meta-analysis. *Early Education & Development, 19*(1), 7–26. doi:10.1080/10409280701838603

Mol, S. E., & Neuman, S. B. (2014). Sharing information books with kindergartners: The role of parents' extra-textual talk and socioeconomic status. *Early Childhood Research Quarterly, 29*(4), 399–410. doi:10.1016/j.ecresq.2014.04.001

Noble, C., Cameron-Faulkner, T., Jessop, A., Coates, A., Sawyer, H., Taylor-Ims, R., & Rowland, C. F. (2020). The impact of interactive shared book reading on children's language skills: A randomized controlled trial. *Journal of Speech, Language, and Hearing Research, 63*(6), 1878–1897. doi:10.1044/2020_JSLHR-19–00288

Noble, C., Sala, G., Peter, M., Lingwood, J., Rowland, C., Gobet, F., & Pine, J. (2019). The impact of shared book reading on children's language skills: A meta-analysis. *Educational Research Review, 28*, 100290. doi:10.1016/j.edurev.2019.100290

Perkins, S. C., Finegood, E. D., & Swain, J. E. (2013). Poverty and language development: Roles of parenting and stress. *Innovations in Clinical Neuroscience, 10*(4), 10–19.

Phillips, B. M., & Lonigan, C. J. (2009). Variations in the home literacy environment of preschool children: A cluster analytic approach. *Scientific Studies of Reading, 13*(2), 146–174. doi:10.1080/10888430902769533

Piasta, S. B., Justice, L. M., McGinty, A. S., & Kaderavek, J. N. (2012), Increasing young children's contact with print during shared reading: Longitudinal effects on literacy achievement. *Child Development, 83*(3), 810–820. doi:10.1111/j.1467-624.2012.01754.x

Seven, Y., Ferron, J., & Goldstein, H. (2020). Effects of embedding decontextualized language through book-sharing delivered by mothers and fathers in co-parenting environments. *Journal of Speech, Language, and Hearing Research, 63*(12), 4062–4081. doi:10.1044/2020_JSLHR-20-00206

Sigel, I. E. (1982). The relation between parental "distancing" strategies and the child's cognitive behavior. In L. M. Laosa & I. E. Sigel (Eds.), *Families as learning environments for children* (pp. 47–86). New York: Plenum.

Sonnenschein, S., & Munsterman, K. (2002). The influence of home-based reading interactions on 5-year-olds' reading motivations and early literacy development. *Early Childhood Research Quarterly, 17*, 318–337. doi:10.1016/S0885-2006(02)00167-9

Sparks, A., & Reese, E. (2013). From reminiscing to reading: Home contributions to children's developing language and literacy in low-income families. *First Language, 33*(1), 89–109. doi:10.1177/0142723711433583

Strang, T. M., & Piasta, S. B. (2016). Socioeconomic differences in code-focused emergent literacy skills. *Reading and Writing, 29*(7), 1337–1362. doi:10.1007/s11145-016-9639-7

van Kleeck, A., Gillam, R., Hamilton, L. S., & McGrath, C. (1997). The relations between middle-class parents book-sharing discussion and their preschoolers abstract language development. *Journal of Speech-Language-Hearing Research, 40*, 1261–1271. doi:10.1044/jslhr.4006.1261

Velthuijs, M. (2000). *Zefardea beyom meuhad meod [Frog in a very special day]*. Tel Aviv, Israel: Zmora Bitan.

Weigel, D. J., Martin, S. S., & Bennett, K. K. (2006). Contributions of the home literacy environment to preschool-aged children's emerging literacy and language skills. *Early Child Development and Care, 176*(3–4), 357–378. doi:10.1080/03004430500063747

Weinfield, N. S., Egeland, B., & Ogawa, J. R. (1998). The affective quality of mother-child interaction. In M. J. Zaslow & C. A. Eldred (Eds.), *Parenting behavior in sample of young mothers in poverty* (pp. 114–169). New York: Manpower Demonstration Research Corporation.

Whitehurst, G. J., Falco, F. L., Lonigan, C. J., Fischel, J. E., DeBaryshe, B. D., Valdez-Menchaca, M. C., & Caulfield, M. (1988). Accelerating language development Through picture book reading. *Developmental Psychology, 24*(4), 552–559. doi:10.1037/0012-1649.24.4.552

Whitehurst, J. W., & Lonigan, C. J. (2001). Emergent literacy: Development from pre-readers to readers. In S. B. Numan & D. K. Dikinson (Eds.), *Handbook of early literacy research* (pp. 11–29(. New York: Guilford.

6 Using Early Caregiver Training to Enhance the Neurodevelopment of Very Young, Vulnerable African Children Exposed to or Living With HIV

Monica K. Gentchev, Michael J. Boivin, and Sarah Murray

6.1 Introduction

Over 25 million individuals in sub-Saharan Africa are living with HIV, 1.5 million of whom reside in Uganda (UNAIDS, 2019). Of the people living with HIV in Uganda, 100,000 are children between 0 and 14 years of age (UNAIDS, 2019). In addition, approximately 1 million children in Uganda are orphans, with one or both parents deceased due to the epidemic, and a new child is orphaned approximately every 14 seconds (Nyamukapa et al., 2008). Within low-income countries such as Uganda, HIV-infected and exposed children (i.e., born to a mother living with HIV but not themselves infected) are more likely to experience cognitive developmental delay (Grantham-McGregor et al., 2007; Walker et al., 2011). Yet, these children live in the context of an underdeveloped social service infrastructure that is limited in its capacity to provide for their developmental, social, and educational needs.

While the pathophysiology has not yet been fully established, the HIV virus places children at an increased risk of developmental and neuropsychological disturbances via direct impacts on brain structures involved in the regulation of emotion, behavior, and cognition (Benton, 2010; Busman, Page, Oka, Giordani, & Boivin, 2013; Scharko, 2006; Sherr, Croome, Castaneda, Bradshaw, & Romero, 2014). Upon reaching school age, children affected by HIV have been shown to have elevated prevalence of behavioral problems associated with impulsivity, hyperactivity, concentration (Mellins et al., 2012), and affect (Musisi & Kinyanda, 2009), as well as compromised executive function and information processing (Wachsler-Felder & Golden, 2002), as compared to unaffected children. Consequently, children living with HIV in sub-Saharan Africa have shown poorer scores in memory, attention, language skills, visual processing, reasoning, and motor skills on average than their unaffected peers (Boivin, Ruisenor-Escudero, & Familiar-Lopez, 2016; Ruel et al., 2012; Van Rie, Mupuala, & Dow, 2008).

DOI: 10.4324/9781003145899-6

By providing high-quality care, caregivers can buffer the effects of biopsychosocial stressors on consequential neuropsychologic stagnation (McCartney, Dearing, Taylor, & Bub, 2007). Studies suggest that improvements in caregiving quality can promote positive developmental outcomes in young children who are already experiencing early signs of cognitive delay (Jaffee, 2007). For instance, a study of rural children aged 1–3 years in low-income areas of India determined that children of mothers who were more involved and provided more stimulation exhibited more positive cognitive development than their counterparts receiving less-responsive care (Agarwal et al., 1992).

However, caregiving quality can be severely impacted by a caregiver's own respective mental and physical health. Within eastern Uganda, the prevalence of depression among patients living with HIV/AIDS is approximately 47% (Chandra, Ravi, Desai, & Subbakrishna, 1998; Tostes, Chalub, & Botega, 2004). Additionally, the physical illness experienced by parents living with HIV can severely disrupt not only their immediate capacity to care for their children but can also contribute to food insecurity and financial instability for the entire family (Klein & Rye, 2004; Klein, 1996). Chronic nutritional hardship is well established as a factor that can severely undermine early childhood development (Grantham-McGregor et al., 2007; Grantham-McGregor, Schofield, & Harris, 1983; Grantham-McGregor, Schofield, & Powell, 1987). As summarized by the UK Millennium Cohort Study, child cognitive development is strongly impacted by economic stability, while behavioral health relies on maternal mental status (Kiernan & Huerta, 2008). The two may interact in complex ways to produce poor health outcomes for some HIV-affected children in sub-Saharan Africa.

6.2 Mediational Intervention for Sensitizing Caregivers

Cognitive and behavioral delays impair children's potential to achieve academic success, which can lead to a cascade of adverse outcomes, including lower future income potential and the subsequent intergenerational transmission of poverty. Evidence-based programs for promoting cognitive development among children living in poverty within low- and middle-income countries aim to interrupt this trajectory and improve a broad spectrum of developmental outcomes for at-risk children. One such program is the Mediational Intervention for Sensitizing Caregivers (MISC), which aims to enhance the development of children by positively impacting the day-to-day interactions between child and caregiver within the home.

MISC was developed by Dr. Pnina Klein and is based on Feuerstein's theory of cognitive modifiability (Feuerstein, 1979, 1980). The fundamental premise of this approach is that mediated learning best occurs interactively, i.e., when the caregiver interprets the environment for the child. To do so, the caregiver must be sensitive to the child's cognitive and emotional needs, interests, and capacities. MISC training teaches the caregiver practical strategies towards this purpose, as discussed later. MISC is implemented biweekly for a year (for a total of approximately 24 sessions).

The approach was shown to be feasible for implementation in a low-income country, first in Addis Ababa, Ethiopia, demonstrating MISC to be a culturally adaptable approach with the potential to enhance cognitive, language, behavioral, and academic outcomes in impoverished children (Klein, 1985, 2001, 2004). This chapter focused on applying MISC within a different low-income setting within sub-Saharan Africa, Uganda, as an approach to buffer the effects of living with or having been exposed to HIV. Thus, in the following, a series of studies conducted with children living with HIV (CLWH) and children who were exposed to but uninfected with HIV (CHEU) in Uganda will be discussed, with a focus on findings related to MISC's potential to promote the cognitive, behavioral, or general well-being of the child, caregiver, and family member. Supplemental Figure 6.1 provides information regarding the caregiver and developmental tests used across these studies to assess changes in these outcomes.

6.2 Ugandan Trials of MISC With Children Living With HIV and Children Exposed to but Uninfected With HIV

6.2.1 Training of MISC Trainers

As a first step, consultants who were experts MISC (i.e., MISC master trainers) led a three-week long workshop with a Ugandan field on how to facilitate and implement the MISC intervention with caregivers of young children. To ensure the existence of a treatment as usual control condition that provided similar attention to mothers in a comparison group, the program director for the Uganda Community Based Organization for Child Welfare (UCBOCW) trained a separate field in a health and nutrition education program for caregivers of young children. UNICEF supported UCBOCW staff who had previously implemented the curriculum for this nutrition education program in 17 other rural Ugandan districts. Local MISC trainers selected to deliver the interventions in Uganda were bachelor's degree graduates, many from Makerere University in either Psychology or Social Work. Local MISC trainers were either fluent in the local languages prevalent in the given district (Luganda, Jopadhola, and Ateso, depending on the study) or, when necessary, accompanied by a local translator.

MISC master trainers were devoted to helping local staff learn how to guide caregivers to become aware and develop practical strategies for engaging in mediational processes with their child:

> *Focusing*—gaining the child's attention and directing them to the learning experience in an engaging manner;
>
> *Exciting*—communicating emotional excitement, appreciation, and affection with the learning experience;

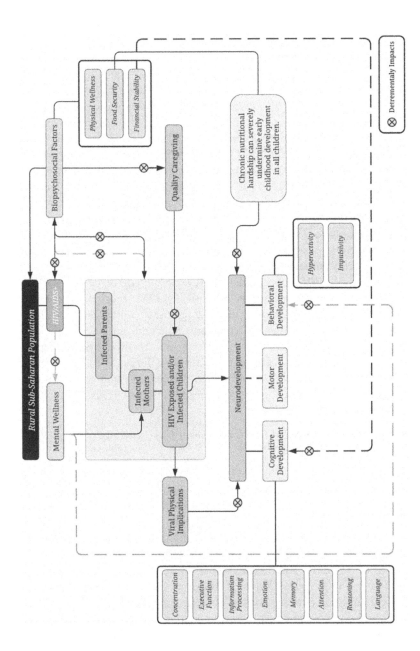

Figure 6.1 Summary model of various factors that mediate early childhood development within the HIV/AIDS-affected family

Expanding—making the child aware of how that learning experience transcends the present situation and can include past and future needs and issues;

Encouraging—emotional support of the child to foster a sense of security and competence; and

Regulating—helping direct and shape the child's behavior in constructive ways with a goal toward self-regulation (Klein, 1985).

The MISC master trainers also taught the locally selected cohort of MISC trainers how to videotape five-minute segments of the caregiver bathing the child, feeding the child, and working with the child. These 15-minute recordings were made for the MISC intervention dyads in the home at the start of training and then at regular intervals through the intervention to be played back to the caregivers as a part of future MISC sessions. Similar recordings were also made with caregiver-child dyads assigned to the control condition, but in this case, they were not shown to caregivers in the sessions as a teaching tool. These videos were still made with caregivers in the control condition because videos in both arms of the trial were scored by an independent observer at a separate study site, using the Observing Mediated Interactions (OMI) rubric (Klein & Rye, 2004; Klein, 1996, 2001) to assess progress in caregiving quality. Specifically, OMI scoring assesses the total number of focusing, exciting, expanding, encouraging, and regulating caregiver/child interactions that occur, consistent with the MISC training. In addition, at baseline and several follow-up points throughout the trial, a trained data collector also visited the caregiver's home to independently administer the (HOME) scale (Caldwell & Bradley, 1979) as an assessment of the quality of the caregiving environment in both trial arms.

6.2.1 Pilot RCTs of MISC With HIV-Exposed Uninfected and Children Living With HIV

MISC was first piloted in eastern Uganda in two randomized controlled pilot studies with different cohorts of children: one with young (aged 2 to 4 years) CHEU and one with young (aged 16 months–5 years of age) CLWH (Boivin et al., 2013a, 2013b). In the Tororo district, 119 dyads comprised of CHEU and their caregivers were assigned to either the MISC or UCBOCW attention control condition. In contrast, in the Kayunga district, 120 dyads composed of a CLHIV and their caregivers were assigned to the same two conditions. In the program's implementation in these settings, the biweekly hour-long caregiver training sessions alternated between home (so MISC trainers could observe and direct caregiver/child interactions) and study office (where videotapes of interactions could be shown to the MISC caregivers). The control condition was structured in the same way for comparability.

In addition to the OMI and HOME measure described earlier, outcomes of interest in the two trials were the Mullen Early Learning Scales (MELS)

to assess multiple domains of child cognitive and motor development (Mullen, 1995); the Color Object Association Test (COAT) to assess memory (Jordan, Johnson, Hughes, & Shapiro, 2008); the Achenbach Child Behavior Checklist (CBCL) for child externalizing and internalizing symptoms (Achenbach et al., 2008); and the Hopkins Symptom Checklist-25 to assess caregiver depression and anxiety symptoms (Hesbacher, Rickels, Morris, Newman, & Rosenfeld, 1980; Winokur, Winokur, Rickels, Rickels, & Cox, 1984). In the Tororo cohort trial, MISC children experienced significantly greater gains compared to controls on the MELS Receptive and Expressive Language development scale and overall MELS composite score of cognitive ability. COAT total memory for MISC children was marginally better than controls. No CBCL differences between the groups were noted. HOME and OMI scores from videotapes measuring caregiving quality also improved significantly more for the MISC group. The MISC enhanced cognitive performance, especially in language development in HEU.

In the Kayunga pilot with the cohort of CLHIV and their caregivers, children assigned to the nutrition education control intervention had higher viral loads than those assigned to MISC (Boivin et al., 2013b) balanced on other characteristics. Of note, children receiving highly active antiretroviral therapy (HAART) on average scored worse on several developmental outcomes relative to those not on HAART. Still, only the difference in MELS Gross Motor Development score was statistically significant between the two cohorts. This may have been an indication of disease severity. The caregiver-child dyads assigned to receive MISC on average scored higher on the MELS Visual Reception scale (visual-spatial memory) and COAT test of memory. Mortality was also less for children given MISC compared with controls during the training year. MISC caregivers significantly improved on the HOME and OMI scales relative to controls, indicating improvement in the quality and nature of caregiving interactions and the caregiver environment. MISC caregivers also experienced greater improvements in depression symptoms relative to caregivers assigned to the control condition.

6.2.2 ECVT Rescoring for Improved Validity

In the aforementioned studies (Boivin et al., 2013a, 2013b), the MSEL was used to assess motor skills and the cognitive development domains of language and visual-spatial analysis skills, while the COAT assessed working memory and learning to document the potential neurodevelopmental benefits of MISC. As neither of these assessments measure attention, both pilot cohorts were initially administered the Early Childhood Vigilance Test (ECVT) to assess attention (Zelinsky, Hughes, Rumsey, Jordan, & Shapiro, 1996). Systematic bias in the scoring of these data was identified, and thus, these results were deemed not yet trustworthy for assessing intervention impact at the time of publication of other trial results. However, the ECVT data for the Tororo and Kayunga pilot trials were later re-evaluated by a single trained researcher masked as to the assigned intervention arm and time point (baseline or one of the follow-ups) of the data collected. The reliability of scoring was also assessed by having this single researcher recode 30 randomly collected videos, resulting in no significant differences in scores.

Having assured data quality and addressed initial problems with scoring and controlling for ECVT baseline performance, age at assessment, and sex, we found in a subsequent analysis that while all CHEU showed benefits in attention across study follow-up regardless of the assigned arm in the Tororo pilot, children in the MISC arm exhibited significantly better scores on the ECVT relative to those in the control condition at six months. This difference had attenuated and was non-significant at 12 months (Ikekwere et al., 2021). The extent to which improved attention during the first six months of caregiver training intervention may reinforce improvements evident in child receptive language acquisition deserving further exploration in the future (Boivin et al., 2016).

6.2.3 Cluster Randomized Control Trial With Children Living With and Children Exposed to but Uninfected With HIV

A subsequent study was conducted that enrolled 120 CLHIV aged 2–5 and their female caregivers and 221 CHEU aged 2–3 and their female caregivers residing in 18 sub-counties within Tororo or Busia district (Bass et al., 2017; Boivin, Nakasujja, et al., 2017). Geographic clusters were generated and used as the unit of randomization to MISC or the same nutrition education control condition as used in the pilot trials (Bass et al., 2017). Local field trainers for this trial underwent a two-week training in their respective intervention. In addition, weekly supervision occurred through the intervention period, and a weeklong refresher training was held during the year-long implementation. During this study, data were collected at baseline, six months, 12 months (immediate post-intervention), and 24 months (one year following completion of the intervention). In a change from the prior pilot studies, the CBCL was not administered. However, the Behavior Rating Inventory of Executive Function (BRIEF) was added to assess the child's executive function (Gioia, Espy, & Isquith, 2011).

Beginning with the cohort of dyads where the child was living with HIV, dyads in the two arms were demographically comparable at baseline. However, the BRIEF inhibitor self-control scale scores were worse on average at baseline among children assigned to MISC relative to those assigned to control. Throughout implementing the interventions and follow-up, children in both arms experienced positive neurological and cognitive developmental changes. Children in MISC experienced significant improvements in receptive language relative to control children immediately post-intervention. At this same time point, MISC children exhibited worse BRIEF meta-cognition, inhibitor self-control, and global executive function scores than those in the control arm—but this difference was not maintained at future follow-ups (Bass et al., 2017). Children whose caregivers were assigned to MISC performed better on the ECVT at six months than those in the control group in the Tororo pilot trial with CHEU-caregiver dyads. This demonstrated moderate effect sizes of MISC on attention. However, this was no longer a significant effect at the 12-month follow-up (at the end of the MISC intervention). In addition, both children whose caregivers were assigned to MISC and the control group exhibited a trend of positive growth in ECVT scores across the yearlong intervention period that was not significantly different by the arm (no other statistically significant effects of MISC on child outcomes were noted) (Boivin, Weiss, et al., 2017).

Caregivers of the children living with HIV in both intervention arms experienced mental health improvements and functionality over time. Yet, MISC caregivers reported fewer depression symptoms and less functional impairment relative to those in the control condition. Additionally, caregivers in MISC consistent and significantly improved average HOME scores across intervention implementation and follow-up compared to caregivers assigned to the control arm. When HOME scores and OMI scores were added to linear mixed-effects models with MSEL receptive language as the outcome, effects of MISC were no longer significant, indicating probable mediation.

In the second cohort of CHEU and their caregivers enrolled in this same Tororo-based RCT, caregiving quality was better in the MISC arm than the control arm at all follow-up time points as measured by the HOME scale. No other significant benefits were noted in child neurodevelopment outcomes in MISC relative to control dyads. Like the cohort with CLHIV in the dyads, the BRIEF score was worse in the MISC arm relative to the control arm at the 24-month follow-up (Boivin, Weiss, et al., 2017) (see Figure 6.2).

6.2.3.1 Assessing Potential Benefits of MISC for Other Children in the Household

While the studies within this review illuminate the various ways by which early childhood development programs can enhance neurocognitive development through caregiver training focused on a specific young child, it is unclear to what extent these potential benefits may extend to other children in the household. Siblings of children targeted by the intervention may benefit from the caregiver using their newly learned skills with children other than the target child or through broader improvements in the family context and family functioning. To test this hypothesis, caregiver-child dyads in the CHEU cohort of the RCT of MISC in Tororo were also invited to enroll up to two additional children aged 0 to 12 years currently living in the same household as the target child (Boivin, Augustinavicius, Familiar-Lopez, et al., 2020). If more than two siblings were living in the household at the time of recruitment, the two siblings closest in age to the

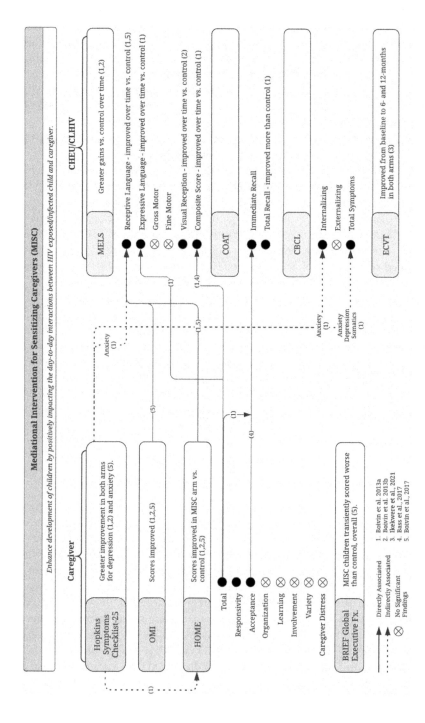

Figure 6.2 Summary model of MISC influence on various neurodevelopmental markers within HIV/AIDS-affected family

target child were included. A total of 294 siblings enrolled from 211 households were enrolled. Depending on their age, they were either administered the same assessments as the target study child in the dyad, or if older, the Kaufman Assessment Battery for Children, Second Edition (KABC) (Kaufman & Kaufman, 2004); Test of Variables of Attention (TOVA) (Dupuy & Greenberg, 1993/2005); the BRIEF School-Age Parent version; and the Attention-Deficit/Hyperactivity Disorder-Rating Scale IV. Data collection with other children in the household followed the same follow up assessment schedule with the target study child and caregiver.

Siblings of children whose caregivers were assigned to MISC performed significantly better at six months on KABC sequential processing (working memory) and simultaneous processing at 12 months compared to the sibling of children whose caregivers were randomized to the control condition. However, the improvement was transient and plateaued by the 24-month assessment, no longer exhibiting a significant difference by treatment arm. Thus, while MISC may have provided some short-term neurocognitive benefits to other children in the house, these were not sustained. Analysis of the BRIEF and ADHD outcomes indicated significant differences by treatment arm across all time points, with MISC mothers scoring their children as having significantly more executive functioning problems than control mothers. This could be due to MISC enhancing caregivers' attention to their children and making them more aware of the child's difficulties.

6.2.3.2 Using Eye Tracking With Computerized Testing for Evaluating MISC Benefits in Infants and Toddlers

Thirty-one HIV-exposed Ugandan infants aged 6–12 months who were siblings of children who had previously been a part of a malaria treatment study in Tororo were enrolled in a separate assessment of the Fagan Test of Infant Intelligence (FTII) (Chhaya et al., 2018). The FTII assesses the duration of an infant's visual engagement with novel versus familiar human faces as an early indicator of neurocognitive development and developmental risk. While children are shown images of faces, a Tobii X2-30 infrared camera assesses eye tracking, including location and duration of visual engagement, through pupil detection and compares these for novel versus familiar faces (Chhaya et al., 2018). We sought to assess this test's feasibility in a low-resource country setting like Uganda and the degree to which the score on the FTII was associated with other measures of child neurocognitive development. We found that infants did exhibit a more sustained gaze when shown images of novel faces. This longer duration of visual engagement with novel faces was generally associated with higher MSEL scores, most strongly with the fine motor score (Chhaya et al., 2018).

Drawing upon children in the Tororo trial with CHEU, 44 children aged 44 to 65 months were also assessed using the same Tobii eye-tracking method while being administered the ECVT test of attention at their 24-month follow-up assessment (Boivin et al., 2020). In this study, the ECVT using the Tobii eye tracking was compared to PROCODER scoring done by a human observer to record the child's gaze taken via a webcam. The results indicated that while the two forms of measurement were highly correlated (rho>0.9), the Tobii was more sensitive and able to capture a greater amount of time the child spent looking at the cartoon played as a part of the ECVT test than was the human coder. ECVT score calculated using neither methodology exhibited a significant association with MSEL and BRIEF scores, assessments of cognitive development (Boivin et al., 2020).

6.3 Conclusions and Future Directions With mHealth and MISC Training

We can conclude from our work with HIV-affected households in Uganda that mothers living with HIV and their children face significant adversity and nearly non-existent access to health services. Parenting interventions delivered by well-trained and supervised paraprofessionals have positively impacted both mothers and children, including preventing perinatal depression and improving child cognitive development (Cooper et al., 1999; Stein et al., 2008). Due to the one-on-one sessions, these programs' long-term delivery structure cannot be feasibly implemented as a broader prevention strategy in LMIC. Human and health resources are limited, and adolescent motherhood is common, and environmental risk factors for poor child development (e.g. poverty, stigma) are prevalent. *An important future direction would be to adopt a skills-focused parenting program for group delivery supported with SMS technology that can efficiently and synergistically improve related maternal and infant health outcomes.* Text messaging is one of the most frequent forms of mobile phone communication and is available on every mobile phone regardless of model or mobile network provider, with minimal costs per message, supporting the utility of text-messaging interventions (TMIs) for disseminating health-related information among adolescents.

The primary goal of this MISC initiative in settings like Uganda would be to test the acceptability and feasibility of adapting a well-established parenting training (PT) program (MISC) to a shorter group-based delivery model, supported by short message service (SMS, or text messages) technology for adolescent mothers in Uganda (PT-SMS). TMI are a scalable strategy that can maximize uptake and participation, capitalizing on adolescents' widespread use of mobile devices and potentially improve the wellbeing of adolescent mothers and their young children in LMIC. Minimizing in-clinic time, interventions that incorporate SMS may particularly benefit high-risk adolescents who lack access to developmentally tailored individualized care but are often pioneers in using new technologies. While published research from higher-income countries on mHealth solutions for adolescents is growing, there is much less documentation of mHealth-based parenting interventions for youth living in LMIC. Therefore, we propose developing an automated, interactive text message platform to provide adolescent mothers with relevant parenting skills and concepts that enhance child development and maternal wellbeing. We propose that the feasibility and acceptability of the PT-SMS intervention will be established with significant scale-up potential to other low-income settings for service delivery among HIV-affected mothers.

The specific aims for this proposal pertaining to future directions would consist of formative research including two focus groups (with adolescent mothers) and 10 key informant interviews (with health providers, peer educators, local leaders, and local digital service providers) that could inform the content development of SMS for HIV-affected mothers to receive the PT intervention in the rural Ugandan cultural context. By the end of this stage, we will have developed an SMS bank based on the MISC curriculum. Adolescent mothers especially are at risk in such settings. Our plan would be that those with a first-born child between 6 and 9 months old will attend four monthly, in-clinic PT group sessions led by a facilitator that will introduce the PT program, rehearse parenting skill exercises, and facilitate sharing of parenting experiences. All participants will receive three text messages (one for each MISC core component) every week during the same four-month PT group sessions period and provide mothers with anonymous, accurate, and non-judgmental information about parenting skills. Messages could be crafted to provide age-appropriate, MISC-based messages integrating emotional support and praise, maternal behaviors to support infant development, and support for infant feeding. After the proposed activities, we would have a fully adapted, feasible, and acceptable PT+SMS intervention ready to be tested at scale in Uganda among adolescent mothers.

6.4 Future Directions: Longitudinal Impact of MISC on School Success Among HIV-Affected Children

School success has been highlighted within the Sustainable Development Goals as "one of the most powerful and proven vehicles for sustainable development." Children from disadvantaged socioeconomic backgrounds often enter school at a disadvantage; these disparities can persist throughout their education, leading to reduced future earnings and adult poverty ((Grantham-McGregor, Cheung, Cueto et al., 2007; Leffel, 2013). However, research from the US indicates that early childhood programming (ages 2–5 years) can promote children's wellbeing through adolescence and adulthood, particularly for those at risk of poor outcomes due to poverty (Ramey et al., 2000; Reynolds, Temple, & Ou, 2003; Schweinhart, 2013). Further, children living with HIV-infected and -affected caregivers are at an even more pronounced disadvantage due to instability in caregiving (Van Rie et al., 2008) and poverty-related stress (Richter, 2003).

Early childhood programming often brings together children, parents, and early childhood educators in school-based settings to provide formal preschool services in high-income countries. In many low- and middle-income countries (LMIC), formal preschool programming lacks opportunities for children to gain skills for entering school ready to learn. Parenting programs that are delivered in the community may be a more appropriate delivery opportunity for supporting early childhood development in these contexts; a recent report by the National Academies of Sciences (2016) noted that parents who are more knowledgeable about child development "are more likely to have quality interactions with their child and to act in ways that support their child's healthy development."

Our MISC ECD intervention trials with Ugandan moms with HIV evaluated the impact of MISC caregiver training programs on neurocognitive development of HIV-affected children (ages 2–5 years) and caregiver wellbeing. The MISC intervention trained caregivers to be more sensitive to their child's developmental needs and react to those needs through enrichment activities using materials available in their own homes. The UCOBAC intervention provided caregivers with education in meeting the health and nutritional needs of their children. The MISC intervention was marginally better than the UCOBAC intervention on outcomes of receptive language skills (HIV-infected) and higher quality home environment (HIV-exposed but uninfected), and caregiver wellbeing (HIV-infected and HIV-exposed). Children in both intervention conditions showed improvement overtime in the other neurocognitive outcomes. Both interventions contain components of parenting programs standardly used throughout LMIC settings.

An important future direction in MISC intervention work in LMICs is to see how well-characterized cohorts of MISC-exposed HIV-affected children are better prepared for formal schooling when they reach school-age compared to children in treatment-as-usual (e.g., UCOBAC) children. We could investigate how language skills variations (as a marker of school readiness) and the quality of home environment impact school performance and child development outcomes as these children progress through their primary school years. We propose a four-year longitudinal follow-up of Ugandan caregivers and children who participated in previous year-long MISC intervention trials *to document how early gains in language skills, improved quality of caregiving, and improved caregiver wellbeing affect school performance and child development in a context of broad adversity*. Such a longitudinal study also provides an opportunity to explore potential distal impacts of the two parenting interventions on child development within the family and school environments. One example is how a small (n=84) study of poor, non-HIV-affected children in Ethiopia who participated in MISC reported greater school attendance rates, higher school achievement, and better behavioral regulation than controls did after six years of follow-up (Klein & Henning, 2004). Such a "future directions" longitudinal follow-up MISC intervention study takes advantage of a well-characterized sample of HIV-affected children with two years of cognitive and neurodevelopment assessment data to build our understanding of child development in the middle-childhood years in contexts of broad adversity. Such a study could describe cognitive development, neurodevelopment, and learning as part of a lifelong process that underlies overall functioning and quality-of-life. Understanding how important language skills and home environment in the preschool years are to primary school success in a resource-poor adverse environment will provide valuable information for program targeting other high-risk populations globally.

6.5 Future Directions: Dissemination and Implementation (D & I) Research for the Scale-Up of Evidence-Based MISC Caregiver Training Interventions

MISC uses trainers to provide caregivers with skills and knowledge to increase recognition of their child's needs and utilize materials in their own environment to enhance the child's regular activities to promote further development. Home-based parenting programs aimed at promoting child health and wellbeing have demonstrated success across various outcomes in rigorous controlled trials. A meta-analysis of 60 home-based parenting programs found that child benefits included enhanced cognitive and socio-emotional outcomes, while parent benefits included improved parenting attitudes and behaviors (Sweet & Appelbaum, 2004). This topic has far-reaching implications for promoting positive youth development and preventing emotional and behavioral problems, particularly in low-resource settings where families are large. Children often face significant adversity, and access to mental and behavioral health services is limited.

An important domain of dissemination and implementation science for future MISC scale-up research is to rigorously evaluate the integration and sustainability of MISC within three different care systems across governmental and non-governmental organizations in a given LMIC, such as Uganda, with varying types of providers. Such a study could generate a roadmap, including the relevant measurement tools, to assess organizational readiness to implement evidence-based child promotion services and monitor organizational progress to achieve service sustainability. Such a D & I research initiative could generate important information on the time and resources needed to integrate and sustain the MISC child development promotion program. Materials generated as part of such a study could then be available to adapt MISC to other LMIC settings.

By studying a multi-stage implementation cycle, from readiness through adoption and into sustainability, this kind of D & I research would evaluate the integration and sustainability of the MISC program into a primary care setting, a non-governmental organization, and a community-based organization, using different provider types, including nurses, community health workers, and peer providers. Such an initiative's key goal would be to evaluate the stages of implementation and related effectiveness of MISC implementation as conducted by providers across three different organization and provider types. We expect that different organization and provider types will need different types of organizational intervention assistance and resources to build sustainability. Another goal of such MISC-related DEI work would be to examine mediators associated with sustainability. Proposed mediators would include acceptability, reach, feasibility, willingness to change, and organizational climate. Finally, a third goal would be to characterize the paths to sustainability across organization types. A series of case studies, such as MISC D & I research, would identify barriers and solutions used to overcome these barriers by organization type. The participating organizations go through the phases of initiating and sustaining mental health services within their ongoing programming.

In so doing, a major future direction for such MISC D & I work would be to inform global health promotion programs in the process, barriers, and facilitators to establishing sustainable evidence-based promotion services. It would do so across 1) diverse service settings and 2) diverse provider types in an LMIC setting. Such D & I research would need to occur with MISC in a real-world scenario likely found in other LMIC. Doing such work in Uganda would do so in a research setting well characterized in terms of different service delivery and workforce samples in serving populations affected by HIV.

Acknowledgements

We acknowledge the contributions of Dr. Judith K Bass, especially with respect to "Future Directions" portions for MISC in the final portion of this chapter. Dr. Bass is an Associate Professor of Global Mental Health in the Department of Mental Health at the Johns Hopkins Bloomberg School of Public Health. She was co-PI with Professor Boivin on the principal NIH funding that supported the Uganda-based work reviewed in this chapter (R01HD070723: MPIs Boivin, Bass), contributing expertise especially in mixed-methods research approaches, trial design and implementation, and capacity building and mentoring related to the study of common mental health problems in low- and middle-income countries. Her early intervention trial studies investigated whether evidence-based and more traditional non-governmental organization (NGO) designed interventions reduced the burden of mental health problems in the populations to which they were targeted. Her expertise and proposals were especially important in Section 6.5 of this review pertaining to Dissemination and Implementation Scientific work for the future scale-up of MISC in LMICs.

We also recognize the contributions of Dr. Cilly Shohet and Deborah Givon of Bar Ilan University, Israel. They were primarily responsible for training our MISC implementation field teams between 2010 and 2017 in Uganda, under Professor Pnina Klein of Bar Ilan University. They were close collaborators of the MISC intervention program under Professor Pnina

Klein's direction, whose life work was dedicated to the origination, conceptual and empirical foundation to MISC, and its implementation globally. In 2011, Professor Klein was the winner of the Israel Prize for these scientific contributions. That is why we dedicate this chapter to Professor Pnina Klein (1920–2014).

References

Achenbach, T. M., Becher, A., Dopfner, M., Heiervang, E., Roessner, V., Steinhausen, H. C., et al. (2008). Multicultural assessment of child and adolescent psychopathology with ASEBA and SDQ instruments: Research fi ndings, applications, and future directions. *Journal of Child Psychology and Psychiatry, 49*, 251–275.

Agarwal, D. K., Awasthy, A., Upadhyay, S. K., Singh, P., Kumar, J., & Agarwal, K. N. (1992). Growth, behavior, development and intelligence in rural children between 1–3 years of life. *Indian Pediatrics, 29*(4), 467–480.

Bass, J. K., Opoka, R., Familiar, I., Nakasujja, N., Sikorskii, A., Awadu, J., Givon, D., . . . Boivin, M. (2017). Randomized controlled trial of caregiver training for HIV-infected child neurodevelopment and caregiver well being. *AIDS (London, England), 31*(13), 1877–1883. https://doi.org/10.1097/QAD.0000000000001563

Benton, T. D. (2010). Psychiatric considerations in children and adolescents with HIV/AIDS. *Child and Adolescent Psychiatric Clinics of North America, 19*(2), 387–x. https://doi.org/10.1016/j.chc.2010.02.004

Boivin, M. J., Augustinavicius, J. L., Familiar-Lopez, I., Murray, S. M., Sikorskii, A., Awadu, J., . . . Bass, J. K. (2020). Early childhood development caregiver training and neurocognition of HIV-exposed Ugandan siblings. *Journal of Developmental and Behavioral Pediatrics: JDBP, 41*(3), 221–229. https://doi.org/10.1097/DBP.0000000000000753

Boivin, M. J., Bangirana, P., Nakasujja, N., Page, C. F., Shohet, C., Givon, D., . . . Klein, P. S. (2013a). A year-long caregiver training program to improve neurocognition in preschool Ugandan HIV-exposed children. *Journal of Developmental and Behavioral Pediatrics: JDBP, 34*(4), 269–278. https://doi.org/10.1097/DBP.0b013e318285fba9

Boivin, M. J., Bangirana, P., Nakasujja, N., Page, C. F., Shohet, C., Givon, D., . . . Klein, P. S. (2013b). A year-long caregiver training program improves cognition in preschool Ugandan children with human immunodeficiency virus. *The Journal of Pediatrics, 163*(5), 1409–16165. https://doi.org/10.1016/j.jpeds.2013.06.055

Boivin, M. J., Nakasujja, N., Familiar-Lopez, I., Murray, S. M., Sikorskii, A., Awadu, J., . . . Bass, J. K. (2017). Effect of caregiver training on the neurodevelopment of HIV-exposed uninfected children and caregiver mental health: A Ugandan cluster-randomized controlled trial. *Journal of Developmental and Behavioral Pediatrics: JDBP, 38*(9), 753–764. https://doi.org/10.1097/DBP.0000000000000510

Boivin, M. J., Ruiseñor-Escudero, H., & Familiar-Lopez, I. (2016). CNS impact of perinatal HIV infection and early treatment: The need for behavioral rehabilitative interventions along with medical treatment and care. *Current HIV/AIDS Reports, 13*(6), 318–327. https://doi.org/10.1007/s11904-016-0342-8

Boivin, M. J., Weiss, J., Chhaya, R., Seffren, V., Awadu, J., Sikorskii, A., & Giordani, B. (2017). The feasibility of automated eye tracking with the early childhood vigilance test of attention in younger HIV-exposed Ugandan children. *Neuropsychology, 31*(5), 525–534. https://doi.org/10.1037/neu0000382

Busman, R. A., Page, C. F., Oka, E., Giordani, B., & Boivin, M. J. (2013). Factors contributing to the psychosocial adjustment of Ugandan preschool children with HIV/AIDS. In M. J. Boivin & B. Giordani (Eds.), *Neuropsychology of children in Africa: Perspectives on risk and resilience.* New York: Springer.

Caldwell, B. M., & Bradley, R. H. (1979). *Home observation for measurement of the environment.* Little Rock, AR: University of Arkansas Press.

Chandra, P. S., Ravi, V., Desai, A., & Subbakrishna, D. K. (1998). Anxiety and depression among HIV-infected heterosexuals—a report from India. *Journal of Psychosomatic Research, 45*(5), 401–409.

Chhaya, R., Weiss, J., Seffren, V., Sikorskii, A., Winke, P. M., Ojuka, J. C., & Boivin, M. J. (2018). The feasibility of an automated eye-tracking-modified Fagan test of memory for human faces in younger Ugandan HIV-exposed children. *Child Neuropsychology: A Journal on Normal and Abnormal Development in Childhood and Adolescence, 24*(5), 686–701. https://doi.org/10.1080/09297049.2017.1329412

Cooper, P. J., Tomlinson, M., Swartz, L., Woolgar, M., Murray, L., & Molteno, C. (1999). Post-partum depression and the mother-infant relationship in a South African peri-urban settlement. *The British Journal of Psychiatry, 175*, 554–558.

Dupuy, T. R., & Greenberg, L. M. (1993/2005). *The T.O.V.A. manual for IBM personal computer or IBM compatible.* Minneapolis, MN: Universal Attention Disorders.

Feuerstein, R. (1979). *The dynamic assessment of retarded performers.* New York: University Park Press.

Feuerstein, R. (1980). *Instrumental enrichment: Redevelopment of cognitive functions of retarded performers.* New York: University Park Press.

Gioia, G. A., Espy, K. A., & Isquith, P. K. (2011). *Behavior rating inventory of executive function preschool version, permissions and licensing.* Psychological Assessment Resources, Inc. Retrieved July 20, 2011, from http://www4.parinc.com/Products/PermsLicensing.aspx?id=8

Grantham-McGregor, S., Cheung, Y. B., Cueto, S., Glewwe, P., Richter, L., Strupp, B., & International Child Development Steering. (2007). Developmental potential in the first 5 years for children in developing countries. *The Lancet, 369*(9555), 60–70.

Grantham-McGregor, S., Schofield, W., & Harris, L. (1983). Effect of psychosocial stimulation on mental development of severely malnourished children: An interim report. *Pediatrics, 72*, 239–243.

Grantham-McGregor, S., Schofield, W., & Powell, C. (1987). Development of severely malnourished children who received psychosocial stimulation: 6-year follow-up. *Pediatrics, 79*, 247–254.

Hesbacher, P. T., Rickels, K., Morris, R. J., Newman, H., & Rosenfeld, H. (1980). Psychiatric illness in family practice. *The Journal of Clinical Psychiatry, 41*, 6–10.

Ikekwere, J., Ucheagwu, V., Familiar-Lopez, I., Sikorskii, A., AwaduPhD, J., Ojuka, J. C., . . . Boivin, M. J. (2021). Attention test improvements from a cluster randomized controlled trial of caregiver training for HIV-exposed/uninfected Ugandan preschool children. *The Journal of Pediatrics*, S0022–3476(21)00313–9. Advance online publication. https://doi.org/10.1016/j.jpeds.2021.03.064

Jaffee, S. R. (2007). Sensitive, stimulating caregiving predicts cognitive and behavioral resilience in neurodevelopmentally at-risk infants. *Development and Psychopathology, 19*(3), 631–647.

Jordan, C. M., Johnson, A. L., Hughes, S. J., & Shapiro, E. G. (2008). The color object association test (COAT): The development of a new measure of declarative memory for 18- to 36-month-old toddlers. *Child Neuropsychology, 14*, 21–24.

Kaufman, A. S., & Kaufman, N. L. (2004). *Manual for the Kaufman assessment battery for children* (2nd ed.). Circle Pines, MN: AGS Publishing.

Kiernan, K. E., & Huerta, M. C. (2008). Economic deprivation, maternal depression, parenting and children's cognitive and emotional development in early childhood. *The British Journal of Sociology, 59*(4), 783–806.

Klein, P. S. (1985). *More intelligent and sensitive child.* Ramat-Gan, Israel: BarIlan University.

Klein, P. S. (Ed.). (1996). *Early intervention: Cross-cultural experiences with a mediational approach.* New York: Garland Press.

Klein, P. S. (Ed.). (2001). *Seeds of hope: 12 years of early intervention in Africa.* Oslo, Norway: Unipub Forlag.

Klein, P. S., & Henning, F. (2004). Interaction-oriented early intervention in Ethiopia: The MISC approach. *Infants and Young Children, 17*(4), 340–354.

Klein, P. S., & Rye, H. (2004). Interaction-oriented early intervention in Ethiopia: The MISC approach. *Infants and Young Children, 17*, 340–354.

Leffel, K., & Dana, S. (2013). Parent-directed approaches to enrich the early language environments of children living in poverty. *Seminars in Speech and Language, 34*(4), 267–278.

McCartney, K., Dearing, E., Taylor, B. A., & Bub, K. L. (2007). Quality child care supports the achievement of low-income children: Direct and indirect pathways through caregiving and the home environment. *Journal of Applied Developmental Psychology, 28*(5–6), 411–426.

Mellins, C. A., Elkington, K. S., Leu, C. S., Santamaria, E. K., Dolezal, C., Wiznia, A., Abrams, E. J. (2012). Prevalence and change in psychiatric disorders among perinatally HIV-infected and HIV-exposed youth. *AIDS Care, 24*(8), 953–962.

Mullen, E. M. (1995). *Mullen scales of early learning: AGS edition.* Minneapolis, MN: American Guidance Service.

Musisi, S., & Kinyanda, E. (2009). Emotional and behavioural disorders in HIV seropositive adolescents in urban Uganda. *East African Medical Journal, 86*(1), 16–24.

National Academies of Sciences, Engineering, and Medicine, Division of Behavioral and Social Sciences and Education, Board on Children, Youth, and Families, Committee on Supporting the Parents of Young Children, Breiner, H., Ford, M., & Gadsden, V. L. (Eds.). (2016). *Parenting matters: Supporting parents of children Ages 0–8.* Washington, DC: National Academies Press (US).

Nyamukapa, C. A., Gregson, S., Lopman, B., Saito, S., Watts, H. J., Monasch, R., & Jukes, M. C. (2008). HIV-associated orphanhood and children's psychosocial distress: Theoretical framework tested with data from Zimbabwe. *American Journal of Public Health, 98*(1), 133–141. https://doi.org/10.2105/AJPH.2007.116038

Ramey, C. T. C., Frances, A., Burchinal, M., Skinner, M., Gardner, D., & Ramey, S. L. (2000). Persistent effects of early childhood education on high-risk children and their mothers. *Applied Developmental Science, 4*(1), 2–14.

Reynolds, A., Temple, J. R., & Ou, S. R. (2003). School-based early intervention and child wellbeing in the Chicago longitudinal study. *Child Welfare, 82*(5), 633–656.

Richter, L. M. (2003). Poverty, underdevelopment and infant mental health. *Journal of Paediatrics and Child Health, 39*(4), 243–248.

Ruel, T. D., Boivin, M. J., Boal, H. E., Bangirana, P., Charlebois, E., Havlir, D. V., et al. (2012). Neurocognitive and motor deficits in HIV-infected Ugandan children with high CD4 cell counts. *Clinical Infectious Diseases, 54*, 1001–1009.

Scharko, A. M. (2006). DSM psychiatric disorders in the context of pediatric HIV/AIDS. *AIDS Care, 18*(5), 441–445.

Schweinhart, L. J. (2013). Long-term follow-up of a preschool experiment. *Journal of Experimental Criminology, 9*(4), 389–409.

Sherr, L., Croome, N., Castaneda, K. P., Bradshaw, K., & Romero, R. H. (2014). Developmental challenges in HIV infected children—an updated systematic review. *Children and Youth Services Review, 45,* 74–89.

Stein, A., Malmberg, L. E., Sylva, K., Barnes, J., Leach, P., & FCCC Team. (2008). The influence of maternal depression, caregiving, and socioeconomic status in the postnatal year on children's language development. *Child: Care, Health and Development, 34*(5), 603–612.

Sweet, M. A., & Appelbaum, M. I. (2004). Is home visiting an effective strategy? A meta-analytic review of home visiting programs for families with young children. *Child Development, 75*(5), 1435–1456. https://doi.org/10.1111/j.1467-8624.2004.00750.x

Tostes, M. A., Chalub, M., & Botega, N. J. (2004). The quality of life of HIV-infected women is associated with psychiatric morbidity. *AIDS Care, 16*(2), 177–186.

UNAIDS. (2019). *Uganda.* Retrieved from http://aidsinfo.unaids.org/

Van Rie, A., Mupuala, A., & Dow, A. (2008). Impact of the HIV/AIDS epidemic on the neurodevelopment of preschool-aged children in Kinshasa, Democratic Republic of the Congo. *Pediatrics, 122*(1), e123–e128.

Wachsler-Felder, J. L., & Golden, C. J. (2002). Neuropsychological consequences of HIV in children: A review of current literature. *Clinical Psychology Review, 22*(3), 441–462.

Walker, S. P., Wachs, T. D., Grantham-McGregor, S., Black, M. M., Nelson, C. A., Huffman, S. L., . . . Richter, L. (2011). Inequality in early childhood: Risk and protective factors for early child development. *The Lancet, 378*(9799), 1325–1338.

Winokur, A., Winokur, D. F., Rickels, K., & Cox, D. S. (1984). Symptoms of emotional distress in a family planning service: Stability over a four-week period. *The British Journal of Psychiatry Journal of Mental Science, 144,* 395–399.

Zelinsky, D., Hughes, S., Rumsey, R. I., Jordan, C., & Shapiro, E. G. (1996). The early childhood vigilance task: A new technique for the measurement of sustained attention in very young children. *Journal of the International Neuropsychological Society, 2,* 23.

7 The Mediational Intervention for Sensitizing Caregivers to Enhance the Neurodevelopment of Children to Prevent Konzo Disease

Monica K. Gentchev, Michael J. Boivin, and Esperance Kashala-Abotnes

7.1 Introduction

Konzo is a permanent and clinically distinct neurologic entity that impacts the upper motor neuron pathways. Due to its resilience in the face of drought, acidic soils, and crop diseases, cassava has become the basic food staple in much of central and western Africa (Tylleskar & Tshala Katumbay, 2015). More than 600 million people around the globe rely on cassava as their primary source of nutrition. Sub-Saharan Africa holds approximately 20% of this estimate, and most people reside within ecological zones that cannot yield enough food outside of cassava to supply the region. Where other nutritional plants or protein sources are available (e.g., certain insects or caterpillars), they tend not to be culturally preferred or acceptable. Outbreaks of this disease frequent during times of food insecurity (e.g., the lean season, drought, and war or conflict-related displacement). The harvesting of cassava increases to account for low food sources of protein and other essential nutrients, or in times of drought and food insecurity. At such times, traditional practices for processing the cassava that might detoxify it (fermentation and drying in the sun) are not followed, allowing cyanide to persist in high concentrations within the plant tubers when prepared into flour food. The term "konzo" translates to "bound" legs (described as abnormal gait and restricted mobility) and originates from the *Yaka* tribe in the Democratic Republic of Congo (DRC) to designate a technique used by hunters to weaken legs and catch wild animals. Konzo results from cyanide toxins in poorly processed high-yield "bitter" cassava, a tuberous root used as a source of flour.

The World Health Organization (WHO) recommends konzo be defined based on the concurrent findings of visible spastic abnormalities in walking, a history of sudden onset in a formerly healthy person, and bilaterally exaggerated knee or ankle jerks without signs of disease of the spine (World Health Organization, 1996). As suggested by these antiquated terms, konzo was initially characterized as a disease confined to motor pathways

DOI: 10.4324/9781003145899-7

in the central nervous system with minimal recognition of the associated cognitive effects. Electrophysiologic and neuropsychiatric evidence later emerged, showing that higher-level brain functioning may be affected as well (Tylleskar & Tshala Katumbay, 2015). Although the global impact of konzo is not yet known, it is perhaps the biggest non-infectious and nutritionally dependent public health threat facing early childhood neurodevelopment in Africa today (Newton, 2017).

This paper discusses implementing a hybrid model for community intervention utilizing the Mediational Intervention for Sensitizing Caregivers (MISC) to prevent konzo. Although the program is still in progress, the use of MISC is an innovative community-based way to help prevent konzo. The chapter outlines the aims, research procedures and initial progress and emphasizes the role of MISC as a community-based response.

7.2 Literature Review

7.2.1 Background

Medical literature first document Konzo in 1938 (Trolli, 1938). Since then, outbreaks occurred in many sub-Sahara African countries like the DRC, the Central African Republic, Mozambique, and Tanzania. Konzo has affected hundreds of thousands of persons, with the majority of cases occurring in the DRC. Accurate prevalence estimates (as high as 5% in some rural regions) have been difficult to obtain due to unreliable demographic data and inadequate surveillance systems (Tshala-Katumbay et al., 2013).

More than 600 million people around the globe rely on cassava as their primary source of nutrition. Sub-Saharan Africa holds approximately 20% of this estimate, and most people reside within ecological zones that cannot yield enough food outside of cassava. Women and children are highly affected, particularly during times of economic hardship due to a lack of access to meat, beans, and other sources of sulfur amino acids necessary for the liver to detoxify cyanide. Children as young as a year old have been afflicted by konzo, suggesting that neurotoxicity may begin when caregivers wean children from breast milk to cassava porridge (Tshala-Katumbay et al., 2013). Outbreaks are frequent during times of food insecurity. While it is possible to extract cyanide from cassava by properly processing the roots before food production, these agricultural methods are time-intensive and minimize crop yield. Consequently, pre-production processing is often insufficient throughout a famine, which can lead to higher dietary cyanogen exposure (Ngudi, Kuo, & Lambein, 2003; Chabwine et al., 2011).

Konzo persists outside of periods of food shortage. A qualitative agronomic study recently evaluated potential factors and their contribution to increased cyanogenic glucoside levels in cassava (Imakumbili, Semu, Semoka, Abass, & Mkamilo, 2019). The researchers interviewed farmers in the Newala district of Tanzania regarding the taste of their cassava crops. Cassava root bitterness is often associated with heightened cyanide levels, which prompted which factors influenced the taste. The research found that red clayey-, fatigued-, sandy-, and red soils were the significant contributors to cassava root bitterness (14.2%). Redness within these soil types indicated the presence of high concentrations of nutrient-poor iron oxides. Plant age (7.5%) at harvest was highly dependent on the cassava variety, with sweet tastes and lower cyanogen levels near 12–18 months after planting; albeit more bitter cassava varieties were consistent between 24–26 months. Harvesting fatigued plants tended to have detrimental effects on the bitterness, which illustrated the impact of poor weeding (0.8%), piecemeal harvesting (0.8%), and branch pruning (0.8%). When framers harvest Cassava in its entirety, the plant appears to contain the lowest level of cyanide.

Konzo is easily recognizable amongst community members in endemic regions due to its peculiar features. The most prominent sign is a symmetric postural abnormality with spastic (cross-legged or scissoring) gait during ambulation. Clinically, deep tendon reflexes of the lower limbs typically exhibit hyperreflexia, extensor plantar response, and frequently ankle clonus. In more severely affected individuals, widespread motor deficits can be illustrated by abnormal reflexes and tetraparesis with weakness of the trunk. More specific fine motor control insufficiencies are present in affected individuals, including impairments in speech, swallowing difficulties, and vision. Further, an inspection may also demonstrate pendular nystagmus and signs of bilateral optic neuropathy (e.g., temporal pallor of the optic discs and visual field defects, suggesting bilateral optic neuropathy) (Mwanza & Tshala-Katumbay, 2005).

Cyanogenic neurotoxicity in konzo is not exclusive to defective motor control. Studies have further associated dietary cyanogen exposure with early child neurodevelopmental and cognitive delay, even in the absence of clinically evident paralysis. Cyanogenic glycosides contained in bitter cassava target neurons in brain structures that are involved in such processes (i.e., thalamus, piriform cortex, hypothalamus, hippocampus, and cerebellum), including the integration of memory, emotions, control of visceral functions, olfaction, and motor skills (Soler-Martín et al., 2010).

Espérance Kashala-Abotnes and colleagues studied konzo-related neurodevelopmental impacts by administering the Mullen Scales of Early Learning (MSEL) and Gensini Gavito Scale (GGS) on children living in and out of konzo-prevalent regions (Kashala-Abotnes et al., 2018). Respectively, these two scales assess cognitive ability and motor development, in addition to psychomotor development and growth in children. The study provided that linear growth and cassava cyanogen exposure were the main predictors of early child development and cognition in this sample. The mechanisms of action of the neurotoxic chemical compounds in cassava have not been completely elucidated.

7.2.2 Prevention of Konzo: A Role for MISC

Several studies using the Mediational Intervention of Sensitizing Caregivers (MISC) training program found that MISC influences the neurodevelopment of very young HIV-affected children and their caregivers' mental health (Boivin et al., 2013a, 2013b, 2017a, 2017b; Bass et al., 2016, 2017; Murray et al., 2017). This MISC caregiver-training intervention is family-oriented, has been specifically adapted for use in low-resource rural African settings, and has proven efficacy in HIV-affected populations. MISC learning takes place by training caregivers in practical day-to-day activities with the child to enhance such mediational processes as *focusing* (gaining the child's attention and directing them to the learning experience in an engaging manner); *exciting* (communicating emotional excitement, appreciation, and affection with the learning experience); *expanding* (making the child aware of how that learning experience transcends the present situation and can include past and future needs and issues, therefore extending beyond the immediate need of the moment); *encouraging* (positive emotional support of the child to foster a sense of security and competence); and *regulating* (helping direct and shape the child's behavior in constructive ways with a goal towards self-regulation).

The Uganda-based clinical trial results found that MISC is both feasible and well-accepted in the impoverished rural subsistence agricultural setting and enhances caregiving quality. It improves neurodevelopment in young children and caregiver mental health and functionality for daily activities of caregiving (Boivin et al., 2013a, 2013b, 2017a, 2017b; Bass et al., 2017). The critical developmental period for children is between 1 to 5 years of age. During this time, they develop the dynamic capacity to benefit from new learning experiences. There is a consensus from developmental research that adult-child interactions are of central importance in this process (Bonnier, 1992; Farah et al., 2009; Rao et al., 2010). The caregiver provides secure emotional attachments in a nurturing environment, creating learning experiences that allow for a child's neurocognitive ability to blossom (Vigotsky, 1978; Feuerstein, 1980). Effective mediational behaviors by caregivers were significantly related to children's social-emotional stability and the willingness to explore and learn about the world around them. (Feuerstein, 1980; Feuerstein, 1979). This premise was foundational to the MISC method (Klein, 1996, 2001; Klein & Rye, 2004).

Considering the positive results of MISC in Uganda, we thought that combining the Wetting Method (WTM) with MISC could have benefits. This health intervention method would enhance efficacy in preventing konzo in at-risk communities exposed to cyanogenic cassava within the DRC and benefit both mother and child (Bass et al., 2016). The research aims to establish a hybrid program to prevent konzo in the population mentioned earlier. Improved safety profiles for cassava consumption are related to the appropriate processing of the shrub and food product. It is possible to consume cassava more safely when the plant tissue integrity is disrupted by soaking the shrub in water for up to four days or grating the tuber. This process is then followed by heating the product, such as by sun drying. These methods consequently hydrolyze linamarin, the main cyanogenic glycoside within bitter cassava, to glucose and cyanohydrins. The latter product spontaneously breaks down into ketones at pH > 5, allowing for hydrogen cyanide (HCN) gas release. Therefore, more acidic conditions deter this process, causing cyanohydrins to persist within the food product. However, the feasibility of such measures may be unrealistic under economic distress.

During the last decade, residents of Kahemba have taken short-cuts in the proper processing of cassava, a phenomenon that has led to an increase in food cyanogenic exposure. These attenuated processing methods typically involve soaking the peeled tubers in water for less than the three days necessary for adequate fermentation and failing to dry the soaked tubers in sunlight for at least a day before pounding the tubers into flour for storage. This modification has led to rising numbers of konzo cases, with prevalence in households up to 20% in some of the Kahemba District Health Zones (Banea, Nahimana, Mandombi, Denton, & Kuwa, 2012). Given these circumstances, an alternative option known as the Wetting Method (WTM) was established, allowing consumers to detoxify cassava post-production.

The WTM approach has been repeatedly demonstrated in this region to reduce cyanogenic levels in poorly processed cassava flour to safe levels, even if the flour is initially very toxic from the inadequate initial processing (Banea et al., 2012, 2013; Tshala-Katumbay et al., 2013; Makila-Mabe et al., 2014). The WTM is a post-production option for removing cyanogens from cassava flour. This process involves adding dry flour to a bowl and marking the inside of the bowl. Water is then added with mixing; the volume of the damp flour initially decreases and then increases with additional water. No more water is added when the level of the wet flour comes up to the mark. The wet flour is then placed in a thin layer not greater than 1 cm thick on a mat and allowed to stand for two hours in the sun or five hours in the shade for the hydrogen cyanide gas to escape. The damp flour is mixed with boiling water to make the thick porridge (fufu) which people eat with pounded, boiled cassava leaves (saka saka) or some other food to give it flavor (Banea et al., 2012).

In the DRC, the WTM for detoxifying cassava flour was taught to rural women to minimize cyanogens in Cassava before human consumption to prevent further outbreaks of konzo in the household (Banea et al., 2012). In collaboration with a DRC Ministry of Health National Nutrition program (PRONANUT), our study launched a village randomized controlled trial (RCT) of non-inferiority, peer-led WTM training of mothers versus community health worker, specialist-led. This study provided evidence that specialist-led WTM training could help minimize cyanogens in cassava before human consumption (Banea et al., 2012). While WTM has proven effective, the study placed extensive consideration on developing a strategy that would enhance mothers' motivation to use this method. We think that a link between the WTM and MISC might fill this gap.

7.3 A Hybrid MISC-WTM Program to Better Prevent Konzo in Younger Children

7.3.1 Aims and Objectives

WTM has the potential to reduce the burden of konzo. However, it is labor-intensive for caregivers preparing food, so consistent and long-term adherence to the WTM may be problematic. Furthermore, it may detract from other essential daily caregiving activities for children in the home, placing them at risk neurodevelopmentally in other ways. Finally, the WTM, while effective in minimizing nutritional risk for konzo when consistently implemented, does not address other risk factors for impaired neurodevelopment of children in impoverished konzo-affected areas (protein and micronutrient deficiencies; lack of clean water; neurodevelopmental and neurological (CNS) risk from pervasive and chronic infectious diseases such as malaria, schistosomiasis, trypanosomiasis, onchocerciasis, and helminth infections).

Based on the results of recent MISC clinical trials in rural Uganda with HIV-affected households, the hypothesis is that strategy will improve child neurodevelopment by increasing the mothers' sensitivity to the development of their children and improving maternal emotional wellbeing and functionality. The enhanced maternal/child attachment fostered by MISC will be synergistic with WTM and enhance adherence to WTM food preparation. With MISC learning, not only are mothers sensitized to caregiving functionality, nutritional support, and the benefit of daily activities as a means of enhancing their child's neurodevelopment, but they become more aware of the necessity of konzo prevention to do so.

Exploring the mediating effects of caregiver emotional wellbeing and functionality is premised on the literature that indicates that down-regulated emotional wellbeing in caregivers may compromise their ability to care for themselves and others, potentially worsening the care recipient's health outcomes. Additionally, caregiver depression may interfere with attention and the processing of information received during the WTM training and significantly reduce motivation to enact the cassava processing strategies during times of emotional or physical duress (Familiar et al., 2016). We give careful consideration to caregiver emotional wellbeing and functionality as mediators of the MISC+WTM intervention on cyanogenic exposure and child neurodevelopmental outcomes from enriched caregiving.

This study is the first scalable, evidence-based ECD program in the DRC. We aim to adapt our MISC caregiver training curriculum to the DRC context, adding WTM training as a part of that curriculum. We do this through a 12-month MISC+WTM caregiver training program. Secondly, we evaluate the "value-added" efficacy of the MISC+WTM intervention compared to WTM alone concerning (a) reduction in Cassava cyanogenic exposure, (b) improved caregiver emotional wellbeing and functionality, and (c) improved neurodevelopmental outcomes of children at 6 and 12 months.

Finally, we explore whether reductions in Cassava cyanogenic exposure and improved child neurodevelopmental outcomes in MISC+WTM arm versus WTM alone are mediated by improvements in caregiver emotional wellbeing and caregiving functionality at 6–12 months.

We are enrolling 100 households where the mother is the principal caregiver and food preparer for one or more children of 4 years of age or younger. However, the primary caregiver cannot be diagnosed with konzo following a full neurological exam at study enrollment. Randomization occurs by geographic location (i.e. village) rather than individually to minimize the likelihood of contamination and diffusion effects within a community.

7.3.2 WTM

The intervention is implementing the WTM cassava processing technique in participating households. Twenty women with leadership and communication skills were already trained to implement WTM. These individuals are conducting the training for WTM-only households in the current cohort. These women are mothers that have mastered the WTM technique and have been certified as trainers to train and support other small groups of other mothers. They must present the cassava cyanogenic content to the lowest achievable level. As part of the program, colorful and durable laminated posters depicting the WTM will be distributed to participating households. Previous experience indicates that these are kept for more than a year on walls in houses.

We are collecting cyanogenic content in household cassava flour, and the mother's and child's urinary-SCN (U-SCN) levels at baseline and months 6 and 12 (Boivin, Okitundu et al., 2013; Boivin et al., 2017b; Kashala-Abotnes et al., 2018). The effectiveness of the processing of cassava flour are being monitored by measuring the cyanogenic content of cassava flour using the picrate paper method. Trainers are receiving training in in-field portable color-assay measure of U-SCN in the urine. This test is a simple, semi-quantitative picrate paper method and color comparison chart designed for field-based use with cassava-dependent populations (Haque & Bradbury, 1999). This is a critical component of the intervention since color change due to higher cyanide exposure, compared to no change when urine from trainers is tested, is conclusive for whether mothers properly process cassava.

7.3.3 MISC

The MISC/WTM trainers are different from the WTM-only trainers (who will not be certified in MISC). The MISC/WTM training is led by 10 women leaders in the Kahemba community (different than the WTM peer or professional trainers) whom the Uganda MISC consultants had already trained in April 2018. These trainers are implementing MISC training in Kahemba with 40 households with younger children as part of a pilot study.

The project team successfully implemented MISC training with konzo-at risk mothers in Kahemba after conducting a one-week training workshop with 10 women leaders from the affected communities and medical and administrative leaders from the Kahemba health zone.

The Ugandan MISC trainers will continue to train the community leader women responsible for MISC until they are MISC-certified. They will also continue quality assurance follow-up for the fidelity of MISC training in Kahemba every six months throughout the study period. There will be an annual MISC refresher training workshops specifically for the community women leaders for the MISC field training. The present pilot uses the training session videos of the 10 Kahemba community leader woman MISC trainers conducting individual training sessions. A Ugandan MISC consultant will evaluate these as part of quality assurance. We shall assess the outcomes at baseline and months 6 (mid-intervention) and 12 (post-intervention).

We have already documented significant improvements in MISC caregiving after just six months in Uganda (Boivin et al., 2013a, 2013b). For WTM training, the dose was established based on previous experience as to the number of months of weekly training for the WTM to be fully adopted at the community level, as evidenced by lower cyanide levels in the surveillance of levels in the household cassava flour used for food in participating households. We are tracking the completed training sessions will be tracked for each household and each trainer. In addition, training and adherence for the study mothers in the MISC+WTM intervention arm will be monitored using the "Observed Mediational Interactions" (OMI) scoring rubric, used in all of our previous Uganda MISC clinical trials.

7.3.4 Outcome Measures

In addition to tracking progress with MISC implementation, we use several measures and technologies to measure neurological development and mental health outcomes. We monitor neurological development using three methods: the Tobii eye-tracking and professional studio software, Mullen Scales of Early Learning (MSEL), and the Early Childhood Vigilance Test (ECVT). The eye-tracking was modified to evaluate attention and working memory of Ugandan HIV-exposed children 6–12 months of age (Chhaya et al., 2018). This test's outcomes are the ratio of time the infant spent looking at the unfamiliar picture to the familiar picture, total time gazing at the familiar face, and total time spent viewing the presentation video screen across all faces (familiar and unfamiliar). We hope to evaluate their working memory for human faces with their eye-tracking responses on the modified Fagan Test of Infant Intelligence (mFTII). When these children reach 2 years of age, they will continue to be evaluated with eye-tracking responses to the Early Childhood Vigilance Test (ECVT) attention measurement animation (Boivin et al., 2017c). The MSEL provides a measure of the general measure of fluid intelligence thought to underlie cognitive ability. Finally, the *Early Childhood Vigilance Test (ECVT)* (Goldman, Shapiro, & Nelson, 2004; Ruff, Capozzoli, Dubiner, & Parrinello, 1990) is an experimental measure of vigilance used in preschool children to evaluate sustained attention (World Health Organization, 1996).

In addition to these previously given measures, we are using the Home Observation for the Measurement of the Environment (HOME) (Caldwell & Bradley, 1979), Hopkins Symptoms Checklist-25 (HSCL), and the caregiver functional impairment for caregiving daily activities (Feuerstein, 1979; Bass et al., 2016, 2017).

7.4 Conclusion and Future Directions for MISC

We are expanding upon our present caregiver-training interventions in Kahemba in konzo at-risk communities with this new project. Early evidence shows that neurotoxicity can begin as soon as they are weaned from breast milk to cyanogenic cassava porridge. Positive results are essential to show the value of MISC in public health interventions in resource-poor communities. Other chapters in this volume have already shown how MISC, community-development, and community-based interventions could benefit from MISC and vice versa. The early signs of applying MISC in the context of preventing konzo are positive. This is an important development as current MISC studies have not necessarily used MISC as a mechanism within public health approaches.

In the next phase of our work there, we hope to procure resources for the needed software development, supporting our capacity for doubling the eye-tracking resolution for our current instrumentation. We hope to use this same technology to longitudinally monitor our konzo prevention's neurodevelopmental integrity for at-risk infants and toddlers in our MISC caregiver-training clinical trial studies to prevent konzo.

References

Banea, J., Bradbury, J., Mandombi, C., C, N., Kuwaa, D., & Katumbay, T. (2013). Control of konzo by detoxification of cassava flour in three villages in the Democratic Republic of Congo. *Food and Chemical Toxicology*, *60*, 506–513.

Banea, J., Nahimana, G., Mandombi, C. B., Denton, I., & Kuwa, N. (2012). Control of konzo in DRC using the wetting method on cassava flour. *Food and Chemical Toxicology*, *50*(5), 1517–1523.

Bass, J., Nakasujja, N., Familiar-Lopez, I., Sikorskii, A., Murray, S., Opoka, R., . . . Boivin, M. (2016). Association of caregiver quality of care with neurocognitive outcomes in HIV-affected children aged 2–5 years in Uganda. *AIDS Care*, *28*, 76–83.

Bass, J., Opoka, R., Familiar, I., Nakasujja, N., Sikorskii, A., Awadu, J., . . . Boivin, B. (2017). Randomized controlled trial of caregiver training for HIV-infected child neurodevelopment and caregiver well being. *AIDS*, *31*(13), 1877–1883.

Boivin, M. J., Bangirana, P., Nakasujja, N., Page, C., Shohet, C., Givon, D., . . . Klein, K. (2013a). A year-long caregiver training program improves cognition in preschool

Ugandan children with human immunodeficiency virus. *The Journal of Pediatrics,* *163*(5), 1409–1416.

Boivin, M. J., Bangirana, P., Nakasujja, N., Page, C., Shohet, C., Givon, D., . . . Klein, K. (2013b). A year-long caregiver training program to improve neurocognition in preschool Ugandan HIV-exposed children. *Journal of Developmental & Behavioral Pediatrics,* *34*(3), 269–278.

Boivin, M. J., Nakasujja, N., Familiar-Lopez, I., Murray, S., Sikorskii, A., Awadu, J., . . . Bass, J. (2017a). Effect of caregiver training on the neurodevelopment of HIV-exposed uninfected children and caregiver mental health: A Ugandan cluster-randomized controlled trial. *Journal of Developmental & Behavioral Pediatrics, 38*(9), 753–764.

Boivin, M. J., Okitundu, D.-M., Makila-Mabe, B., Sombo, M., Mumba, D., Sikorskii, A., & Mayambu, T.-K. D. (2017b). Cognitive and motor performance in Congolese children with konzo during 4 years of follow-up: A longitudinal analysis. *Lancet Global Health, 5*(9), e936–e947.

Boivin, M. J., Okitundu, D.-M., Mumba, D., Tylleskar, T., Page, C., Muyembe, J., & Tshala-Katumbay, D. (2013). Neuropsychological effects of konzo: A neuromotor disease associated with poorly processed Cassava. *Pediatrics, 131*(4), e1231–1239.

Boivin, M. J., Weiss, J., Chhaya, R., Seffren, V., Awadu, J., Sikorskii, A., & Giordani, B. (2017c). The feasibility of automated eye tracking with the early childhood vigilance test of attention in younger HIV-exposed Ugandan children. *Neuropsychology, 31*(5), 525–534.

Bonnier, C. (1992). Evaluation of early stimulation programs for enhancing brain development. *Acta Paediatrica, 97*(7), 853–858.

Caldwell, B., & Bradley, R. (1979). *Home observation for measurement of the environment.* Fayetteville: University of Arkansas Press.

Chabwine, J., Masheka, C., Balol'ebwami, Z., Maheshe, B., Belegamire, S., & Rutega, B. (2011). Appearance of konzo in South-Kivu, a wartorn area in the Democratic Republic of Congo. *Food and Chemical Toxicology, 49*(3), 644–649.

Chhaya, R., Weiss, J., Seffren, V. S., Winke, P., Ojuka, J., & Boivin, M. (2018). The feasibility of an automated eye-tracking-modified Fagan test of memory for human faces in younger Ugandan HIV-exposed children. *Child Neuropsychology, 24*(5), 686–701.

Familiar, I., Murray, S., Ruisenor-Escudero, H., Sikorskii, A., Nakasujja, N., & Boivin, M. (2016). Socio-demographic correlates of depression and anxiety among female caregivers living with HIV in rural Uganda. *AIDS Care, 28*(12), 1541–1545.

Farah, M., Betancour, L., Shera, D., Savage, J., Giannetta, J., Brodsky, N., . . . Hurt, H. (2009). Environmental stimulation, parental nurturance and cognitive development in humans. *Developmental Sciences, 11*(5), 793–801.

Feuerstein, R. (1979). *The dynamic assessment of retarded performers.* New York: University Press Park.

Feuerstein, R. (1980). *The dynamic assessment of retarded performers.* New York: University Park Press.

Goldman, D., Shapiro, E., & Nelson, C. (2004). Measurement of vigilance in 2-year-old children. *Developmental Neuropsychology, 25*(3), 337–250.

Haque, M., & Bradbury, J. (1999). Simple method for determination of thiocyanate in urine. *Clinical Chemstry, 45*(9), 1459–1464.

Imakumbili, M., Semu, E., Semoka, J., Abass, A., & Mkamilo, G. (2019). Farmers' perceptions on the causes of cassava root bitterness: A case of konzo-affected Mtwara region, Tanzania. *Plos One, 14*(4), e0215527.

Kashala-Abotnes, E., Sombo, M.-T., Okitundu, D., Kunyu, M., Makila-Mabe, G., Tylleskär, T., . . . Boivin, M. (2018). Dietary cyanogen exposure and early child neurodevelopment: An observational study from the Democratic Republic of Congo. *Plos One, 13*(4), e0193261.

Klein, P. (1996). *Early intervention: Cross cultural experiences with a mediational approach.* New York: Garland Publications.

Klein, P. (2001). *Seeds of hope: Twelve years of early intervention in Africa.* Oslo: Unipub forlag.

Klein, P., & Rye, H. (2004). Interaction-oriented early intervention in Ethiopia: The MISC approach. *Infants and Young Children, 17,* 340–354.

Makila-Mabe, B., Kikandau, K., Sombo, T., Okitundu, D., Mwanza, J., Boivin, M., . . . Tshala-Katumbay, D. (2014). Serum 8,12-iso-iPF2α-VI isoprostane marker of oxidative damage and cognition deficits in children with konzo. *Plos One, 9*(9), e107191.

Murray, S., Familiar, I., Nakasujja, N., Winch, P., Gallo, J., Opoka, R., . . . Bassi, K. (2017). Caregiver mental health and HIV-infected child wellness: Perspectives from Ugandan caregivers. *AIDS Care, 29*(6), 793–799.

Mwanza, J.-C., & Tshala-Katumbay, D. T. (2005). Neuro-ophthalmologic manifestations of konzo. *Environmental Toxicology and Pharmacology, 19*(3), 491–496.

Newton, C. (2017). Cassava, konzo, and neurotoxicity. *Lancet Global Health, 5*(9), e853–e854.

Ngudi, D., Kuo, Y.-H., & Lambein, F. (2003). Cassava cyanogens and free amino acids in raw and cooked leaves. *Food and Chemical Toxicology, 41*(8), 1193–1197.

Rao, H., Betancourt, L., Giannetta, J., Brodsky, N., Korczykowski, M., Avants, B., . . . Farah, M. (2010). Early parental care is important for hippocampal maturation: Evidence from brain morphology in humans. *NeuroImage, 49*(1), 1144–1150.

Ruff, H., Capozzoli, M., Dubiner, K., & Parrinello, R. (1990). A measure of vigilance in infancy. *Infant Behavior & Development, 13*(1), 1–20.

Soler-Martín, C., Riera, J. S. A., Cutillas, B., Ambrosio, S., Boadas-Vaello, P., & Llorens, J. (2010). The targets of acetone cyanohydrin neurotoxicity in the rat are not the ones expected in an animal model of konzo. *Neurotoxicology and Teratology, 32*(2), 289–294.

Trolli, G. (1938). Paraplegie spastique epidemique, "Konzo" des indigenes du Kwango. In G. Troli (Ed.), *Resume des observations reunies, au Kwango, au sujet de deux affections d'origine indeterminee* (pp. 1–36). Brussels: Fonds reine Elisabeth.

Tshala-Katumbay, D., Mumba, N., Okitundu, L., Kazadi, K., Banea, M., Tylleskär, T., . . . Muyembe-Tamfum, J. (2013). Cassava food toxins, konzo disease, and neurodegeneration in sub-Sahara Africans. *Neurology, 80*(10), 949–951.

Tylleskar, T., & Tshala Katumbay, D. (2015). Konzo: A permanent, non-progressive, motor neuron disease. In J. Chopra & I. Sawhney (Eds.), *Neurology in the tropics* (pp. 377–386). Chennai: Eslevier.

Vygotsky, L. (1978). *Mind in society: The development of higher mental functions.* Boston, MA: Harvard University Press.

World Health Organization. (1996). Konzo, a distinct type of upper motoneuron disease. *The Weekly Epidemiological Record, 71*(30), 225–232.

8 The Mediational Intervention for Sensitizing Caregivers for Community-Based Organizations to Address the Needs of Orphans and Vulnerable Children (OVC) in South Africa

Carla Sharp, Madeleine Allman, Jan Cloete, and Lochner Marais

8.1 The Impact of HIV/AIDS on Children: Orphanhood, Mental Health, and Attachment Disruption

Despite significant advances in fighting the HIV/AIDS pandemic over the last few decades, approximately 26 million people are living with HIV/ AIDS in sub-Saharan Africa (SSA; United Nations, 2016). The extensive prevalence and associated mortality rates mean that children continue to be at risk of HIV infection, living with a parent with chronic illness, orphanhood, and related vulnerability factors, including poverty, lack of basic resources and access to services, and impaired caregiving. These intersecting factors related to the effects of HIV/AIDS on children has led to the operational term "orphans and vulnerable children" (OVC; Foster, 2016). Globally, there are over 16 million OVC, the vast majority in SSA (Allison, 2012; UNAIDS, 2012), with over 10 million children having lost one or both parents to the HIV/AIDS epidemic (Blevins & Kawata, 2019; Pillay, 2014; Sewpaul & Matthias, 2013). In South Africa, estimations are between 1.9 million (UNAIDS, 2010) to 3.7 million (UNICEF, 2013).

OVC suffer many negative consequences, including malnutrition, school dropout, poor psychosocial wellbeing, early sexual debut (younger than 14 years of age), lack of family support, homelessness, child labor, increased violence or sexual abuse exposure, and heightened stress (Cluver, 2011; Doku, 2009; Foster, 2006), which together confer significant risk for short- and long-term mental health problems (Betancourt et al., 2014; Cluver & Gardner, 2007; Sharp, Jardin, Marais, & Boivin, 2015). We recently undertook a systematic literature review of the detrimental impact of orphanhood on child mental health (Sharp et al., 2015), which confirmed the conclusions of other systematic reviews (Chi & Li, 2013; Cluver, Gardner, &

DOI: 10.4324/9781003145899-8

Operario, 2007; Wild, 2001) that HIV affected children suffer from high rates of mental health problems. Our review also demonstrated the effect of orphan status on school and cognitive functioning. For example, AIDS-orphans in SA are less likely to be attending school (Skinner, Sharp, Jooste, Mfecane, & Simbayi, 2013) and more likely to be delayed in school (Cluver, Orkin, Boyes et al., 2012; Cluver, Orkin, Gardner et al., 2012), with detrimental effects on educational and cognitive developmental outcomes (Jenkins, Baingana, Ahmad, McDaid, & Atun, 2011). Risk factors are further compounded by stigma and lack of social support, leading to increased rates of psychological disorders and other mental health sequelae (Cluver & Gardner, 2007). Clearly, addressing the mental health needs of HIV-affected children is crucial for both emotional and cognitive development.

The recent impact of COVID-19 stands to further exacerbate these factors with potentially devastating effects on the psychosocial wellbeing of HIV/AIDS-affected communities (Spaull et al., 2020). Preliminary evidence in South Africa suggests significant job losses (47%), concentrated among the already vulnerable, and increased household and child hunger, exacerbated by the closure of schools and their feeding schemes. Problems experienced during the national lockdown, including accessing medication, antiretroviral treatment (ART), condoms, and contraception, will likely have long-term impacts on the population outcomes of HIV/AIDS with downstream effects on child developmental outcomes, including mental health (Spaull et al., 2020).

Adding to the complex array of adverse factors mentioned previously, OVC may experience the additional trauma of becoming the caretaker of a chronically ill parent or the loss of a parent to HIV/AIDS, living in a child-headed household, or living in institutionalized care (Skinner et al., 2006; Thurman & Kidman, 2011). Therefore, attachment trauma is common among OVC, with orphaned children at increased risk due to the loss of their attachment figure(s) (Kang'ethe & Makuyan, 2014). Indeed, several studies in SSA support the link between OVC status and attachment disruption in South Africa. For instance, in a study of peri-urban mother-infant dyads (n = 147) in South Africa and using the Strange Situation procedure 18-months post-partum (Tomlinson, Cooper, & Murray, 2005), infant attachment was characterized as attached (62%), resistant (8%), avoidant (4%), and disorganized (26%). While a rate of around 60% secure attachment is typical for other (Western) populations, the rate of 26% as disorganized is much higher than recorded rates in other populations, which typically shows a rate of around 15% (Van Ijzendoorn, Schuengel, & Bakermans-Kranenburg, 1999). In this study, insecure attachment was associated with maternal depression and specific parenting behaviors (intrusiveness, remoteness). Barenbaum and Smith (2016) compared attachment, psychological wellbeing, and living environment of children in SSA. Children, regardless of living environment (with extended family or institution), who reported having at least one trusting relationship with an adult had increased psychological wellbeing. No formal attachment measure was utilized in this study. Rather, a self-report measure of presence of a trusting relationship with an adult was used. Other studies also examined the importance of attachment figures. A review of children affected by HIV/AIDS named the presence of a trusting relationship with a caregiver as a strong protective factor against negative mental health outcomes. Additionally, adequate child coping skills modeled after caregiver coping skills was reported as a global protective factor (Chi & Li, 2013).

8.2 Social-Cognitive Development in Children Affected by HIV/AIDS

While attachment disruption has a profound impact on many domains of socio-emotional function, it appears to be particularly important for social-cognitive development (Fonagy, Gergely, Jurist, & Target, 2002). Social-cognitive development, in turn, has a profound impact on mental health in children and adolescents (Sharp, Fonagy, P., & Goodyer, 2008). This is because social cognition undergirds our relational functioning. Put differently, social cognition allows us to have productive, collaborative, and mutually rewarding and loving relationships, in which absence we become vulnerable for all forms of psychopathology (Sharp & Hernandez Ortiz, 2021).

Prominent approaches to understanding the development of social cognition emphasize the role of attachment security in providing an "early laboratory" for children to engage in the "serve-and-return" between parent and child to stimulate social-cognitive development (Sharp et al., 2020). Already in the late 1980s and 1990s, it became abundantly clear that children's social-cognitive development does not occur in a vacuum, but is embedded within intimate family interactions (Dunn, 1988, 1993, 1994; Dunn, Brown, & Beardsall, 1991; Dunn, Brown, Slomkowski, Tesla, & Youngblade, 1991; Perner, Ruffman, & Leekam, 1994). The fact that family interactions were shown to play a role in the development of mentalizing suggested that attachment security may be an important longitudinal but also a concurrent predictor of social-cognitive development. A landmark study in this regard was the study by Fonagy et al. (1991), who assessed 100 first-time mothers and 100 first-time fathers before the birth of their child. Attachment classification was coded for the frequency of parents' references to mental states in their descriptions of childhood relationships—that is, mentalizing capacity. Families were followed up at 12 and 18 months after the babies' birth, during which the Strange Situation procedure (Ainsworth, Blehar, Waters, & Wall, 1978) was administered. Findings demonstrated that the social–cognitive capacity of mothers as measured by a mentalizing measure (the frequency of parents' references to mental states in their accounts of their own childhood during the administration of the attachment interview), predicted the likelihood of their children being securely attached at follow-up, even when controlling for verbal IQ. Moreover, when children were followed up at age 5½, security of attachment in infancy predicted performance on a cognitive-emotion task (Harris, 1989). Taken together, these longitudinal findings suggest that attachment plays a critical role in affecting social-cognitive development and that attachment is related to a caregiver's capacity to make sense of her own mental states and those of her children, which in turn affects the child's developing social-cognitive function. The caregiver's role as "mediator" of her child's nascent understanding of self and the world is clear: to assist her child in building a realistic and adaptive account of her social reality, which is flexible to the impact of a constantly changing environment.

While many children will automatically receive mediated learning from adults, there are many for whom external economic and social conditions disrupt caregiving practices in dramatic ways, most notably war, poverty, malnutrition, discrimination, and the effects of HIV/AIDS (Klein & Rye, 2004). Especially in the case of losing primary caregivers, as is the case with the majority of OVC, children may experience mental starvation of any cultural transmission of mediation from an adult caregiver, alongside actual physical deprivation (Klein & Rye, 2004), negatively affecting social-cognitive development and mental health outcomes.

While research on theory of mind and/or mentalizing is still nascent in SSA, studies are beginning to emerge (Goodman & Dent, 2019; Malcolm-Smith, Woolley, & Ward, 2015) and do indeed show atypical development of social-cognitive capacity in OVC. Children's Theory of Mind scores have been shown to positively correlate with caregiver support, and mentalizing scores were inversely correlated with aggression and externalizing behavior, as well as interpersonal difficulties. In other studies, emotion recognition has been utilized to examine empathy function with adversity-exposed youth and found these youth to be more likely to interpret stronger emotions from stimuli and show stronger response bias to negative emotions (da Silva Ferreira, Crippa, & de Lima Osório, 2014; Quas, Dickerson, Matthew, Harron, & Quas, 2017).

Another recent study examined mental perspective taking with the false belief task in school-aged children in the Western Cape of South Africa. A large subset (nearly one quarter of the sample) scored at chance level or worse, indicating difficulty with mentalizing. Subjects with the lowest perspective-taking ability also exhibited increased aggressive, externalizing behavior and interpersonal difficulties (Malcolm-Smith et al., 2015). In a study of Swaziland youth, researchers compared adversity-exposed youth to controls in an emotion recognition and empathy function task. Adversity-exposed youth perceived stronger anger, sadness, and happiness in ambiguous and negative images. Researchers found that perceptions of sadness mediated the relationship between adversity exposure and empathic concern (Quas et al., 2017). This finding is consistent with other literature that shows maltreated children's tendency to interpret facial emotions less accurately and show greater reactivity, response bias, and brain activation of regions associated with anger and other negative emotions (da Silva Ferreira et al., 2014).

Conversely, it appears that caregiving quality can buffer the negative effects of social-cognitive development in children. For instance, a recent study in rural Uganda examining preschool-aged children's school readiness found that increased theory of mind (mentalizing) scores in children were correlated with caregiver social support, caregiver education level, and caregiver time spent reading aloud to children (Goodman & Dent, 2019). These findings reflect that in vulnerable populations with risk factors, including poverty and high adversity, caregiver support may positively contribute to children's social-cognitive development. Neither of these studies was longitudinal, nor did they examine attachment trauma directly.

8.3 Quality Caregiving as Central Focus for WHO Global Strategy for Women's, Children's, and Adolescents' Health

Several factors have been identified to effectively address the negative impact of HIV/AIDS on children and increase resilience. The World Health Organization (WHO) developed the Global Strategy for Women's, Children's, and Adolescents' Health to guarantee children the right to survive and transform health and human potential. The WHO emphasizes the need for multi-level action to meet its goals, from high-level policies to targeted interventions for high-risk families. The strategy includes three initiatives: Survive (eliminate preventable deaths), Thrive (promote good health), and Transform (enhance environments and communities), and a central focus on Nurturing Care. Nurturing care is conceptualized as conditions that promote health, safety, early learning, and responsive caregiving within families and other caregivers. Nurturing care's function is to promote healthy physical, social, emotional, and cognitive development in children while protecting them from the harmful effects of adversity. Responsive caregiving is the basis of building trust and social relationships where a child builds an emotional bond with their caregiver to understand more about others and relationships (WHO, 2018). As discussed earlier, a child's relationship with their primary attachment figure(s) is also the most important source of developing social cognition (Bowlby, 1979).

The WHO's strategy also includes specific guidance on the impact of HIV/AIDS on early childhood development, emphasizing the need to address social issues such as stigma and interpersonal support (WHO, 2018). The concept of nurturing care is important for OVC as it promotes emotion regulation and social-cognitive development (Sharp et al., 2008). Thus, the WHO recommends that in low-access areas where medical and psychological services are not readily available, interventions should be implemented to improve caregiving quality (Friedli, 2009).

8.4 Community-Based Organizations (CBOs) as Strategic Points of Intervention to Address the Mental Health Needs of OVC

Further compounding negative outcomes is the global crisis in the scarcity of mental health workers in the developing world (Eaton et al., 2011; Kakuma et al., 2011). One solution is to build caregiver and community capacity by enhancing traditional community-based support systems (Schenk & Michaelis, 2010; Schenk, 2009; Skeen et al., 2017), which are more cost-effective than care provided in clinical settings. Community-based care is also more consistent with African cultural values of shared care for the community (Eze, 2010). CBOs (Community Based Organizations) offer strategic points of intervention in this regard (Marais et al., 2013; Marais et al., 2018), and are attended by children who have a higher likelihood of living in overcrowded households, being orphaned, and undergoing greater exposure to community violence (Yakubovich et al., 2016). CBOs are grassroots-level organizations that are developed by members of the community with the help of non-governmental organizations and some government support. They are community-led and community-driven and provide various forms of support to OVC, including meals, counselling services, financial assistance, and healthcare counseling (Marais et al., 2013; Richter et al., 2009). OVC uses CBOs because legal guardians (which may include extended family members in the case of orphanhood) cannot always provide meals and emotional and other material support at home—aspects that may be particularly lacking in child-headed households.

While CBOs provide critical community support, CBO careworkers rarely receive specialized training in caregiving or child mental health and suffer the same disparities OVC do. CBO careworkers themselves ask for training in effective ways to improve the mental health of OVC (Marais et al., 2013; Schenk, Michaelis, Sapiano, Brown, & Weiss, 2010). A community development approach (Christens, 2012) recommends an emphasis on human care (Jordans & Tola, 2013) and task shifting ("task sharing"), defined as delegating tasks to existing but untrained cadres—an essential response to shortages in human resources for mental health (Kakuma et al., 2011).

Recently, our team published a systematic review of studies published between 2008–2019 that evaluated community-based caregiver interventions to support the mental health of OVC in SSA (Penner et al., 2020). Ten studies were identified, and while these studies represent a marked improvement on where the field was 10 years ago, several limitations remain, also articulated in other recent reviews (Han et al., 2019; Sikkema et al., 2015; Skeen et al., 2017). Only five randomized control trials (RCTs) have been conducted (Bell et al., 2008; Bhana et al., 2014; Eloff et al., 2014; Puffer et al., 2016; Ward et al., 2020). Of those that have been conducted, studies do not typically focus specifically on improving mental health. Of the five RCTs previously conducted, three (Bell et al., 2008; Bhana et al., 2014;

Puffer et al., 2016) were combination HIV risk behavior prevention and mental health interventions that did not show significantly improved mental health. The other two (Eloff et al., 2014; Ward et al., 2020) demonstrated significant effects for child externalizing problems (6–10 year olds; Eloff et al., 2014) and child problem behavior (2–9 year olds; Ward et al., 2020). Even so, in general, across studies, effect sizes for mental health outcomes are modest. Moreover, interventions are typically home-visiting programs, thereby not fully leveraging the CBO care environment where children spend up to 50% of their waking time and impeding scalability due to the costs involved in home visiting. Importantly, not a single intervention had been designed to improve the quality of caregiving provided by CBO care-workers specifically. Training CBO careworkers in the principles of quality caregiving offers a new role for CBO careworkers beyond simply taking care of the physical needs of OVC. Expanding the CBO careworker's role has significant scale-up potential as this knowledge can be transferred and generalized to legal guardians of OVC. Together, these factors justified our adaptation of MISC for the CBO environment, which we discuss next.

8.5 The Mediational Intervention for Sensitizing Caregivers for Community-Based organizations (MISC-CBO)

8.5.1 Rationale for Choosing MISC for CBO Adaptation

We decided to choose MISC adaptation for the CBO environment, first, on its strong evidence base in Africa. Four randomized controlled trials support the effectiveness of MISC. The first was conducted in 68 mother-infant dyads of a low-SES, urban, high-crime-rate community in Israel. Results at post-intervention and up to six years later showed increased and sustained maternal mediation, in addition to positive child outcomes. Similar results were demonstrated in an RCT with 120 rural Ugandan child-caregiver dyads with HIV/AIDS (Boivin et al., 2013a) and an RCT of 119 uninfected HIV-exposed children and their caregivers (Boivin et al., 2013b). These results were replicated in larger RCTs of HIV-exposed, but uninfected (Boivin et al., 2017) and HIV/AIDS-affected (Bass et al., 2017) children in Uganda where children showed significant cognitive gains, especially in language development, which has clear implications for mental health problems in OVC.

The second reason for choosing MISC for adaptation to the CBO environment was its value as a cultural and developmental transportable intervention and its relevance for both cognitive and socio-emotional outcomes (Sharp et al., 2021). MISC is a strengths-based intervention that does not impose a model of parenting on the caregiver. Instead, it ascribes to an implicit change model that facilitates reflective capacity so that the caregiver enhances her caregiving capacity independently and consistent with her own culture (Sharp et al., 2020). Because MISC does not use any materials or worksheets, but utilizes the everyday interactions between caregiver and child (cleaning up, doing homework, discussing daily events, etc.), MISC is highly suitable for low-resource settings (Klein, 1996; Sharp, Shohet, Givon, Marais, & Boivin, 2018). It teaches a set of principles common to high-quality caregiving that can be applied to any developmental age, culture, or setting of the child, making MISC highly adaptable and scalable cross-culturally and cross-developmentally (Klein, 1996; Sharp et al., 2018; Shohet & Jaegermann, 2012).

8.5.2 Study Design

We present an abbreviated version of our main research outcomes paper (Sharp et al., 2021), which can be referred to for full details of the study design and results. We elected to conduct a quasi-experimental design that includes a control group and process evaluation with strong foci on qualitative and community participatory methods in acknowledgement. We first had to evaluate MISC for feasibility and acceptability in the CBO environment. Accordingly, we followed intervention adaptation approaches (Matthews & Hudson, 2001; Wingood & DiClemente, 2008) to include an initial formative research phase (qualitative interviews and focus groups) with community stakeholders, a Community Advisory Board (CAB), CBO careworkers, and service users to adapt MISC to its unique context. A quasi-experimental study followed the formative phase to compare MISC with Treatment as Usual (TAU) (Trial registration: University of Houston ClinicalTrials.gov Identifier: NCT04359043, MISC-CBO in Children Affected by HIV/AIDS).

8.5.3 Study Setting and Population

The study was conducted in the Free State, with an HIV prevalence rate of 15% (compared to 13.2% for SA). The Free State is the third-largest province and the third-most-urbanized province in SA, with the Mangaung Metropolitan Municipality the most densely populated. Of the 752,906 people living in Mangaung, 618,408 (82%) are Black (mostly Sesotho), 32,071 (4%) are Coloured, 1,257 (0.2%) are Indian/Asian, and 101,170 (13%) are White (the SA term "Coloured" is used by the SA census and widely accepted to categorize individuals of mixed race). Currently, 31% of children in the Mangaung Metropolitan Municipality are orphaned. The population from which the sample was drawn is poor: 38.2% did not have adequate clothing; more than 60% of household income emanated from grants. The mean average household monthly expenditure was 1,518 rand/R (approx. $115 based on R13.2 to $1 exchange rate at the time of the survey), with 11.9% of total expenditure spent on clothing and 75.6% on food. We recruited 88 OVC and their CBO careworkers (n = 18) across four CBOs. Two CBOs (45 children; 9 careworkers) received MISC, and two CBOs (43 children;

9 careworkers) received TAU. Recruitment flow, retention, and baseline characteristics of the sample are discussed in the Results section.

8.5.4 MISC Adaptation

Please refer to Chapters 2 and 3 for clear descriptions of the basic format and content of MISC (Chapter 2) as well as the MISC training model (Chapter 3). To organize the adaptation process, we make use of the Framework for Reporting Adaptations and Modifications-Expanded (Stirman, Baumann, & Miller, 2019), which is also summarized in the supplemental online material in Sharp et al. (2021):

1. Timing of adaptation: Regarding the question of timing, adaptations to MISC were made in the year preceding the implementation of the study, which required iterative adaptation until acceptability was reached.
2. Planned or reactive adaptations: Modifications were planned and proactive based on hypothesized fit with the culture and context, but included continuous feedback and approval from the community advisory board (CAB).
3. Who determined adaptations: Because we were following community-based participatory research practices (Matthews & Hudson, 2001; Penchansky & Thomas, 1981), modifications were determined collaboratively through a series of iterative steps. First, we established a CAB to provide participatory community input on all aspects of adaptation. The CAB included the directors (not involved in the intervention) of the two CBOs, two community religious leaders, and two representatives from a well-established NGO working with children rights. We also invited a member of the local municipality and a representative from the Department of Social Development. These community stakeholders were selected based on their knowledge of and legitimacy in the community. MISC workshop presentations were conducted, followed by focus groups, including community religious leaders, CBO careworkers, and OVC and their caregivers to incorporate the perspective of those that will use MISC. Feedback from the CAB was integrated with feedback from the focus groups, and the investigative team, with input from MISC consultants who helped finalize adaptations.
4. Types of modifications made: Topics for adaptations included cultural (Sesotho), context (CBO), and mental health adaptations. While MISC was considered culturally agile due to its implicit change model, focus group participants highlighted that authoritarian instruction is often the accepted mode of adult-child interaction in the Sesotho culture. Focus group participants acknowledged that the culture is modernizing, but foresaw that the affective component of eye contact and the cognitive component of Expansion in MISC might be hardest to integrate

with their ways of working as these components require higher levels of agency in children and collaboration in dyads, which, according to focus group participants, was inconsistent with the child's passive role in interactions with adult caregivers. It was decided not to modify these components but to evaluate their relevance through implementation. The strengths-based nature of MISC was a particularly attractive feature for both CBO careworkers and legal guardians, in that MISC was viewed as sensitizing them to what they were already doing well, and helping them to do more of it, and therefore not culturally intrusive. Regarding context (CBO) adaptations, the study team had to build stronger managerial support for careworkers taking on MISC training and consideration of how MISC should be managed in a group setting. Recommendations were made regarding the format of MISC to alternate individual video-feedback sessions with in-service training on a bi-weekly basis as they fit better with CBO schedules. Mental health adaptations required the incorporation of socio-emotional examples during MISC training sessions with careworkers. Thus, instead of using traditional "learning" examples (e.g. "This is a butterfly"), the use of socio-emotional learning events had to be incorporated (e.g. "You have tears in your eyes. Are you feeling sad?"). In addition, provisions for children with severe trauma and emotional problems and consideration that children will be going back to potentially adverse environments after receiving MISC were discussed. While these discussions did not lead to any modifications, they highlighted the importance of MISC trainers' sensitivity to the vulnerability of the population they work with. Child participants expressed interest in MISC and were primarily interested in whether MISC would help them resolve peer conflict at the CBO.

5. Level of modifications: The modifications previously discussed reflect modifications at different levels, including the child level (consideration of trauma histories), system's level (managerial support; scheduling), and treatment foci (socio-emotional context).

6. Type and nature of content-level modifications: Adaptations reflected modification to the format (alternating in-service and video-feedback sessions).

7. Were modifications fidelity-consistent? Modifications were fidelity-consistent in that they preserved the core elements of the intervention that are needed for the intervention to be effective.

8. Rationale for the modifications: The main reason behind the adaptation process was to ensure cultural fit between MISC and the Sesotho CBO context, consistent with (Schenk & Michaelis, 2010) recommendations for community-based service development for OVC.

These adaptations resulted in approval from the CBO to proceed with the adapted version, thereafter named MISC-CBO.

8.5.5 MISC-CBO Training and Supervision

Two Sesotho-speaking MISC trainers underwent a three-day workshop by the MISC co-developers, followed by a period of observation and supervision using videos and roleplay until the MISC trainers were deemed adherent. The MISC trainers were supervised bi-weekly and as needed, via Skype by two MISC co-developers (Cilly Shohet and Deborah Givon) and the principal investigator, a clinical psychologist (Carla Sharp). MISC trainers maintained log diaries on intervention progress and session attendance.

8.5.5 Treatment as Usual (TAU)

The two CBOs assigned to TAU received standard CBO services consisted of assisting OVC with the identification process of being an OVC, helping them obtain birth certificates, helping them obtain and administer medication if they were sick, leading a recreational program, and assisting children with their homework. Child attendance in the MISC and TAU CBOs were equivalent in terms of time spent at the CBO.

8.6 Outcome Measures

We used a standardized measure of mental health outcomes Strengths and Difficulties Questionnaire (SDQ; Goodman, 2001), which has been validated for use Sesotho-speaking populations in SA (Sharp et al., 2014).

The second outcome was caregiving quality, and for that, we used the Observing Mediational Interaction (OMI; Klein, 2014). The OMI is an observational coding scheme specifically developed to evaluate the extent to which a caregiver's interactions show evidence of MISC affective and cognitive components. The OMI was used in three prior MISC RCTs (Bass et al., 2017; Boivin et al., 2013a, 2013b, 2017). Following their approach, a standard five-minute interaction task between careworker and child was video-recorded, and the same task was repeated at 6 and 12 months post-baseline. Specifically, the careworker interacted with the child in a coloring exercise. The affective components were each rated on a five-point scale (1—none; 2—rarely; 3—sometimes; 4—most of the time; 5—all of the time) and summed to derive a total score of competence in affective components across the full five-minute interaction task. The cognitive (mediational) components were tallied in terms of the frequency that they occurred during the five-minute task interaction: Focusing, Affecting (providing or requesting meaning), Expanding, Regulating, and Rewarding. Two Sesotho coders were trained by the OMI co-developers and brought to coding reliability through standard reliability procedures (Haidet et al., 2009). These procedures included (1) the use of a predetermined coding or rating scheme (in this case, the OMI), which allows for manualized procedures and decision rules to assign codes to emotional and cognitive components, (2) three-day training in OMI coding, (3) practice until deemed competent, (4) competency test and approval as a trained coder by the OMI developers, and (5) quarterly supervision and con-sensus meetings with the OMI co-developers to maintain fidelity in coding, including calibration reliability checks evaluating whether the coder was still reliable based on supervisor assessment.

In our analyses, we controlled for effects of age, gender, socio-economic status, and the child's home environment, which was assessed through the Caldwell Home Observation for the Measurement of the Environment (HOME; Bradley et al., 1992).

8.7 Results

8.7.1 Feasibility and Acceptability

A qualitative approach was used to assess feasibility and acceptability using Penchansky and Thomas (1981) model of "access" to care that covered Acceptability, Accessibility, Affordability, Availability, and Accommodation of MISC in the CBO context. This framework assesses the fit between intervention characteristics and its context and offers a helpful model to evaluate feasibility and acceptability. CBO careworkers were interviewed post-intervention face-to-face by a female Sesotho research team member at the CBO. A directed content analysis (Hsieh & Shannon, 2005) of post-intervention interviews revealed several themes supporting the feasibility and acceptability of MISC, which we summarize in Table 8.1.

8.7.2 The Effect of MISC-CBO on Mental Health Outcomes in Children

As depicted in Figure 8.1—Panel A, the interactive effect of MISC and post-baseline timepoints was statistically significant for the SDQ outcome ($F(1, 86) = 13.43$, $p < .001$,), over and above other terms in the model. MISC participants had lower SDQ at 12 months follow-up ($M = 34.02$, $SD = 2.69$) relative to TAU participants ($M = 39.21$, $SD = 3.06$).

8.7.3 The Effects of MISC-CBO on the Quality of Caregiving

The interactive effect of MISC and post-baseline timepoints was statistically significant for the MISC affective components ($F(1, 73) = 11.15$, $p = .001$,) and the Expanding cognitive component ($F(1, 81) = 12.24$, $p < .001$,). As depicted in Figure 8.1—Panels B and C, the interactive effects were domi-nated by the main effects of MISC, such that MISC had higher affective and Expanding scores, regardless of time (6- and 12-month follow-ups). Although the interactive effect of MISC and post-baseline timepoints was not statistically significant for the Rewarding component of OMI, there was a statistically significant main effect of MISC ($F(1, 81) = 6.37$, $p = .014$,), with higher Rewarding scores ($M = 4.07$, $SD = 0.84$) for MISC participants

Table 8.1 Representative quotes from the directed qualitative content analyses

Acceptability — *Is MISC acceptable as an intervention in terms of cultural and needs fit?*	And even these videos, you get scared you understand . . . but as time went on, I ended up seeing myself being okay feeling free to act naturally.
	It taught me being in the children's shoes or a person who can act on behalf of a child.
	Eye contact is not part of our culture, but I now believe that eye contact is essential to see whether the child is listening to you.
	I feel that I truly now know how to reward and touch. I make sure that the children do not get bored during our interactions. I give them affect. I also use eye contact to see if they understand.
	We are now more aware of the children's emotions. The children feel more welcome at the centre.
	In the beginning, the eye contact part of the programme gave me problems because I had never done it before. Even when you look them in the eyes, indeed there's no longer that thing. We're not ashamed anymore to look them in the eyes.
	MISC has brought joy for both the children and myself.
	I feel great after this training because I have learnt a lot.
	With the MISC training, I know I have to be sensitive in how I do things with the children. I have to do things intentionally. If I want to make a child focus, I need to do this intentionally.
	It has changed to a point now they . . . they know that we're not only an organisation who's focusing on maybe assisting only children on homeworks, educational activities but we go beyond.
	Mhm. All I can say is yes, the MISC has worked for me, right? I was harsh on children and I didn't know that like . . . okay sometimes we have to . . . to know a child by looking at them and see how different they are, whether they are happy, has problems, and so on.
	The children would show up being dirty, but after MISC they come to the center clean. You see that the MISC has an impact at home.
Affordability — *How affordable was MISC in the context of the CBO?*	So we didn't have extra costs as an organization to say we're gonna spend over, on this. We did not need anything extra for the MISC.
	Huh-uh, mm-mhm. I don't see them. We did not encounter [extra cost]. The cost was fine.
Availability — *Were adequate resources available to support the CBO's delivery of MISC?*	The trainer let you talk when there was a problem, or if you did not quite understand.
	More or less, we were communicating regular with the trainers and also with the team.
	Our concerns, they were quite taken seriously.
	What can I say though? Sister Sister Kholisa [the MISC trainer], she was like . . . iyoh! I really miss her. Yes, it was good.
	We were able to pinpoint what was happening here and I was able to say "Ous'Kholisa okay, I messed up here but I am doing my very best" so that she can correct me.
	We knew we were going to have a meeting which we are going to discuss some of the issues, of which the trainers would be available.
	I would ask, may I please speak about something that challenges me in this and that. She was able to listen attentively.
	When we talked I would be free. She supported me and cared.

Accommodation — *Was the CBO organized in such a way to accommodate MISC?*	It was easy because MISC was part of our daily work.
	We were doing MISC before but not knowing that we were doing the MISC.
	They implemented the training of MISC in-between, so it was part of our daily routine.
	Because sometimes it's difficult to join something you have no understanding about, but as time went on it ended up being easy.
	It did not take too much of my time and energy.

relative to TAU participants (M = 0.73, SD = 0.99) across post-baseline timepoints. There was also a statistically significant main effect of MISC on Provision of meaning ($F(1, 81)$ = 4.02, p = .048,), with MISC participants had scores (M = 59.91, SD = 5.71) relative to TAU participants (M = 44.93, SD = 4.70) across post-baseline timepoints.

8.8 Conclusions and Future Directions

Against the background of a critical need to equip community-based care workers with the skills to address OVC' mental health needs, we conducted a quasi-experimental feasibility trial in South Africa to adapt and evaluate MISC for the CBO environment. Our study represents a novel adaptation of MISC in that it was the first time that MISC was explicitly evaluated for the 7–11 age range based on the importance of building mental health resilience against the adolescent onset of psychiatric problems, often coinciding with sexually risky behaviors in OVC (Cluver, 2011). This was also the first application of MISC in OVC with mental health as the primary outcome and the CBO careworker (instead of home caregiver/parent) as unit of intervention. It is also the first adaptation of MISC for the South African Sesotho cultural context. We showed that MISC-CBO was deemed acceptable and feasible in terms of attendance and post-intervention qualitative interviews. Furthermore, quantitative outcomes suggested improvement of child mental health (multi-informant SDQ total difficulties scores) in MISC relative to TAU by post-intervention and improved quality of caregiving at post-intervention MISC affective components and the cognitive components of Expanding. The main effect for the cognitive component of Provision of Meaning and Rewarding were also demonstrated.

As the first adaptation of MISC to the CBO care environment, our work should, however, be seen as a first step, and the full adaptation of MISC for the CBO environment and several limitations should be acknowledged. Our study was a quasi-experimental feasibility trial with associated limitations: (1) limitations on the causal conclusions we can draw from the results, (2) reduced statistical power to detect the mediational effects of purported mechanisms of action and expected moderating variables, (3) lack of careful monitoring of treatment-as-usual (TAU), and (4) lack of follow up beyond post-intervention.

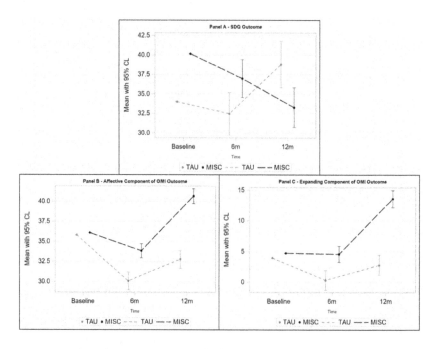

Figure 8.1 Effect of MISC vs. TAU on child mental health and caregiving quality

Note: Panels A through C represent line plots depicting interactions of MISC and post-baseline timepoints for (A) SDQ outcome, (B) Affective components of OMI outcome, and (C) Expanding component of OMI outcome. Please note that the 6m and 12m means are adjusted (conditional on covariates in the estimated models) while the baseline mean is unadjusted. Error bars for the baseline means are therefore not included as they inaccurately present variability in the data due to their unadjusted nature.

The next step would be a larger-scale randomized-controlled trial to fully evaluate the direct, interactive, and mediating factors associated with MISC effectiveness. The current study introduces a culturally appropriate, developmentally transportable, sustainable, and scalable evidence-based CBO intervention that can be readily and effectively implemented globally in low-resource settings, and our team looks forward to further evaluation.

References

Ainsworth, M. D., Blehar, M., Waters, E., & Wall, S. (1978). *Patterns of attachment.* Hillsdale, NJ: Erlbaum.

Allison, S. (2012). The role of families among orphans and vulnerable children in confronting HIV/AIDS in Sub-Saharan Africa. In W. Pequegnat (Ed.), *Family and HIV/AIDS: Cultural and contextual issues in prevention and treatment* (pp. 173–194). New York: Springer Science + Business Media.

Barenbaum, E., & Smith, T. (2016). Social support as a protective factor for children impacted by HIV/AIDS across varying living environments in southern Africa. *AIDS Care, 28*(suppl.2), 92–99, doi: 10.1080/09540121.2016.1176683.

Bass, J. K., Opoka, R., Familiar, I., Nakasujja, N., Sikorskii, A., Awadu, J., . . . Boivin, M. (2017). Randomized controlled trial of caregiver training for HIV-infected child neurodevelopment and caregiver well being. *AIDS, 31*(13), 1877–1883.

Bell, C. C., Bhana, A., Petersen, I., Mckay, M. M., Gibbons, R., Bannon, W., & Amatya, A. (2008). Building protective factors to offset sexually risky behaviors among black youths: A randomized control trial. *Journal of the National Medical Association, 100*(8), 936–944.

Betancourt, T., Scorza, P., Kanyanganzi, F., Fawzi, M. C., Sezibera, V., Cyamatare, F., . . . Kayiteshonga, Y. (2014). HIV and child mental health: A case-control study in Rwanda. *Pediatrics, 134*(2), e464–472.

Bhana, A., Mellins, C. A., Petersen, I., Alicea, S., Myeza, N., Holst, H., . . . McKay, M. (2014). The VUKA family program: Piloting a family-based psychosocial intervention to promote health and mental health among HIV infected early adolescents in South Africa. *AIDS Care, 26*(1), 1–11.

Blevins, B. K., & Kawata, K. (2019). The orphan impact: HIV-AIDS and student test scores from sub-Saharan Africa. *Educational Review*, 1–24.

Boivin, M. J., Bangirana, P., Nakasujja, N., Page, C. F., Shohet, C., Givon, D., . . . Klein, P. S. (2013a). A year-long caregiver training program improves cognition in preschool Ugandan children with human immunodeficiency virus. *Journal of Pediatrics, 163*(5), 1409–1416.

Boivin, M. J., Bangirana, P., Nakasujja, N., Page, C. F., Shohet, C., Givon, D., . . . Klein, P. S. (2013b). A year-long caregiver training program to improve neurocognition in preschool Ugandan HIV-exposed children. *Journal of Developmental and Behavioral Pediatrics, 34*(4), 269–278.

Boivin, M. J., Nakasujja, N., Familiar-Lopez, I., Murray, S. M., Sikorskii, A., Awadu, J., . . . Bass, J. K. (2017). Effect of caregiver training on the neurodevelopment of HIV-exposed uninfected children and caregiver mental health: A Ugandan cluster-randomized controlled trial. *Journal of Developmental and Behavioral Pediatrics, 38*(9), 753–764.

Bowlby, J. (1979). The Bowlby-Ainsworth attachment theory. *Behavioral and Brain Sciences, 2*(4), 637–638.

Bradley, R. H., Caldwell, B. M., Brisby, J., Magee, M., Whiteside, L., & Rock, S. L. (1992). The home inventory—a new scale for families of preadolescent and early adolescent children with disabilities. *Research in Developmental Disabilities, 13*(4), 313–333.

Chi, P. L., & Li, X. M. (2013). Impact of parental HIV/AIDS on children's psychological well-being: A systematic review of global literature. *AIDS and Behavior, 17*(7), 2554–2574.

Christens, B. (2012). Targeting empowerment in community development: A community psychology approach towards enhancing local power and well-being. *Community Development Journal, 47*(4), 538–554.

Cluver, L. (2011). Children of the AIDS pandemic. *Nature, 474*(7349), 27–29.

Cluver, L., & Gardner, F. (2007). The mental health of children orphaned by AIDS: A review of international and southern African research. *Journal of Child and Adolescent Mental Health, 19*(1), 1–17.

Cluver, L., Gardner, F., & Operario, D. (2007). Psychological distress amongst AIDS-orphaned children in urban South Africa. *Journal of Child Psychology and Psychiatry, 48*(8), 755–763.

Cluver, L. D., Orkin, M., Boyes, M. E., Gardner, F., & Nikelo, J. (2012). AIDS-Orphanhood and caregiver HIV/AIDS sickness status: Effects on psychological symptoms in South African Youth. *Journal of Pediatric Psychology, 37*(8), 857–867.

Cluver, L. D., Orkin, M., Gardner, F., & Boyes, M. E. (2012). Persisting mental health problems among AIDS-orphaned children in South Africa. *Journal of Child Psychol and Psychiatry, 53*(4), 363–370.

da Silva Ferreira, G. C., Crippa, J. A., & de Lima Osório, F. (2014). Facial emotion processing and recognition among maltreated children: A systematic literature review. *Frontiers in Psychology, 17*(5), 1460.

Doku, P. N. (2009). Parental HIV/AIDS status and death, and children's psychological wellbeing. *International Journal of Mental Health Systems, 3*(1), 26.

Dunn, J. (1988). *The beginnings of social understanding.* Boston, MA: Harvard University Press.

Dunn, J. (1993). *Young children's close relationships: Beyond attachment.* New York: Sage.

Dunn, J. (1994). Changing minds and changing relationships. In C. Lewis & P. Mitchell (Eds.), *Children's early understanding of mind: Origins and development* (pp. 297–310). Mahwah, NJ: Lawrence Erlbaum Associates.

Dunn, J., Brown, J., & Beardsall, L. (1991). Family talk about feeling states and children's later understanding of others' emotions. *Developmental Psychology, 27*(3), 448–455.

Dunn, J., Brown, J., Slomkowski, C., Tesla, C., & Youngblade, L. (1991). Young children's understanding of other people's feelings and beliefs: Individual differences and their antecedents. *Child Development, 62*(6), 1352–1366.

Eaton, J., McCay, L., Semrau, M., Chatterjee, S., Baingana, F., Araya, R., . . . Saxena, S. (2011). Scale up of services for mental health in low-income and middle-income countries. *Lancet, 378*(9802), 1592–1603.

Eloff, I., Finestone, M., Makin, J. D., Boeving-Allen, A., Visser, M., Ebersohn, L., . . . Forsyth, B. W. (2014). A randomized clinical trial of an intervention to promote resilience in young children of HIV-positive mothers in South Africa. *AIDS, 28*(3), S347–357.

Eze, M. O. (2010). *Intellectual history in contemporary South Africa.* London: Palgrave Macmillan.

Fonagy, P., Steele, M., Steele, H., Moran, G. S., & Higgitt, A. C. (1991). The capacity for understanding mental states: The reflective self in parent and child and its significance for security of attachment. *Infant mental health journal, 12*(3), 201–218.

Fonagy, P., Gergely, G., Jurist, E. L., & Target, M. (2002). *Affect regulation, mentalization, and the development of self.* New York: Other Press.

Foster, G. (2006). Children who live in communities affected by AIDS. *Lancet, 367*(9511), 700–701.

Friedli, L. (2009). *Mental health, resilience and inequalities.* Geneva: World Health Organization.

Goodman, G., & Dent, V. F. (2019). Studying the effectiveness of the storytelling/story-acting (STSA) play intervention on Ugandan preschoolers' emergent literacy, oral language, and theory of mind in two rural Ugandan community libraries. In *Early childhood development: Concepts, methodologies, tools, and applications* (pp. 1174–1205). Hershey, PA: IGI Global.

Goodman, R. (2001). Psychometric properties of the strengths and difficulties questionnaire. *Journal of the American Academy of Child and Adolescent Psychiatry, 40*(11), 1337–1345.

Haidet, K. K., Tate, J., Divirgilio-Thomas, D., Kolanowski, A., & Happ, M. B. (2009). Methods to improve reliability of video-recorded behavioral data. *Research in Nursing & Health, 32*(4), 465–474.

Han, H. R., Floyd, O., Kim, K., Cudjoe, J., Warren, N., Seal, S., & Sharps, P. (2019). Intergenerational interventions for people living with HIV and their families: A systematic review. *AIDS and Behavior, 23*(1), 21–36.

Harris, P. L. (1989). *Children and emotion.* New Jersey: Basil Blackwell.

Hsieh, H., & Shannon, S. E. (2005). Three approaches to qualitative content analyses. *Qualitative Health Research, 15*(9), 1277–1288.

Jenkins, R., Baingana, F., Ahmad, R., McDaid, D., & Atun, R. (2011). Social, economic, human rights and political challenges to global mental health. *Mental Health and Family Medicine, 8*(2), 87–96.

Jordans, M., & Tola, W. (2013). Mental health in humanitarian settings: Shifting focus to care systems. *International Health, 5*, 9–10.

Kakuma, R., Minas, H., van Ginneken, N., Dal Poz, M. R., Desiraju, K., Morris, J. E., . . . Scheffler, R. M. (2011). Human resources for mental health care: Current situation and strategies for action. *Lancet, 378*(9803), 1654–1663.

Kang'ethe, S., & Makuyan, A. (2014). Orphans and vulnerable children (OVC) care institutions: Exploring their possible damage to children in a few countries of the developing world. *Journal of Social Sciences, 38*(2), 117–124.

Klein, P. S. (1996). *Early intervention: Cross-cultural experiences with a mediational approach.* London: Routledge.

Klein, P. S. (2014). *OMI—observing mediational interaction manual* (Unpublished manuscript).

Klein, P. S., & Rye, H. (2004). Interaction-oriented early intervention in Ethiopia—The MISC approach. *Infants and Young Children, 17*(4), 340–354.

Malcolm-Smith, S., Woolley, D., & Ward, C. L. (2015). Examining empathy and its association with aggression in young Western Cape children. *Journal of Child & Adolescent Mental Health, 27*(2), 135–147.

Marais, L., Rani, K., Sharp, C., Skinner, D., Serekoane, J., Cloete, J., . . . Lenka, M. (2018). What role for community? Critical reflections on state-driven support for vulnerable children and orphans in South Africa. In P. Westoby & L. Shevellar (Eds.), *Routledge research companion to community development* (pp. 71–83). London: Routledge.

Marais, L., Sharp, C., Pappin, M., Sigenu, K., Skinner, D., Lenka, M., . . . Serekoane, J. (2013). Community-based support for the mental health of orphans and vulnerable children in South Africa: A triangulation study. *Vulnerable Children and Youth Studies, 9*(2), 151–158.

Matthews, J. M., & Hudson, A. M. (2001). Guidelines for evaluating parent training programs. *Family Relations, 50*(1), 77–86.

Penchansky, R., & Thomas, J. W. (1981). The concept of access—definition and relationship to consumer satisfaction. *Medical Care, 19*(2), 127–140.

Penner, F., Sharp, C., Marais, L., Shohet, C., Givon, D., & Boivin, M. (2020). Community-based caregiver and family interventions to support the mental health of orphans and vulnerable children: Review and future directions. *New Directions for Child and Adolescent Development, 171*, 77–105.

Perner, J., Ruffman, T., & Leekam, S. R. (1994). Theory of mind is contagious: You catch it from your sibs. *Child Development, 65*, 1228–1238.

Pillay, J. (2014). Challenges educational psychologists face working with vulnerable children in Africa: Integration of theory and practice. In *Psychology in education* (pp. 95–111). Leiden: Brill Sense.

Puffer, E. S., Green, E. P., Sikkema, K. J., Broverman, S. A., Ogwang-Odhiambo, R. A., & Pian, J. (2016). A church-based intervention for families to promote mental health and prevent HIV among adolescents in rural Kenya: Results of a randomized trial. *Journal of Consulting and Clinical Psychology, 84*(6), 511–525.

Quas, J. A., Dickerson, K. L., Matthew, R., Harron, C., & Quas, C. M. (2017). Adversity, emotion recognition, and empathic concern in high-risk youth. *PloS one, 12*(7), e0181606.

Richter, L. M., Sherr, L., Adato, M., Belsey, M., Chandan, U., Desmond, C., . . . Wakhweya, A. (2009). Strengthening families to support children affected by HIV and AIDS. *AIDS Care, 21*(1), 3–12.

Schenk, K. D. (2009). Community-based interventions providing care and support to orphans and vulnerable children: A review of evaluation evidence. *AIDS Care, 21,* 918–942.

Schenk, K. D., & Michaelis, A. (2010). Community interventions supporting children affected by HIV in sub-Saharan Africa: A review to derive evidence-based principles for programming. *Vulnerable Children and Youth Studies, 5*(1), 40–54.

Schenk, K. D., Michaelis, A., Sapiano, T. N., Brown, L., & Weiss, E. (2010). Improving the lives of vulnerable children: Implications of Horizons research among orphans and other children affected by AIDS. *Public Health Reports, 125*(2), 325–336.

Sewpaul, V., & Matthias, C. (2013). *Child rights in Africa.* London: Sage.

Sharp, C., Fonagy, P., & Goodyer, I. (2008). *Social cognition and developmental psychopathology.* Oxford: Oxford University Press.

Sharp, C., & Hernandez Ortiz, J. (2021). Mindreading and psychopathology in middle childhood and adolescence. In S. Lecce & R. T. Devine (Eds.), *Theory of mind in middle childhood and adolescence: Integrating multiple perspectives.* London: Taylor and Francis.

Sharp, C., Jardin, C., Marais, L., & Boivin, M. (2015). Orphanhood by AIDS-related causes and child mental health: A developmental psychopathology approach. *Journal of HIV & AIDS, 1*(3). doi:10.16966/2380-5536.114

Sharp, C., Kulesz, P., Marais, L., Shohet, C., Rani, K., Lenka, M., . . . Boivin, M. (2021). Mediational intervention for sensitizing caregivers to improve mental health outcomes in orphaned and vulnerable children. *Journal of Clinical Child & Adolescent Psychology,* 1–16. doi:10.1080/15374416.2021.1881903

Sharp, C., Shohet, C., Givon, D., Marais, L., & Boivin, M. I. M. E. (2018). Early childhood interventions: A focus on responsive caregiving. In M. Tomlinson, A. Stevenson, & C. Hanlon (Eds.), *Child and adolescent development in Africa in the context of the sustainable development goals* (pp. 245–270). Cape Town: UCT Press.

Sharp, C., Shohet, C., Givon, D., Penner, F., Marais, L., & Fonagy, P. (2020). Learning to mentalize: A mediational approach for caregivers and therapists. *Clinical Psychology: Science and Practice, 27*(3), e12334.

Sharp, C., Venta, A., Marais, L., Skinner, D., Lenka, M., & Serekoane, J. (2014). First evaluation of a population-based screen to detect emotional-behavior disorders in orphaned children in Sub-Saharan Africa. *Aids and Behavior, 18*(6), 1174–1185.

Shohet, C., & Jaegermann, N. (2012). Integrating infant mental health into primary health care and early childhood education settings in Israel. *Zero to Three, 33*(2), 55–58.

Sikkema, K. J., Dennis, A. C., Watt, M. H., Choi, K. W., Yemeke, T. T., & Joska, J. A. (2015). Improving mental health among people living with HIV: A review of intervention trials in low- and middle-income countries. *Global Mental Health, 2,* e19.

Skeen, S., Sherr, L., Tomlinson, M., Croome, N., Ghandi, N., Roberts, J. K., & Macedo, A. (2017). Interventions to improve psychosocial wellbeing for children affected by HIV and AIDS: A systematic review. *Vulnerable Children and Youth Studies, 12*(2), 91–116.

Skinner, D., Sharp, C., Jooste, S., Mfecane, S., & Simbayi, L. (2013). A study of descriptive data for orphans and non-orphans on key criteria of economic vulnerability in two municipalities in South Africa. *Curationis, 36*(1), 1–8.

Skinner, D., Tsheko, N., Mtero-Munyati, S., Segwabe, M., Chibatamoto, P., Mfecane, S., . . . Chitiyo, G. (2006). Towards a definition of orphaned and vulnerable children. *AIDS and Behavior, 10*(6), 619–626.

Spaull, N., Ardington, C., Bassier, I., Bhorat, H., Bridgman, G., Budlender, J., . . . Casale, D. (2020). *NIDS-CRAM wave 1 synthesis report: Overview and findings*. Data First Open Data Portal. Retrived from https://www.datafirst.uct.ac.za.

Stirman, S. W., Baumann, A. A., & Miller, C. J. (2019). The FRAME: An expanded framework for reporting adaptations and modifications to evidence-based interventions. *Implementation Science, 14*(1), 1–10.

Thurman, T., & Kidman, R. (2011). Child maltreatment at home: Prevalence among orphans and vulnerable children in KwaZulu-Natal, South Africa. *New Orleans: Tulane University School of Public Health, 201*(1).

Tomlinson, M., Cooper, P., & Murray, L. (2005). The mother-infant relationship and infant attachment in a South African peri-urban settlement. *Child Development, 76*(5), 1044–1054.

UNAIDS. (2010). *Report on global AIDS epidemic*. Geneva, Switzerland: UNAIDS.

UNAIDS. (2012). *Report on the global AIDS epidemic*. Geneva, Switzerland: UNAIDS.

UNICEF. (2013). *National plan of action children in South Africa 2012–2017*. New York: UNICEF.

United Nations. (2016). *Fact sheet: Joint United Nations programme on HIV/AIDS*. New York: United Nations.

Van Ijzendoorn, M. H., Schuengel, C., & Bakermans-Kranenburg, M. J. (1999). Disorganized attachment in early childhood: Meta-analysis of precursors, concomitants, and sequelae. *Development and Psychopathology, 11*(2), 225–250.

Ward, C. L., Wessels, I. M., Lachman, J. M., Hutchings, J., Cluver, L. D., Kassanjee, R., . . . Gardner, F. (2020). Parenting for lifelong health for young children: A randomized controlled trial of a parenting program in South Africa to prevent harsh parenting and child conduct problems. *Journal of Child Psychology and Psychiatry, 61*(4), 503–512.

Wild, L. (2001). The psychological adjustment of children orphaned by AIDS. *Southern African Journal of Child and Adolescent Mental Health, 13*(1), 3–22.

Wingood, G. M., & DiClemente, R. J. (2008). The ADAPT-ITT model: A novel method of adapting evidence-based HIV Interventions. *Journal of Acquired Immune Deficiency Syndrome, 47*, S40–46.

World Health Organizations. (2018). *Nurturing care for early childhood development: A framework for helping children survive and thrive to transform health and human potential*. Geneva, Switzerland: World Health Organizations.

Yakubovich, A. R., Sherr, L., Cluver, L. D., Skeen, S., Hensels, I. S., Macedo, A., & Tomlinson, M. (2016). Community-based organizations for vulnerable children in South Africa: Reach, psychosocial correlates, and potential mechanisms. *Children and Youth Services Review, 62*, 58–64.

9 Mediational Intervention for Sensitizing Caregivers of Toddlers With Sensory Processing and Self-Regulation Disorders

Nurit Jaegermann and Ornit Freudenstein

9.1 Sensory Processing

During pregnancy, the womb serves as an optimal environment that protects the fetus from overstimulation and allows the gradual development of the sensory systems (Tocchio, Kline-Fath, Kanal, Schmithorst, & Panigrahy, 2015). Immediately after birth, the newborn is exposed to different sensory stimulations in various intensities. The newborn's first developmental challenge is twofold: He needs to be able to take in the sensory richness of the environment, and at the same time maintain an optimal arousal state wherein he is calm and attentive (Lewkowicz & Turkewitz, 1981; Stern, 2018; Williamson & Anzalone, 2001). The newborn gradually learns to balance his growing awareness of the environmental stimuli—touch, motion, smells, tastes, sights and sounds—with the developing capacity to be interested and focused and explore and to enjoy the world around him. According to Greenspan and Wieder (2006), these abilities constitute the foundation of the child's developing self-regulation.

There are innate individual differences in the ability of infants to process sensory information from their body and the environment and to respond to it in a regulated and adapted manner (Aron, Aron, & Jagiellowicz, 2012; Ayres & Robbins, 2005; Jaegermann & Klein, 2010; Smith, 2019). Most of these differences are of a genetic origin (Mueller, Brocke, Fries, Lesch, & Kirschbaum, 2010; Popova, Lange, Probst, Gmel, & Rehm, 2017), and they are visible in the behavioral patterns of infants and toddlers. Some babies are calmer while others tend to be more active, some are noisier while others are quieter and more introverted (Brazelton & Nugent, 1995; Dunn, 2007; Thompson & Raisor, 2013).

From birth, neuro-typical infants can regulate themselves to an optimal arousal state in which they may lie calmly and be attentive, interested and responsive (Feldman, 2003, 2007; Geeraerts, Backer, & Stifter, 2020). Optimal arousal state supports interactions with the human and the physical environment and supports learning and development (Williamson & Anzalone, 2001). At first, the

DOI: 10.4324/9781003145899-9

infant's optimal arousal state is short and quite fleeting. Gradually, along with his parents' ongoing sensitive and adaptive caregiving patterns, the length and stability of the infant's optimal arousal states extend (Candilis-Huisman, 2019; de Barbaro, Clackson, & Wass, 2017; Feldman, 2007).

The term "Sensory Processing" explains these innate differences, using neurophysiological concepts that describe the neural processes of intake, registration, processing, integrating, decoding and reacting to sensory stimuli (Bundy & Murray, 2002; Dunn, 2007; Smith, 2019). It should be noted that "Temperament" is another leading concept that describes behavioral characteristics of infants and refers to an innate component in the development of the ability to self-regulation (Rothbart, Ellis, & Posner, 2004). There are studies that offer a conceptual and clinical overlap between the two concepts (temperament and sensory processing) (for example, DeSantis, Harkins, Tronick, Kaplan, & Beeghly, 2011). Using the concept of sensory processing in the context of developmental risk is beneficial mainly due to the clinical and interventional reference that sensory processing contributes.

9.2 Self-Regulation

Self-regulation serves as a critical human capacity that functions as a cornerstone for optimal development (Mahoney, Boyce, Fewell, Spiker, & Wheeden, 1998; Posner & Rothbart, 2000; Bronson & Bronson, 2001; Vohs & Baumeister, 2016). A recent meta-analysis showed that self-regulation in childhood predicts academic and employment achievement, interpersonal behavior, mental health and healthy living in later life (Robson, Allen & Howard., 2020). Self-regulation is based on the ability to plan socially accepted responses from internal and interpersonal discourse (Als, 1989; Bronson & Bronson, 2001; Cicchetti, 1996). Moreover, self-regulation refers to the developing ability to control and adapt the quality and intensity of the responses to external and internal stimuli/events (e.g., sudden barking of a dog, disturbing thoughts or emotions) (Dunn, 2007; Dunn, Little, Dean, Robertson, & Evans, 2016; Williamson & Anzalon, 2001). Fonagy and Target (2002) refer to self-regulation as the main mediator between genetic predispositions, early experiences and adult functioning. Self-regulation refers to children's ability to control their responses to stress, maintain attention and interpret their own and others' mental states. The ability to self-regulate develops rapidly throughout the first years of life and is based on both innate and acquired aspects (Bronson & Bronson, 2001). The innate aspect refers to the child's neurophysiological foundation, expressed by the child's sensory profile (Dunn et al., 2016; Jaegermann & Klein, 2010; Porges, 2011; Willamson & Anzalone, 2001). The acquired aspect refers to the child's experiences with the environment, especially the quality of parent-child day-to-day interactions (Eisenberg et al., 2001, 2003; Kochanska, Coy, & Murray, 2001; Lobo & Lunkenheimer, 2020).

Sameroff (2009) and Sameroff and Fiese (2000a, 2000b) focused on the relationship of the infant with his caregivers, who provide for his needs and support his physical and mental development. The development of self-regulation is perceived as a process in which the balance between external regulation by the caregiver and the child's self-regulation changes from dependence on external regulation in infancy, to independent self-regulation, as the toddler develops and achieves the ability for self-control and self-care. In other words, there is a transition from total reliance on the caregiver as an external regulator to independent self-regulation in the first years of life.

Indeed, infants depend on excessive, devoted and sensitive care based on external regulation of their caregivers in the first months of life (Feldman, Greenbaum, & Yirmiya, 1999; Winnicott, 1960). The role of the parent is to regulate the baby's emotions and behavior as well as to provide for his physiological needs: to soothe in distress, to feed, to change diapers and clothes, to bathe, to regulate the room temperature, to pick up a fallen pacifier, to cover when it's cold etc. In typical development, each infant, in his own pace, begins to develop patterns of self-regulation until he can become more and more independent in controlling his behavior, less helpless and less dependent on his caregivers (Calkins, Perry, & Dollar, 2016). Behaviors such as calming down when the mother enters the room, reaching out and taking a desired toy or putting the pacifier that has fallen into his mouth are examples that represent the developing ability to self-regulate.

9.3 Sensory Processing and Self-Regulation

According to Williamson and Anzalon's model (Schaaf & Anzalone, 2001; Williamson & Anzalon, 2001), the innate sensory processing ability influences the infant's behavior and self-regulation of his responses through four basic observable functional components: *Arousal, Attention, Affect* and *Action*. In their view, individual differences between infants and toddlers in their innate ability for sensory processing will be reflected in behavioral patterns that represent these four basic components. The four components together contribute to the behavioral organization and form the core of self-regulation in young children.

9.3.1 Arousal

Arousal refers to the child's ability to maintain optimal arousal through activity and to move through different states of sleep and wakefulness. Brazelton and Nugent (1995) defined six states of arousal in infants: deep sleep, light sleep, drowsiness, quiet wakefulness (optimal arousal), active wakefulness (fussiness) and crying. The various arousal states are related to sensory processing. For example, a hug may be pleasant to a child in a drowsiness state or a quiet wakefulness state. In contrast, a hug may be rejected or irritate a child in a state of stress or a state of active wakefulness.

9.3.2 Attention

Attention refers to the ability to selectively focus on a stimulus or task, while filtering stimuli irrelevant to the situation. It also refers to the ability to effortlessly shift attention from one stimulus to another when needed. Most children can maintain attention relatively easily in a state of quiet wakefulness. However, for children who tend to be more active, the state of active wakefulness is more appropriate for attention regulation.

Children with challenges in sensory processing have difficulty maintaining optimal arousal and therefore face a challenge to focus and respond adaptively. For example, infants with sensory processing challenges have difficulty relating to input from multiple sensory systems simultaneously. They can look and smile at a caregiver during a face-to-face interaction, as long as the caregiver is not talking. When the auditory stimulus is combined with a visual stimulus, the infant may feel "overwhelmed" with the stimuli and have difficulty maintaining attention. He may look away from the caregiver.

9.3.3 Affect (the Expression of Emotion)

Sensations and emotions are profoundly related. Sensation usually creates emotional responses, which express how a child experiences and copes with a specific sensory stimuli or event, subjectively. For example, does the child laugh with pleasure and get excited while playing an intensive motor game? Or, does he suddenly look tense and dissatisfied when his mother turns on a vacuum cleaner?

Affect is an important component of social relationships, which involve a large and varied quantity of dynamic sensory stimulation. For example, the day-to-day interactions between a mother and her infant often involve touch, movement, sights, sounds, smells and tastes. In addition, playing actively with peers involves intensive vestibular and proprioceptive stimulation. A challenge to cope with these sensations affects interpersonal relationships. Children who have difficulty organizing regulated adaptive responses to sensory stimuli tend to show increased or flattened emotional responses. Such emotional responses in infancy may influence the formation of the early attachment relationship. For example, an irritable baby with tactile defensiveness (sensitivity to touch) becomes "stiff" and resists when held and hugged. His mother may interpret this behavior as rejection, and in response, she may prefer to leave her child alone and calm rather than interfere with the baby's fragile regulation through dyadic interactions. Thus, fewer and fewer opportunities for positive and enjoyable mutual interactions can, over time, affect the bonding between the infant and the parent.

9.3.4 Action

Action refers to a planned and well-organized goal-directed motor behavior that is executed for the first time or in a new way. Such a motor action involves sensory perception and cognition to function purposefully. Although motor movements are the basis for action, action is much more complex than just movements. Play is a good example of action. Play depends on neuro–motor maturity; however, it is also affected by a large number of variables. To play in an adaptive way, a child must set himself a goal for an action related to the environment (idea) and be able to plan and perform a sequence of actions to achieve the goal. For example, a toddler imagining a traveling train arranges a line of small cars and carefully pushes them onto the mountain formed from the sofa cushions while making a train.

According to Williamson and Anzalone (2001), these four fundamental components of functioning—Arousal, Attention, Affect and Action—are interrelated and affect each other in complex interactions.

9.4 Sensory Processing and Self-Regulation Disorders in Infants and Toddlers (SPD)

In the general population, the prevalence of sensory profiles that are related to functioning difficulties is approximately 5–16% in full-term infants with no other developmental diagnosis (Ahn, Miller, Milberger, & Mcintosh, 2004; Ben-Sasson, Carter, & Briggs-Gowan, 2009; Gouze, Hopkins, Lebailly, & Lavigne, 2009; Miller, Anzalone, Lane, Cermak, & Osten, 2007). Social-emotional, motor performance, cognitive and learning or attention difficulties, and communication challenges may appear and put the child at developmental risk (Dale et al., 2011; DeGangi, 2017; Flanagan, Schoen, & Miller; 2017; Germani et al., 2014). When the family is confronting additional risk factors, child's developmental risk becomes even more severe.

Children with such challenging sensory profiles are considered to have Sensory Processing Disorder (SPD) (Ahn et al., 2004; Ben-Sasson et al., 2009; Miller et al., 2007; Zero to Three, 2016). SPD in infants and toddlers was first clinically recognized under the diagnosis "Regulatory Disorders" in "Zero to Three's Diagnostic Classification of Mental Health and Developmental Disorders of Infancy and Early Childhood" (Zero to Three, 1994). In the revision of Zero to Three (Zero to Three, 2005), the disorder was renamed "Regulation Disorders of Sensory Processing" to highlight the sensory basis of the behaviors included in the diagnosis. In the last revision—the DC:0–5 (2016)—the diagnosis was renamed again to "Sensory Processing Disorders".

In children with sensory processing disorder (SPD), the ability of the nervous system to effectively take in sensory information, to organize it, to process and to interpret the information is affected. These children are missing clear and precise information about their body and the environment around them (Dunn et al., 2016; Porges, 2011). Due to the misinterpretation of situations, the child may show unregulated and maladapted responses (Ayres & Robbins, 2005; Schaaf et al., 2010; Smith, 2019). In other words, the child may be faced with difficulty taking in information, acting on, learning and enjoying various stimuli, social interactions and experiences (Bundy & Murray, 2002; Smith, 2019).

Infants and toddlers with SPD show unregulated behavioral patterns, such as irritability, lack of interest in their surroundings, difficulty in self-soothing, attention difficulties and motor-functioning difficulties. Sleeping and eating difficulties may appear as well (DeGangi, 2017; Stalker & Reebye, 2007; Williamson & Anzalone, 2001; Zero to Three, 2005, 2016). Parents of children with SPD experience and report feelings of confusion, stress and depression and difficulties in interacting with the child (DeGangi, 2017; Jaegermann & Klein, 2010). A recent study showed that mothers of toddlers with SPD were less sensitive and less regulating, used less teaching behaviors and were more intrusive than were mothers of toddlers without sensory challenges (Jaegermann, Pinto, & Adi-Japha, in preparation).

Dunn (Dunn & Daniels, 2002; Dunn et al., 2016) developed a model to explain how sensory processing disorders affect infants, toddlers and their families' daily lives. The model referred to the behavioral patterns mentioned previously and organized them into four patterns:

1. Sensitivity to Stimuli—characterized by restlessness, irritability, anger and frustration, or a defensive reaction to sensory stimuli.
2. Sensation Avoiding—characterized by behaviors that minimize the exposure to unexpected stimuli, such as isolation, withdrawal, preference for familiar activities etc.
3. Poor/Low Registration—related to slow or imperceptible responses to sensation and characterized by self-absorption, lack of connectedness, lack of emotional expressions of enthusiasm and enjoyment, or slow responses.
4. Sensation Seeking—children with sensation-seeking profile derive pleasure from a rich sensory environment and behaviors that create rigorous sensations, such as hyper motor activity or creating loud noise with toys and other objects.

Dunn (Dunn, 2007; Dunn et al., 2016) noted that the clinical picture of the behavioral categories characterizing children with SPD is not always consistent and accurate. Children with SPD may seem unresponsive in some situations and over-reactive in other situations. They may be hypersensitive to touch and hypersensitive to taste. In addition, Dunn noted that sensory processing is also affected by the toddler's physiological state (fatigue, hunger, illness etc.).

Miller, Reisman, McIntosh and Simon (2001) proposed an ecological model in which a child's responsiveness is affected by the environmental context. In addition, Miller et al. (2007) suggested a model intended to classify individual profiles of children with SPD. Her classification included three categories:

1. Sensory Modulation Disorder—refers to the child's responses to sensory stimuli and includes over-responsivity, under-responsivity or Sensation Seeking.

2. Sensory Discrimination Disorder—characterized by having a difficulty recognizing and interpret correctly sensory stimuli.
3. Sensory-Based Motor Disorder—includes both a lack of postural control and difficulty in planning and organizing a motor response (Dyspraxia).

When the infant's innate ability for sensory processing is atypical, his ability to develop self-regulation is challenged and he needs extra sensitive and adapted care, for a longer period, to be calm, attentive and interactive and to ensure better developmental outcomes (Dunn, 2007; Pluess & Belsky, 2013). Some parents can intuitively respond to these needs and provide the child with interactions tailored to their challenging, sensory-based, regulatory needs. However, empirical and clinical evidence shows that infants and toddlers with SPD interactions with their parents are not optimal (DeGangi, 2017; Jaegermann & Klein, 2010; Jaegermann et al., in preparation).

Jaegermann and Klein (2010) examined 30 mothers and toddlers with SPD at two times of about eight weeks apart. The study's findings showed that there was a decrease in the mother's ability to behave in a regulated manner with a child and support mutual communication with him between the first and second evaluation. Other maternal behaviors such as focusing the child's attention, mediating behavior regulation and regaining the child's attention also showed a declining trend within this short time. These findings are particularly important because the decline in the quality of the mother's responses when interacting with her child occurs mainly concerning the toddler's behavioral regulation and attention. This finding, obtained over a short period (approximately eight weeks), highlights the importance of early intervention to improve the quality of parent-child interaction with toddlers coping with SPD.

9.5 Parental Guidance for Toddlers with Sensory Processing and Self-Regulation Disorders

The relationship between young children and their parents has a crucial impact on the child's emotional, social, cognitive and linguistic development. These relationships promote optimal developmental growth when they are warm, nurturing, sensitive to the child's needs, characterized by reciprocal responsiveness, a high level of "adaptability" and "synchrony" (Feldman, 2007; Shonkoff, Phillips, & National Research Council, 2000; Thomas, Abell, Webb, Avdagic, & Zimmer-Gembeck, 2017). Moreover, a quality learning experience is a crucial component of the parent-child relationship that predicts optimal development (Klein, 1996).

One of the main goals in early intervention programs with at-risk infants and toddlers is promoting the quality of the parent-child relationships (Bronfenbrenner, 1974; Cramer et al., 1990; Gilkerson & Stott, 2000; Hanzlik, 1998; Thomas, Letourneau et al., 2017). Intervention programs intended to support the parent-child relations are based on the assumption that the parent's behavior serves as a primary pathway for influencing the child's development (Hembree-Kigin & McNeil, 2013).

9.6 Mediational Intervention for Sensitizing Caregivers for Toddlers With Sensory Processing and Self-Regulation Disorder

The MISC-SP (Jaegermann & Klein, 2010) is an evidence-based parental guidance program that focuses on enhancing the quality of interaction between parents and young children with SPD. The MISC-SP program is based on the basic MISC model (Mediational Intervention for Sensitizing Caregivers; Klein, 1996, 2003), of which the efficacy was proven in a series of studies (Klein, 1996, 2003; Klein & Alony, 1993).

In an efficacy trial, the effects of the MISC-SP intervention were compared to those of another intervention designed to enhance children's sensory functioning (the SI group) and to a control group receiving no intervention and received general developmental parental guidance post-study. Participants were 86 toddlers (12–18 months old) with SPD and their mothers, who were randomly assigned to the aforementioned three research groups. Following the intervention period, mothers in the MISC-SP group showed more sensitive behavior, supported their toddlers' communication and regulated behavior better, and used teaching behaviors more appropriately than mothers in the two other groups (Jaegermann & Klein, 2010).

The MISC-SP program targets the understanding of the mutual influence between the child's behavioral and emotional regulation difficulties and parental responsiveness. The program is focused on raising the parents' awareness of their child's sensory and regulatory individual profile and explaining the child's behavioral challenges in light of his sensory profile.

The assumption that underlies the MISC-SP program is that a sensitive parent-child interaction adapted to the toddler's special sensory/regulatory needs (sensory profile) can moderate and even prevent the potential negative effects of SPD on the toddler's development.

The MISC-SP program integrates into the basic MISC model components of three leading therapeutic models for social-emotional, sensory and self-regulation development: (1) **DIR**—*Developmental, Individual-differences & Relationship-based model* (Greenspan & Wieder, 2006); (2) **MBT**—the *Metallization-based Treatment* (Bateman & Fonagy, 2013); and (3) **SI**—*Sensory Integration* (Ayres & Robbins, 2005; Smith, 2019). The MISC-SP program consists of three main goals:

Reframing—Redefining the parental perception of the child's behavioral challenges through evaluating and explaining his sensory profile.
Reflecting and Metallizing—Supporting the ability of parents to observe the child's behavior and interpret their child's and own mental states sensitively.

Mediating—Encouraging parents to use learning opportunities that occur during daily interactions with the child.

During the intervention, parents are encouraged when they are sensitive, adapted to the child's sensory and regulatory needs and using teaching behaviors such as Expansion (giving additional information to the child regarding an object or event) or Meaning (naming objects and events and adding to it emotional expressions). According to Klein (1996), by being exposed to teaching behaviors, the child's ability to gain more from further learning experience is enhanced.

The MISC-SP addresses diverse aspects of parent-child interaction that support optimal development, including **emotional, communication** and **teaching** aspects as mentioned earlier. Jaegermann and Klein (2010) found that the MISC-SP intervention program significantly promoted measures relating to the quality of parent-child interactions and measures relating to the development of the toddler with SPD. That is, various aspects of the mothers' behavior in the interaction improved as a result of the intervention and, consequently, the developmental abilities of the toddlers improved as well. Following the mothers' guidance and the change in their behavior, their children could regulate attention more maturely and be partners in longer and more varied and enriching interactions. The children also responded in a more organized and planned manner and reacted less defensively to sensory stimuli.

The program has been implemented for about two decades within the Harris Program Clinic at the School of Education, Bar-Ilan University. In addition, special training programs are being implemented for professionals working with young children and their families in different settings. For the past decade, the program has been applied in community projects with high-risk populations in collaboration with public systems such as the Ministry of Health, the Ministry of Education, municipalities, health care systems etc. Over the years, research has been conducted with our students within the Harris university clinic to further refine the intervention components. For example, in an unpublished thesis, David (David, 2017) found that maternal encouraging behavior that includes a simple explanation of the action and its consequences ("Very good! You did it now slowly and carefully. . . . Look what a tall tower you built!") is significantly related to improved toddler motor planning abilities. Research findings like the latter support our clinical ability to adapt the parental guidance we offer, deferring sensory and regulatory child profiles and deferring personal and cultural parent and family characteristics.

9.7 Conclusion

The MISC-SP intervention targets both existing behavioral challenges and potential developmental difficulties of young children who are at developmental risk due to neurological inborn difficulties to process sensory information. The MISC-SP intervention integrates a clinical understanding of SPD with a developmental understanding of the fundamental role of parent—child interactions in child development, particularly in the development of the ability to regulate emotions and behaviors.

During the past decade, there have been significant efforts to enhance professional awareness to the importance of early identification and intervention with infants and toddlers with SPD and their parents. Additional efforts need to be made to ensure that more and more infants and toddlers with SPD are identified and treated, especially among families facing additional risk factors.

We suggest conducting studies that focus on parental behaviors that support the self-regulation of children with various SPD symptoms and with other populations that struggle with SPD, such as children diagnosed with Autism Spectrum Disorder.

References

Ahn, R. R., Miller, L. J., Milberger, S., & McIntosh, D. N. (2004). Prevalence of parents' perceptions of sensory processing disorders among kindergarten children. *American Journal of Occupational Therapy, 58*(3), 287–293.

Als, H. (1989). Self regulation and motor development in preterm infants. In J. Lockamn & N. Hazem (Eds.), *Action in social context: Perspectives on early development* (pp. 65–97). Los Angeles and New York: Plenum Press.

Aron, E. N., Aron, A., & Jagiellowicz, J. (2012). Sensory processing sensitivity: A review in the light of the evolution of biological responsivity. *Personality and Social Psychology Review, 16*(3), 262–282.

Ayres, A. J., & Robbins, J. (2005). *Sensory integration and the child: Understanding hidden sensory challenges.* Los Angeles: Western Psychological Services.

Ben-Sasson, A., Carter, A. S., & Briggs-Gowan, M. J. (2009). Sensory over-responsivity in elementary school: Prevalence and social-emotional correlates. *Journal of Abnormal Child Psychology, 37*(5), 705–716.

Bateman, A., & Fonagy, P. (2013). Mentalization-based treatment. *Psychoanalytic Inquiry, 33*(6), 595–613.

Brazelton, T. B., & Nugent, J. K. (1995). *Neonatal behavioral assessment scale.* Cambridge: Cambridge University Press.

Bronfenbrenner, U. (1974). *A report on longitudinal evaluation of preschool programs: Vol 2. Is early intervention effective?* Washington, DC: Department of Health and Welfare.

Bronson, M. B., & Bronson, M. (2001). *Self-regulation in early childhood: Nature and nurture.* New York: Guilford Press.

Bundy, A. C., & Murray, A. E. (2002). Sensory integration: A. Jean Ayres' theory revisited. In A. C. Bundy, S. J. Lane, & E. A. Murray (Eds.), *Sensory integration: Theory and practice* (pp. 3–33). Philadelphia: F. A. Davis.

Calkins, S. D., Perry, N. B., & Dollar, J. (2016). A biopsychosocial model of the development of self-regulation in infancy. In L. Balter & C. Tamis-LeMonda (Eds.), *Child psychology: A handbook of contemporary issues* (pp. 3–20). London: Routledge.

Candilis-Huisman, D. (2019). The NBAS: Supporting the newborn and its family at birth. In G. Apter, E. Devouche, & M. Gratier (Eds.), *Early interaction and developmental psychopathology* (pp. 181–193). Berlin: Springer.

Cicchetti, D. (1996). Regulatory processes in development and psychopathology. *Development and Psychopathology, 8,* 1–3.

Cramer, B., Robert-Tissot, C., Stern, D. N., Serpa-Rusconi, S., Demuralt, M., Besson, G., . . . D'Arcis, U (1990). Outcome evaluation in brief mother-infant psychotherapy: A preliminary report. *Infant Mental Health Journal, 11*(3), 278–300.

De Barbaro, K., Clackson, K., & Wass, S. V. (2017). Infant attention is dynamically modulated with changing arousal levels. *Child Development, 88*(2), 629–639.

Dale, L. P., O'Hara, E. A., Schein, R., Inserra, L., Keen, J., Flores, M., & Porges, S. W. (2011). Measures of infant behavioral and physiological state regulation predict 54-month behavior problems. *Infant Mental Health Journal, 32*(4), 473–486.

David, A. (2017). *Effects of maternal behavior in parent-child interaction with toddlers with SPD, on toddlers' motor planning abilities* (Unpublished thesis). School of Education. Bar-Ilan University, Israel.

DeGangi, G. A. (2017). *Pediatric disorders of regulation in effect and behavior: A therapist's guide to assessment and treatment.* Cambridge, MA: Academic Press.

DeSantis, A., Harkins, D., Tronick, E., Kaplan, E., & Beeghly, M. (2011). Exploring an integrative model of infant behavior: What is the relationship among temperament, sensory processing, and neurobehavioral measures? *Infant Behavior and Development, 34*(2), 280–292.

Dunn, W., & Daniels, D. B. (2002). Initial development of the infant/toddler sensory profile. *Journal of Early Intervention, 25*(1), 27–41.

Dunn, W. (2007). Supporting children to participate successfully in everyday life by using sensory processing knowledge. *Infants & Young Children, 20*(2), 84–101.

Dunn, W., Little, L., Dean, E., Robertson, S., & Evans, B. (2016). The state of the science on sensory factors and their impact on daily life for children: A scoping review. *OTJR: Occupation, Participation and Health, 36*(Suppl 2), 3S–26S.

Eisenberg, N., Gershoff, E. T., Fabes, R. A., Shepard, S. A., Cumberland, A. J., Losoya, S. H., . . . Murphy, B. C. (2001). Mother's emotional expressivity and children's behavior problems and social competence: Mediation through children's regulation. *Developmental Psychology, 37*(4), 475–490.

Eisenberg, N., Valiente, C., Morris, A. S., Fabes, R. A., Cumberland, A., Reiser, M., . . . Losoya, S. (2003). Longitudinal relations among parental emotional expressivity, children's regulation, and quality of socioemotional functioning. *Developmental Psychology, 39*(1), 3–19

Feldman, R. (2003). Infant-mother and infant-father synchrony: The coregulation of positive arousal. *Infant Mental Health Journal, 24*(1), 1–23.

Feldman, R. (2007). Parent-infant synchrony and the construction of shared timing; Physiological precursors, developmental outcomes, and risk conditions. *Journal of Child Psychology and Psychiatry, 48*(3–4), 329–354.

Feldman, R., Greenbaum, C. W., & Yirmiya, N. (1999). Mother-infant affect synchrony as an antecedent of the emergence of self-control. *Developmental Psychology, 35*(1), 223–231.

Flanagan, J., Schoen, S., & Miller, L. J. (2017). Early identification of sensory processing challenges in infants at risk for sensory processing challenges. *American Journal of Occupational Therapy, 71*(4), 7111515260.

Fonagy, P., & Target, M. (2002). Early intervention and the development of self-regulation. *Psychoanalytic Inquiry, 22*(3), 307–335.

Geeraerts, S. B., Backer, P. M., & Stifter, C. A. (2020). It takes two: Infants' moderate negative reactivity and maternal sensitivity predict self-regulation in the preschool years. *Developmental Psychology, 56*(5), 869–879.

Germani, T., Zwaigenbaum, L., Bryson, S., Brian, J., Smith, I., Roberts, W., . . . Vaillancourt, T. (2014). Brief report: Assessment of early sensory processing in infants at high-risk of autism spectrum disorder. *Journal of Autism and Developmental Disorders*, *44*(12), 3264–3270.

Gilkerson, L., & Stott, F. (2000). Parent-child relationship in early intervention with infants and toddlers with disabilities and their families. In H. C. Zeanah Jr. (Ed.), *Handbook of infant mental health* (pp. 457–471). New York: Guilford Press.

Gouze, K. R., Hopkins, J., LeBailly, S. A., & Lavigne, J. V. (2009). Re-examining the epidemiology of sensory regulation dysfunction and comorbid psychopathology. *Journal of Abnormal Child Psychology*, *37*(8), 1077–1087.

Greenspan, S. I., & Wieder, S. (2006). *Engaging autism: Using the floortime approach to help children relate, communicate, and think*. Cambridge, MA: Da Capo Press.

Hanzlik, J. R. (1998). Parent-child relations: Interaction and intervention. In J. Case-Smith (Ed.), *Pediatric occupational therapy and early intervention* (pp. 207–222). Boston: Butterworth-Heinemann.

Hembree-Kigin, T. L., & McNeil, C. B. (2013). *Parent-child interaction therapy*. Berlin: Springer Science & Business Media.

Jaegermann, N., & Klein, P. S. (2010). Enhancing mothers' interactions with toddlers who have sensory-processing disorders. *Infant Mental Health Journal*, *31*(3), 291–311.

Jaegermann, N., Pinto, R., & Adi-Japha, E. (in preparation). *Do they get what they need? Mother-child interaction with toddlers with a sensory processing disorder*.

Klein, P. S. (1996). *Early interventions: A cross-cultural application of mediational approach*. New York: Garland.

Klein, P. S. (2003). Early intervention: Mediational intervention for sensitizing caregivers (MISC). In A. S. H. Seng, L. K. H. Pou, & O. S. Tan (Eds.), *Mediated learning experience with children: Applications across contexts* (pp. 68–84). Singapore: McGraw Hill.

Klein, P. S., & Alony, S. (1993). Immediate and sustain effects of maternal mediating behaviors in infancy. *Journal of Early Intervention*, *17*(2), 177–193.

Kochanska, G., Coy, K. C., & Murray, K. T. (2001). The development of self-regulation in the first four years of life. *Child Development*, *72*(4), 1091–1111.

Lewkowicz, D. J., & Turkewitz, G. (1981). Intersensory interaction in newborns: Modification of visual preferences following exposure to sound. *Child Development*, *52*(3), 827–832.

Lobo, F. M., & Lunkenheimer, E. (2020). Understanding the parent-child coregulation patterns shaping child self-regulation. *Developmental Psychology*, *56*(6), 1121–1134.

Mahoney, G., Boyce, G., Fewell, R., Spiker, D., & Wheeden, C. A. (1998). The relationship of parent-child interaction to the effectiveness of early intervention services for at-risk children and children with disabilities. *Topics in Early Childhood Special Education*, *1*(1), 5–17.

Miller, L. J., Reisman, J. E., McIntosh, D. N., & Simon, J. (2001). An ecological model of sensory modulation: Performance of children with fragile X syndrome, autistic disorder, attention-deficit/hyperactivity disorder, and sensory modulation dysfunction. In *Understanding the nature of sensory integration with diverse populations* (pp. 57–88). Cambridge, MA: Academic Press.

Miller, L. J., Anzalone, M. E., Lane, S. J., Cermak, S. A., & Osten, E. T. (2007). Concept evolution in sensory integration: A proposed nosology for diagnosis. *American Journal of Occupational Therapy*, *61*(2), 135–140.

Mueller, A., Brocke, B., Fries, E., Lesch, K.-P., & Kirschbaum, C. (2010). The role of the serotonin transporter polymorphism for the endocrine stress response in newborns. *Psychoneuroendocrinology*, *35*(2), 289–296.

Pluess, M., & Belsky, J. (2013). Vantage sensitivity: Individual differences in response to positive experiences. *Psychological Bulletin, 139*(4), 901–916.

Popova, S., Lange, S., Probst, C., Gmel, G., & Rehm, J. (2017). Estimation of national, regional, and global prevalence of alcohol use during pregnancy and fetal alcohol syndrome: A systematic review and meta-analysis. *The Lancet Global Health, 5*(3), e290–e299.

Porges, S. W. (2011). *The Norton series on interpersonal neurobiology. The polyvagal theory: Neurophysiological foundations of emotions, attachment, communication, and self-regulation.* New York: W. W. Norton & Co.

Posner, M. I., & Rothbart, M. K. (2000). Developing mechanisms of self-regulation. *Development and Psychopathology, 12*(3), 427–441.

Robson, D. A., Allen, M. S., & Howard, S. J. (2020). Self-regulation in childhood as a predictor of future outcomes: A meta-analytic review. *Psychological Bulletin, 146*(4), 324–354.

Rothbart, M. K., Ellis, L. K., & Posner, M. I. (2004). Temperament and self-regulation. In R. F. Baumeister & K. D. Vohs (Eds.), *Handbook of self-regulation: Research, theory, and applications* (pp. 357–370). New York: The Guilford Press.

Sameroff, A. J. (2009). Conceptual issues in studying the development of self-regulation. In S. L. Olson & A. J. Sameroff (Eds.), *Biopsychosocial regulatory processes in the development of childhood behavioral problems* (pp. 1–18). Cambridge: Cambridge University Press.

Sameroff, A. J., & Fiese, B. H. (2000a). Models of development and developmental risk. In C. H. Zeanah Jr. (Ed.), *Handbook of infant mental health* (pp. 3–19). New York: The Guilford Press.

Sameroff, A. J., & Fiese, B. H. (2000b). Transactional regulation: The developmental ecology of early intervention. In J. P. Shonkoff & S. J. Meisels (Eds.), *Handbook of early childhood intervention* (pp. 135–159). Cambridge: Cambridge University Press.

Schaaf, R. C., & Anzalone, M. E. (2001). Sensory integration with high-risk infants and young children. In *Understanding the nature of sensory integration with diverse populations* (pp. 275–311). Austin, TX: Pro-Ed.

Schaaf, R. C., Benevides, T., Blanche, E. I., Brett-Green, B. A., Burke, J. P., Cohn, E., . . . Schoen, S. A. (2010). Parasympathetic functions in children with sensory processing disorder. *Frontiers in Integrative Neuroscience, 4*, 4.

Shonkoff, J. P., Phillips, D. A., & National Research Council. (2000). Rethinking nature and nurture. In *From neurons to neighborhoods: The science of early childhood development.* Washington, DC: National Academies Press.

Smith, M. C. (2019). *Sensory integration: Theory and practice.* Philadelphia: FA Davis.

Stalker, A., & Reebye, P. (2007). *Understanding regulation disorders of sensory processing in children: Management strategies for parents and professionals.* London: Jessica Kingsley Publishers.

Stern, D. N. (2018). *The interpersonal world of the infant: A view from psychoanalysis and developmental psychology.* London: Routledge.

Thomas, R., Abell, B., Webb, H. J., Avdagic, E., & Zimmer-Gembeck, M. J. (2017a). Parent-child interaction therapy: A meta-analysis. *Pediatrics, 140*(3), 1–2.

Thomas, J. C., Letourneau, N., Campbell, T. S., Tomfohr-Madsen, L., Giesbrecht, G. F., & APrON Study Team. (2017b). Developmental origins of infant emotion regulation: Mediation by temperamental negativity and moderation by maternal sensitivity. *Developmental Psychology, 53*(4), 611–628.

Tocchio, S., Kline-Fath, B., Kanal, E., Schmithorst, V. J., & Panigrahy, A. (2015). MRI evaluation and safety in the developing brain. *Seminars in Perinatology, 39*(2), 73–104.

Thompson, S. D., & Raisor, J. M. (2013). Meeting the sensory needs of young children. *Young Children, 68*(2)34.

Vohs, K. D., & Baumeister, R. F. (Eds.). (2016). *Handbook of self-regulation: Research, theory, and applications*. New York: Guilford Publications.

Williamson, G. G., & Anzalone, M. (2001). Sensory integration: A key component of the evaluation and treatment of young children with severe difficulties in relating and communicating. In S. I. Greenspan, B. Kalmanson, R. Shahmoon-Shanok, S. Weider, G. G. Williamson, & M. Anzalone (Eds.), *Assessing and treating infants and young children with severe difficulties in relating and communicating* (pp. 29–36). New York: Zero to Three.

Winnicott, D. W. (1960). The theory of the parent-infant relationship. *International Journal of Psycho-Analysis, 41*, 585–595.

Zero to Three. (1994). *Diagnostic classification, 0–3: Diagnostic classification of mental health and developmental disorders of infancy and early childhood*. Washington, DC: Zero to Three.

Zero to Three. (2005). *Diagnostic classification, 0–3r: Diagnostic classification of mental health and developmental disorders of infancy and early childhood*. Washington, DC: Zero to Three.

Zero to Three. (2016). DC: 0–5™: Diagnostic classification of mental health and developmental disorders of infancy and early childhood: A briefing paper. Washington, DC: Zero to Three.

10 Caregivers With Borderline Personality Disorder

The Promise of MISC

Kiana Wall, Sophie Kerr, and Carla Sharp

10.1 Borderline Personality Disorder and the Caregiver-Child Relationship

Borderline personality disorder (BPD) is a complex mental illness characterized by a variety of symptoms. These symptoms include difficulties with impulsivity (e.g., substance use, risky sexual behavior), emotional dysregulation (e.g., intense anger, and frequent, extreme shifts in mood), turbulent interpersonal relationships (e.g., relationships with many "ups and downs", or on and off again relationships), chronic feelings of emptiness, and deficits in "self-functioning" (e.g., having little self-direction or coherent sense of one's identity; American Psychiatric Association (APA), 2013). This disorder often results in significant, chronic, psychosocial impairment (Álvarez-Tomás, Ruiz, Guilera, & Bados, 2019).

Prevalence estimates for the dramatic-erratic personality disorders, which includes BPD, suggest that 1.6–3.7% of the world population meet diagnostic criteria, with higher prevalence rates in higher-income countries (Winsper et al., 2020). BPD symptoms present equally in males and females in community settings but are most often diagnosed in females in clinical settings (APA, 2013, p. 666). A significant number of women diagnosed with BPD are or will become mothers, and peak symptom severity is often present during late adolescence and young adulthood (Winsper, 2020), substantially overlapping with the age at which many women have children. Therefore, this population represents a unique set of caregiver-child dyads where the mother may experience significant additional parenting challenges.

Prior research has demonstrated that mothers with BPD report low levels of parenting satisfaction and parenting competency (Newman, Stevenson, Bergman, & Boyce, 2007), and high levels of stress related to parenting (Zalewski, Stepp, Whalen, & Scott, 2015). Children of mothers with BPD demonstrate greater rates of BPD, suicidality, depression, externalizing psychopathology, and overall psychosocial impairment than the children of mothers without BPD (Eyden, Winsper, Wolke, Broome, & MacCallum, 2016). These poor outcomes are likely the result of an interaction between both biological and environmental risk factors. Specifically, the caregiving

DOI: 10.4324/9781003145899-10

behaviors of mothers with BPD may be an important environmental factor that, if left unaddressed, could perpetuate the intergenerational transmission of BPD (Stepp, Whalen, Pilkonis, Hipwell, & Levine, 2012). Subsequently, parenting interventions have been developed for mothers with BPD to remediate poor outcomes for their children and interrupt the intergenerational transmission of BPD. Such interventions may reduce mothers' feelings of caregiving-related stress and increase feelings of caregiving competency. The exact mechanisms by which BPD affects caregiver-child interactions, thereby potentially perpetuating the intergenerational transmission of BPD, are discussed later. As we will show, these mechanisms can be organized according to MISC components that form the targets of treatment. In showing the relevance of these components for the typical interaction patterns observed in mothers with BPD and their children, the rationale for the MISC intervention in this population is built.

10.2 Caregiver Behaviors in Mothers With BPD: The Emotional Components of MISC

As described in previous chapters, the emotional components of MISC, including appropriate eye contact and facial expressions, positive affect, physical affection, and interpersonal synchrony, form the foundation of a secure attachment relationship. Grounded in Bowlby's (1969, 1973, 1980) theory of attachment, these emotional components communicate basic messages to the child, including "I love you," "I'm with you," and "It's worthwhile to act," which allow mediated learning (see next section) to take place. Using video-taped unstructured interactions (e.g., free play), semi-structured interactions (e.g., puzzle tasks), and structured interaction paradigms (e.g., the Strange Situation procedure and still-face paradigm) and a variety of behavioral coding schemes, prior research has demonstrated that mothers with BPD often do not exhibit these foundational emotional components in interactions with their children and, in contrast, demonstrate "disrupted affective communication" (Hobson et al., 2009, p. 325).

Most studies have used coding schemes that aim to assess disorganized attachment-behavior and general "parental sensitivity", both of which are relevant to the specific behaviors associated with the emotional components of MISC and speak to the lack of synchrony in these behaviors between mother and child. For example, through behavioral coding of the Strange Situation paradigm (used to assess attachment styles in infancy), Hobson and colleagues (2009) found that mothers with BPD exhibited "disrupted communication" with their infants characterized by frightened behavior (e.g., "hesitant or deferential towards the [child]") or disoriented behavior characterized by sudden or unsynchronized changes in affect, movement, or voice tone (Hobson et al., 2009, p. 328). Macfie, Kurdziel, Mahan, and Kors (2017) found that mothers with BPD were more likely to demonstrate fearful and disoriented behaviors, and behaviors consistent with role reversal (when a parent seeks care from a child), than mothers without BPD. Broadly, fearful and disoriented behavior, and behaviors consistent with role reversal, suggest a severe lack of synchrony, as they are characterized by lack of empathy for the child's perspective, and the inappropriate presence or lack of the emotional components of MISC.

At a more specific, behavioral level, prior research has also found that the behavior of mothers with BPD during both structured (Hobson, Patrick, Crandell, Garcia-Perez, Lee, 2005; Macfie et al., 2017) and unstructured (Crandell, Patrick, & Hobson, 2003; Newman et al., 2007) play interactions have been rated as less sensitive (Crandell et al., 2003; Hobson et al., 2005; Newman et al., 2007; Macfie et al., 2017) and more intrusive compared to healthy control mothers (Crandell et al., 2003; Hobson et al., 2005). Further, Newman and colleagues (2007) also found that the children of mothers with BPD were rated as being less behaviorally and affectively responsive to their parent and less involved in the interaction than the children of mothers without BPD. Kiel, Gratz, Moore, Latzman, and Tull (2011) found no significant group differences in maternal sensitivity between mothers with and without BPD symptoms in response to infant emotional distress during the Strange Situation paradigm, but showed that mothers with high levels of BPD symptoms were more likely to display insensitive behaviors (e.g., ignoring child's crying) *over time* as their child's distress persisted. This increase in insensitivity over time also predicted infants' immediate increase in likelihood of distress. These findings speak to the lack of synchrony that characterizes these mother-child dyad interactions—as the infants' distress increased, mothers with BPD missed the opportunity to "meet with child where they were at" and use the emotional components of MISC to communicate to the child that they were safe and loved.

Further evidence illuminating the emotional components of MISC in BPD mother-child dyads suggests difficulties with mutual attention or engagement, eye contact, shared positive affect, vocalizations, and touch. For example, during an unstructured baseline interaction before a still-face task, Apter and colleagues (2017) found that compared to controls, mothers with BPD spent significantly less time exhibiting social engagement behaviors (e.g., attending to and looking at the child), suggesting less appropriate eye contact, and the children of mothers with BPD exhibited significantly less positive vocalizations (e.g., neutral sounds or laughs), suggestive of less shared positive affect. Further, during the unstructured interaction after the still-face period, mothers with BPD demonstrated more intrusive touch behaviors (e.g., poking, pulling, or pinching) than did mothers without BPD. Given that this finding emerged after the still-face interaction, when children are often emotionally dysregulated given the demands of the still-face task, this may speak to mothers' increased difficulty to embody MISC emotional components when faced with their child's expressions of negative emotions, in particular. Lastly, although most studies have found that mothers with BPD exhibit insensitivity characterized by disconnected or cold behavior, some authors have found evidence of more hostile interactions characterized by overt anger or impatience (Kluczniok et al., 2018; Macfie et al., 2017). For example, Kluczniok et al. (2018) coded maternal behavior of mothers with BPD, depression, and with no diagnosis during a free play period and a puzzle task, and in regression analyses, maternal BPD was found to be a significant predictor of greater hostility but did *not* significantly predict insensitivity.

In summary, years of observational qualitative coding research has demonstrated that mothers with BPD appear to exhibit difficulties with most forms of affective communication with their children. Specifically, the interactions of BPD mother-child dyads are characterized by a lack of positive affect and, at times, the presence of increased negative affect, insensitivity, and possibly even hostility. When the emotional components of MISC are present, they are often misplaced or inappropriate, suggesting a significant lack of synchrony.

10.3 Caregiver Behaviors in Mothers With BPD: The Mediational Components of MISC

The caregiving challenges faced by mothers with BPD can also be understood within the context of the cognitive or mediational components of MISC which were identified and described in Feuerstein's (1979) theory of cognitive modifiability and expanded and operationalized by Klein (1996) for the MISC intervention. These components of learning include focusing, providing meaning, expanding, regulating, and rewarding, and may be compromised in mothers with BPD due to mentalizing deficits associated with the disorder. Specifically, the mentalization-based theory of BPD posits that a core feature of the disorder is a reduced or unstable capacity for mentalization, which is the ability to reflect on one's own and others' mental states and to understand the relationships between mental states and behaviors (Fonagy & Bateman, 2008). To engage in the MISC components, the caregiver must be aware of what the child knows and does not know and structure the interaction in a way that is matched to the child's capacities, mental states, and needs (Sharp et al., 2020; Sharp, 2021). This requires the caregiver to step into the child's shoes and view the child as their own psychological agent. Therefore, individuals who have problems with mentalization will likely have difficulty mediating their child's experience. Also consistent with this notion, Linehan's biosocial model (1993) characterizes BPD as a disorder of emotion dysregulation, with individuals showing high emotional sensitivity, intense emotional responses, and a slow return to baseline emotional states. It can be inferred that constructing mediated learning experiences (MLEs), which require the caregiver to slow down, regulate their own emotions, and match the pace of the interaction, would be particularly difficult for mothers with BPD.

Previous findings on caregiving behaviors and experiences in mothers with BPD do indeed map onto the specific mediational components of MISC (e.g., focusing, affecting, expanding, rewarding, and regulating).

Focusing is defined as an act or sequence of acts directed toward changing the child's perception or behavior and communicates the intention to teach. To be considered mediation, the attempt to focus the child must be intentional, not accidental, and must show reciprocity. Preliminary evidence suggests that mothers with BPD may struggle to focus their child effectively. Newman et al. (2007) coded free-play interactions between mothers and offspring. They found that infants of mothers with BPD were less attentive and less responsive to the mother's attempts to engage them in the interaction. Research also suggests that caregivers with BPD struggle to respond to a child's attempt to focus them. In a community sample of caregiver-child dyads, caregiver BPD features were associated with lower quality of responses to "bids" (an overture or signal that had the potential for response) during structured tasks, illustrating difficulty with responding appropriately to signals for attention from their child (Wilson & Durbin, 2012). These findings can be understood in the context of the caregiver's emotion dysregulation: to effectively focus the child to the present situation, the caregiver must be able to focus themselves, which may be particularly difficult for mothers who are emotionally overwhelmed or dysregulated.

Affecting (provision of, or request for, meaning) occurs when a caregiver names, describes, and gives meaning (without interpretation) to a child's experience. Additionally, the statement or behavior must meet one of the following requirements: convey meaning, express excitement, or identify objects or people by name. Like focusing, mothers with BPD may struggle to slow down and tune in to the present situation through labeling and identifying objects and people. Moreover, mothers with BPD may find it particularly difficult to request or provide meaning related to their child's internal experiences due to problems in mentalizing. Hypermentalizing, defined as the over-attribution of mental states to others beyond observable data, is particularly implicated in BPD (Sharp & Vanwoerden, 2015). Further, individuals with BPD show a negative social-cognitive bias and are more likely to misinterpret mental states as negative, malevolent, or rejecting (Preibler, Dziobek, Ritter, Heekeren, & Roepke, 2010). Research suggests that mothers with BPD struggle to "give meaning" to their child's mental experience or do so in an inaccurate way, reflecting this tendency to hypermentalize. For example, in an infant emotion recognition task, mothers with BPD were more likely to label neutral faces as sad than control mothers (Elliot et al., 2014). Another study found that mothers with BPD referred to their infant's mental states just as often as mothers without BPD, but mothers with BPD were significantly more likely to make non-attuned mind-related comments (Marcoux, Bernier, Séguin, Boike Armerding, & Lyons-Ruth, 2017). Similarly, mothers with high levels of BPD symptoms perceived their infants as more angry than mothers with low levels of BPD symptoms despite no actual differences in anger between infant groups (Kiel et al., 2017). Finally, in a sample of mothers with 3–5-year-old children, maternal BPD was associated with fewer references to children's mental states as well as poorer levels of mental state understanding in their children (Schacht, Hammond, Marks, Wood, & Conroy, 2013).

Expanding is defined as a statement or behavior directed toward extending the child's awareness beyond what is necessary to satisfy the immediate need of the interaction. The act must either expand the child's awareness beyond the immediate context, connect present, past, or future experiences, relate to a general principle or process, or concern things not seen or heard at the moment. Expanding is the metacognitive component of mediation, and it requires the caregiver to carefully scaffold and stretch the child. An emotionally overwhelmed caregiver would likely have difficulty transcending from their immediate situation, senses, and perspective. Additionally, drawing on the research we related to affecting, we hypothesize that maladaptive mentalizing would inhibit effective expanding. While hypomentalizing (reduced mentalizing) could lead to a lack of expanding overall, hypermentalizing may lead mothers to over-interpret situations and expand in rigid or inaccurate ways. The lack of curiosity and rigidity associated with hypermentalizing does not foster mental flexibility or teach the child to use this metacognitive strategy themselves.

Rewarding describes verbal or nonverbal behavior that expresses satisfaction with a child's behavior and identifies specific components of the child's behavior that contribute to the experience of success. Through rewarding, children begin to reflect on how to achieve success and can generalize this to new situations. Research has documented a lack of positive, warm, and encouraging behaviors in caregivers with personality pathology, suggesting a lack of rewarding. For example, in interactions with infants, mothers with BPD used less touch and smiled less often than mothers with depression or no psychiatric problems (White, Flanagan, Martin, & Silvermann, 2011). Furthermore, one study found that caregivers with personality disorders reported using less praise and encouragement with their children (Johnson, Cohen, Kasen, Ehrensaft, & Crawford, 2006).

Regulation refers to behaviors or statements that model, demonstrate, and/or verbally suggest that the child regulate their behavior to the specific requirements of a task. Regulating raises the child's awareness to the possibility of thinking before doing and of planning steps of behavior towards a goal. Research suggests that mothers with BPD have difficulty engaging in this behavior, including findings that mothers with BPD are less effective in structuring interactions with their infants (Newman et al., 2007). In studies with children and adolescents, it appears that mothers with BPD tend to show more controlling behaviors and inhibit independence and autonomy rather than scaffolding and guiding their child's behavior toward goals. Macfie and colleagues (2017) found that mothers with BPD were less likely to support their child's autonomy and more likely to engage in role reversal during puzzle-solving tasks with 4–7-year-old children. Similarly, other studies have found that mothers with BPD were more likely to inhibit autonomy (Frankel-Waldheter, Macfie, Strimpfel, & Watkins, 2015) and use psychological control (Mahan, Kors, Simmons, & Macfie, 2018) during problem-solving interactions with adolescents. It is possible that emotional and behavioral dysregulation in mothers with BPD may impact their ability to regulate their children and lead them to rely on controlling and intrusive strategies to maintain control in the interaction, thereby inhibiting the development of emotion regulation abilities in the child. Indeed, research has demonstrated relationships between maternal BPD and self-regulation problems in infant (Apter et al., 2017), child (Macfie et al., 2017), and adolescent offspring (Frankel-Waldheter et al., 2015). Additionally, in a large community sample, maternal BPD was associated with low self-control in 15–17-year-old daughters and maternal affective and behavioral dysregulation uniquely accounted for maladaptive caregiving behaviors (Zalewski et al., 2015). In sum, research suggests that the interactions of mothers with BPD and their children may be characterized by difficulties with each of the mediational components of MISC.

10.4 Parenting Interventions for Mothers With BPD

To our knowledge, there have been four parenting interventions specifically developed for use with mothers with BPD. These include a specialized 24-week Dialectical Behavior Therapy group (DBT; Linehan, 1993) that includes parenting-specific content (Williams, Yelland, Hollamby, Wigley, & Aylward, 2018), and a group-format intervention based on DBT skills training (Renneberg & Rosenbach, 2016). Over 12 weeks, participants of the latter program complete 10 psychoeducational and skills-based modules relevant to the parent-child relationship. Two interventions that use one-on-one or individual sessions include the Project Air Parenting with Personality Disorder Intervention (McCarthy, Lewis, Bourke, & Grenyer, 2016), based in Australia, and the Helping Families Programme (Day et al., 2017), based in the United Kingdom. The Parenting with Personality Disorder Intervention may last as little as three sessions, but up to 16 sessions to strengthen skills. This intervention prioritizes psychoeducation about child safety and development and explicitly focuses on preventing the intergenerational transmission of psychopathology. The skills reviewed include talking openly about the BPD diagnosis, strategies to avoid children seeing problematic behavior, skills to enhance "mindful parenting", and how to regulate children's behavior. The Helping Families Programme is a psychoeducational parenting intervention consisting of 16 sessions with the parent and other family members as necessary. Sessions include a focus on exploring how the emotional and interpersonal difficulties of the parent impact their child's functioning and identifying goals to remediate this impact. Skills to reach these goals include "evidence-based parenting and self-care strategies" (Day et al., 2017, p. 68).

As illustrated earlier in this chapter, mothers with BPD have significant difficulty with the emotional components of MISC, or the affective behaviors, which contribute to the development of secure caregiver-child attachment relationships. Therefore, attachment-based parenting interventions are also very relevant for use with this population (Cassidy & Shaver, 2016). Four evidence-based attachment interventions include Child-Parent Psychotherapy (CPP), the Attachment and Biobehavioral Catch-up (ABC) program, the Video-Feedback Intervention to Promote Positive Parenting (VIPP) program, and the Circle of Security (COS) program (Berlin, Zeanah, & Lieberman, 2016). CPP has the largest evidence base and is a manualized intervention that consists of parent-child sessions over at least one year. The goals of CPP are to help the parent understand painful childhood memories and experiences and how these experiences influence their current parenting. The ABC and VIPP programs are briefer than CPP, consisting of only 10 and 4–6 sessions, respectively. Each utilizes video-feedback to encourage supportive parenting behaviors (ABC), or to promote parental sensitivity by bringing children's cues into awareness of the parent, helping them interpret these cues accurately, and then respond (VIPP). The COS program has a more limited evidence base and focuses on psychoeducation and enhancing reflection on one's own experiences and parenting through video-feedback that facilitates conceptualization of children's attachment needs and what parenting behaviors support these needs.

Also relevant for use with mothers with BPD are mentalization-based parenting interventions, which are rooted in attachment theory and focus on increasing the parent's reflective capacity. A recent review (Byrne, Murphy, & Connon, 2020) listed randomized control trials for Minding the Baby (MTB; e.g., Slade et al., 2020) as well as the Mothers and Toddlers Program (MTP; now called Mothering from the Inside Out (MIO); e.g., Suchman et al., 2017). Parents First (now Families First) is currently being evaluated in first-time parents using a matched control group design in Sweden (Kalland, Fagerlund, von Koskull, & Pajulo, 2016). Each of these interventions has targeted parents with psychopathology (e.g., substance abuse, PTSD, depression), or low reflective function capacities, but none were specifically developed for parents with BPD, nor have they been evaluated with parents with personality pathology. However, mentalization-based treatment for parents (MBT-P; Nijssens, Luyten, & Bales, 2012) was specifically designed for caregivers with BPD and their infants. While it has not been evaluated in parents with BPD, it was adapted and evaluated among parents of adolescents with BPD in an uncontrolled, pre- and post-study design in Denmark (Bo et al., 2017).

10.5 Limitations of Existing Interventions for Mothers With BPD

The BPD-specific parenting interventions summarized in the previous section have several notable limitations. Firstly, unlike most attachment-based interventions, the parenting programs developed specifically for mothers with BPD are quite short, lasting as few as three weeks or sessions, but no more than 24. Although briefer interventions are becoming increasingly more popular in the field of mental health given their reduced client cost and burden, these interventions may be less appropriate, or less effective in the long-term, for mothers with BPD given that attachment behaviors are often deeply embedded and difficult to change in the short term, particularly in higher-risk populations. For example, two of the very brief attachment-based interventions, the ABC and VIPP programs, are typically only used with lower-risk families (Berlin et al., 2016). Therefore, a longer intervention length, as is typical in attachment-based interventions and many BPD psychotherapies, may be more appropriate for mothers with BPD.

Secondly, most of the interventions developed explicitly for use with mothers with BPD are psychoeducational or focus on maternal skills training (e.g., emotion regulation skills, development of a child safety plan, mindfulness, daily structure and scheduling). Although broadly useful, psychoeducation and skills training cannot provide parents with specific, behavioral instruction on how to interact with their children. They also rely on a level of awareness of self-other interaction patterns that may be lacking in mothers with BPD, who by virtue of their personality challenges may have difficulty in seeing themselves from the outside in, and others from the inside out. Video-based or in vivo observation and feedback on parent–child interactions, which are critical to increase awareness of interaction patterns, as well as teaching the affective aspects of interactions that often go awry in BPD caregiver–child relationships, are not a component of these therapies, unlike most attachment-based interventions.

Thirdly, only two of these interventions (Project Air and Helping Families) use an individual therapy or one-on-one format. None explicitly include the child or other involved parties unless necessary. Although useful, group format interventions, and those that do not include the child in any capacity, may be significant limitations for a parenting intervention for this population. As a highly vulnerable group of patients, seeking support for a highly vulnerable issue (parenting), at least some one-on-one support may be ideal. Additionally, as already noted, feedback that "involves the child" is critical to teaching the affective components of secure attachment relationships.

Lastly, BPD-specific parenting interventions were each developed relatively recently and therefore have limited evidence regarding their efficacy. Specifically, only one has examined maternal outcomes after treatment (Williams et al., 2018). Some evidence exists regarding the feasibility and acceptability of these interventions from the perspective of the clinician (Day et al., 2020; Gray, Townsend, Bourke, & Grenyer, 2019) and the patient (Wilson, Weaver, Michelson, & Day, 2018), but further evidence regarding the clinical utility and effectiveness of these interventions is still needed.

Although existing attachment-based parenting interventions can address many of the limitations of recently developed BPD interventions, the four most well-known attachment-based parenting programs have limitations of their own. For example, both CPP and the COS program focus on reflection on the parents' own attachment histories and experiences. This type of "insight" focus in therapy can be contraindicated for individuals with BPD (Fonagy & Luyten, 2009). Secondly, as already mentioned, the ABC and VIPP programs are relatively brief for an attachment-based intervention and are typically only used in lower-risk settings as preventative interventions. Such brief interventions may not be as effective for BPD mother-child dyads who are often conceptualized as high-risk, and for individuals with BPD who simply have difficulties with trust, rooted in attachment insecurity, which often extends to the therapeutic relationship (Fonagy, Luyten, & Allison, 2015). To have time to build the therapeutic alliance and to get the most out of their parenting program, a longer intervention period may be required for mothers with BPD. Finally, and perhaps most importantly, MISC authors often reiterate that "attachment is not enough" (Sharp et al., 2020). As Klein (1996, p. 5) cogently put it: "In a way, one can say that the affectionate bond between a child and her caregiver opens the gate to the child's mental development, but does not, in itself, determine what will pass through the gate." Therefore, in addition to the attachment-based emotional components, for children to fully realize their socioemotional and cognitive potential, the mediational components of MISC must be present to facilitate learning from the social environment. It may be argued that attachment-based parenting interventions address the emotional components of parent-child interactions but not the mediational or learning components. Unlike MISC, they do not include explicit integration of any learning theory such as Feuerstein's theory of cognitive modifiability.

Mentalization-based caregiver interventions suffer from very similar limitations as those outlined earlier for attachment-based interventions. Many of these interventions are very brief, and mothers are often encouraged to reflect on their own prior attachment experiences (Camoirano, 2017). Additionally, mentalization-based treatments, and their related therapeutic assessment tools, rely heavily on the client's linguistic abilities and propensity to use mental-state talk as indices of adequate mentalization (Camoirano, 2017). They may not fully acknowledge behavioral and kinesthetic responsivity as also being indicative of parental mentalization. As pointed out a decade ago by Shai and Belsky (2011), such an over-reliance on verbal processes may limit an intervention's capacity to bring about change. Because MISC is behaviorally focused and does not rely on the discussion of mental representations of attachment or relationships, it offers a "royal road to epistemic trust" (Sharp et al., 2020) that may be lacking in current mentalization-based interventions. We elaborate further on this idea next.

10.6 MISC as a Feasible and Acceptable Alternative to Existing Parenting Interventions

Against this background, we propose that MISC may be a feasible and acceptable alternative to existing parenting interventions for mothers with

BPD. Firstly, similarly to CPP and many BPD psychotherapies, MISC is not brief but takes time to allow for the modification of long-standing attachment-related caregiving behaviors and interaction patterns. Secondly, the MISC program combines the best structural aspects of each of the interventions summarized. MISC trainers take time at the beginning of therapy, one on one, to simply watch and reflect on video-recorded interactions to bond as a therapist-client dyad. This is highly appropriate for individuals with BPD who, as mentioned, have difficulty with security and trust in all relationships. Only after a therapeutic alliance has been established will a MISC trainer prompt how a caregiver might change their behavior and provide feedback on an interaction, first for pre-recorded videos and later in real-time. Finally, MISC concludes with a group component at the end of the program so that caregivers may have an opportunity to reflect on their MISC experiences with others.

MISC also embodies the most critical aspects of empirically based attachment interventions—specifically, a focus on the affective components of caregiver-child interactions, the "inclusion" of the child through video and observation, and, similarly to the COS program, being conceptualized around a simplistic but comprehensive graphic (the MISC tree) that is approachable for caregivers and helpful in internalizing key concepts. Further, MISC also addresses the weaknesses of some attachment interventions. It shares a length similar to CPP, which is more appropriate for the BPD population than are the ABC or VIPP programs, which are quite brief. However, unlike CPP, MISC does not focus on re-connecting with traumatic childhood experiences to understand current attachment relationships. In our experience, and consistent with the most current mentalization-based approaches (Bateman & Fonagy, 2016), an over-focus on the past may be iatrogenic for mothers with BPD. Instead, a focus on the here-and-now by merely stepping back and observing and mentalizing current interactions between caregivers and children may be a much less threatening and more productive way to repair maladaptive interaction patterns. In MISC, we talk about "the literacy of interaction" whereby the actual interaction (rather than a representation of attachment relationships) is emphasized. Through video feedback, the MISC trainer sensitizes the caregiver to the affective and cognitive components present in their everyday interactions with the child, enhancing the caregiver's literacy of interaction. In so doing, the representational aspects take care of themselves, thus adhering to an implicit change model (Sharp et al., 2020).

Finally, because "attachment is not enough," MISC goes beyond the emotional components of caregiving, which all attachment-based parenting interventions address, to support caregivers in mediating experiences for their children to help ensure that they reach their full potential. The importance of going beyond attachment-based components has also been articulated in recent extensions of mentalization-based theory of BPD through the introduction of the construct of epistemic trust (Fonagy & Allison, 2014; Fonagy & Luyten, 2016). Epistemic trust is understood to foster the child's ability to discern the safety of the social context for learning. Grounded in 30 years of developmental research (e.g. Csibra & Gergely, 2009, 2011; Gergely & Csibra, 2003; Sperber et al., 2010), epistemic trust is defined as "an individual's willingness to consider communication conveying the knowledge from someone as trustworthy, generalizable and relevant to the self" (Fonagy & Luyten, 2016, p. 766). Epistemic trust catalyzes learning. It is a biological signal that conveys that knowledge about to be passed on is reliable since it comes from a trusted source. Elsewhere we have argued that MISC, with its emphasis on learning experiences, offers a critical set of specific methods for extending attachment- and mentalization-based interventions by enhancing communication between caregiver and child in the interest of establishing a context of epistemic trust. MISC is implicitly focused on establishing the communicator (caregiver) as reputable and obliges the communicator to regard the interaction partner (child) as a similarly valid, competent, and interesting agent, which opens a collaborative teaching-learning relationship between the two parties. Its tools of focusing, affecting, expanding, regulating, and rewarding slow down the interaction between caregiver and child to allow for a collaborative exchange of knowledge to take place, which, in turn, fosters epistemic trust and attachment.

10.7 Future Directions

Researchers have designated mothers with BPD and their children as "high-risk" dyads. They have called for parenting interventions to improve the parent-child relationship and minimize negative outcomes in offspring. In this chapter, we have put forward the argument that existing BPD-, attachment-, and mentalization-based caregiver interventions may provide mothers with BPD information about best-practice parenting techniques, psychoeducation about the impact of their symptoms on their children, and may even provide direct feedback on their affective communication with their child; however, they are limited in certain aspects. These limitations include brevity, lack of concrete behavioral instruction or interaction feedback, and a focus on reflection on prior attachment experiences. MISC is a promising alternative caregiving program for this population because of its explicit focus on both the affective behaviors important to secure attachment *and* the behaviors necessary for mediating learning. The format, length, and simplicity of MISC also appear appropriate for this population with unique intervention needs. However, for MISC to reach its full potential, an evidence-based intervention adaptation process must be followed to adapt MISC for the BPD population. As demonstrated in other parts of this edited volume, the randomized controlled trial evidence for MISC is most strongly established for populations affected by HIV/AIDS. Our group is currently funded by the NIH to begin the process of adapting MISC for mothers with BPD. To this end, we will be applying Wingood and DiClemente's (2008) ADAPT-ITT model for adapting MISC to this novel

Table 10.1 Steps of the ADAPT-ITT model and study design for MISC-BPD adaptation

ADAPT-ITT Steps	*MISC-BPD Adaptation Study Underway*
1. **Assessment**—increase understanding of target population (e.g. intervention needs, risk profile, intervention preferences)	1. **Mixed-method assessment** (quantitative surveys and qualitative interviews) of risk factors for poor child outcomes, caregiving behaviors relevant to MISC components, and perceived need for support among mothers with BPD
2. **Decision**—decide whether to adopt or adapt the intervention	2. **Decision** to adopt or adapt MISC based on the results of step 1
3. **Adaptation**—use theatre testing to determine how to adapt the intervention	3. **Theatre testing** with mothers with BPD including a summary of preliminary step 1 results and MISC presentation and examples, and **focus group sessions** to elicit feedback from participants
4. **Production**—produce the first draft of the adapted intervention	4. Steps 4–8 to be completed in a follow-up study
5. **Topical Experts**—receive feedback on the first draft from intervention experts	
6. **Integration**—produce the second draft by incorporating expert feedback; and the third draft for further refinement/ease of use	
7. **Training**—train relevant staff needed for pilot testing	
8. **Testing**—pilot test adapted intervention with 20 participants	

Note: ADAPT-ITT steps as summarized in NCCMT (2017)

context. The proposed steps of this model are summarized in Table 10.1. Currently, work on steps 1–3 is underway.

In conclusion, we argue that MISC targets important aspects of caregiver-child interactions that are particularly relevant for this population and addresses the shortcomings of existing parenting interventions for mothers with BPD. With continued research and adaptation, we believe that MISC offers a promising alternative to improve the lives of both mothers with BPD and their children.

References

Álvarez-Tomás, I., Ruiz, J., Guilera, G., & Bados, A. (2019). Long-term clinical and functional course of borderline personality disorder: A meta-analysis of prospective studies. *European Psychiatry*, *56*(1), 75–83.

American Psychiatric Association. (2013). *Diagnostic and statistical manual of mental disorders (DSM-5®)*. Washington, DC: American Psychiatric Pub.

Apter, G., Devouche, E., Garez, V., Valente, M., Genet, M.-C., Gratier, M., . . . Tronick, E. (2017). The still-face: A greater challenge for infants of mothers with borderline personality disorder. *Journal of Personality Disorders*, *31*(2), 156–169. https://doi. org/10.1521/pedi_2016_30_243

Bateman, A., & Fonagy, P. (2016). *Mentalization-based treatment for personality disorders: A practical guide*. Oxford: Oxford University Press.

Berlin, L. J., Zeanah, C. H., & Lieberman, A. F. (2016). Prevention and intervention programs to support early attachment security: A move to the level of the community. In J Cassidy & P. R. Shaver (Eds.), *Handbook of attachment: Theory, research, and clinical applications* (Vol. 3, pp. 739–758). New York: The Guilford Press.

Bo, S., Sharp, C., Beck, E., Pedersen, J., Gondan, M., & Simonsen, E. (2017). First empirical evaluation of outcomes for mentalization-based group therapy for adolescents with BPD. *Personality Disorders: Theory, Research, and Treatment*, *8*(4), 396–401.

Bowlby, J. (1969). *Attachment and loss: Volume I: Attachment*. New York: Basic Books.

Bowlby, J. (1973). *Attachment and loss: Volume II: Separation, anxiety and anger*. London: The Hogarth Press and the Institute of Psycho-analysis.

Bowlby, J. (1980). *Attachment and loss: Volume III: Loss, sadness, and depression*. London: The Hogarth Press and the Institue of Psycho-analysis.

Byrne, G., Murphy, S., & Connon, G. (2020). Mentalization-based treatments with children and families: A systematic review of the literature. *Clinical Child Psychology and Psychiatry*, *25*(4), 1022–1048.

Camoirano, A. (2017). Mentalizing makes parenting work: A review about parental reflective functioning and clinical interventions to improve it. *Frontiers in Psychology*, *8*, 14.

Cassidy, J., & Shaver, P. (2016). *Handbook of attachment: Theory, research, and clinical applications*. New York: Guilford Press.

Crandell, L. E., Patrick, M. P., & Hobson, R. P. (2003). 'Still-face'interactions between mothers with borderline personality disorder and their 2-month-old infants. *The British Journal of Psychiatry*, *183*(3), 239–247.

Csibra, G., & Gergely, G. (2009). Natural pedagogy. *Trends in Cognitive Sciences*, *13*, 148–153. https://doi.org/10.1016/j.tics.2009.01.005

Csibra, G., & Gergely, G. (2011). Natural pedagogy as evolutionary adaptation. *Philosophical Transactions of the Royal Society of London. Series B, Biological Sciences*, *366*(1567), 1149–1157. https://doi. org/10.1098/rstb.2010.0319

Day, C., Briskman, J., Crawford, M. J., Foote, L., Harris, L., Boadu, J., . . . Mosse, L. (2020). An intervention for parents with severe personality difficulties whose children have mental health problems: A feasibility RCT. *Health Technology Assessment (Winchester, England)*, *24*(14), 1.

Day, C., Briskman, J., Crawford, M. J., Harris, L., McCrone, P., McMurran, M., . . . Ramchandani, P. (2017). Feasibility trial of a psychoeducational intervention for parents with personality difficulties: The helping families programme. *Contemporary Clinical Trials Communications*, *8*, 67–74.

Elliot, R.-L., Campbell, L., Hunter, M., Cooper, G., Melville, J., McCabe, K., . . . Loughland, C. (2014). When I look into my baby's eyes . . . Infant emotion recognition by mothers with borderline personality disorder. *Infant Mental Health Journal*, *35*(1), 21–32. https://doi.org/10.1002/imhj.21426

Eyden, J., Winsper, C., Wolke, D., Broome, M. R., & MacCallum, F. (2016). A systematic review of the parenting and outcomes experienced by offspring of mothers with borderline personality pathology: Potential mechanisms and clinical implications. *Clinical Psychology Review*, *47*, 85–105.

Feuerstein, R. (1979). The ontogeny of learning in man. In M. A. B. Brazier (Ed.), *Brain mechanisms in memory and learning* (pp. 361–371). New York: Raven Press.

Fonagy, P., & Allison, E. (2014). The role of mentalizing and epistemic trust in the therapeutic relationship. *Psychotherapy, 51*(3), 372–380. https://doi.org/10.1037/a0036505

Fonagy, P., & Bateman, A. (2008). The development of borderline personality disorder—
a mentalizing model. *Journal of Personality Disorders, 22*(1), 4–21. https://doi.
org/10.1521/pedi.2008.22.1.4

Fonagy, P., & Luyten, P. (2009). A developmental, mentalization-based approach to the
understanding and treatment of borderline personality disorder. *Development and Psychopathology, 21*(4), 1355–1381.

Fonagy, P., & Luyten, P. (2016). A multilevel perspective on the development of borderline personality disorder. In D. Cicchetti (Ed.), *Developmental psychopathology: Malad-
aptation and psychopathology* (3rd ed., pp. 726–792). Hoboken, NJ: John Wiley & Sons.

Fonagy, P., Luyten, P., & Allison, E. (2015). Epistemic petrification and the restoration
of epistemic trust: A new conceptualization of borderline personality disorder and its
psychosocial treatment. *Journal of Personality Disorders, 29*(5), 575–609.

Frankel-Waldheter, M., Macfie, J., Strimpfel, J. M., & Watkins, C. D. (2015). Effect of
maternal autonomy and relatedness and borderline personality disorder on adolescent
symptomatology. *Personality Disorders: Theory, Research, and Treatment, 6*(2), 152–160.
https://doi.org/10.1037/per0000109

Gergely, G., & Csibra, G. (2003). Teleological reasoning in infancy: The naive theory
of rational action. *Trends in Cognitive Sciences, 7,* 287–292. https://doi.org/10.1016/
S1364-6613(03)00128-1

Gray, A. S., Townsend, M. L., Bourke, M. E., & Grenyer, B. F. (2019). Effectiveness
of a brief parenting intervention for people with borderline personality disorder:
A 12-month follow-up study of clinician implementation in practice. *Advances in Mental Health, 17*(1), 33–43.

Hobson, R. P., Patrick, M. P., Crandell, L., Garcia-Perez, R., & Lee, A. (2005). Personal
relatedness and attachment in infants of mothers with borderline personality disorder. *Development and Psychopathology, 17*(2), 329–347.

Hobson, R. P., Patrick, M. P., Hobson, J. A., Crandell, L., Bronfman, E., & Lyons-Ruth,
K. (2009). How mothers with borderline personality disorder relate to their year-old
infants. *The British Journal of Psychiatry, 195*(4), 325–330.

Johnson, J. G., Cohen, P., Kasen, S., Ehrensaft, M. K., & Crawford, T. N. (2006).
Associations of parental personality disorders and Axis I disorders with childrearing
behavior. *Psychiatry: Interpersonal and Biological Processes, 69*(4), 336–350. https://doi.
org/10.1521/psyc.2006.69.4.336

Kalland, M., Fagerlund, Å., von Koskull, M., & Pajulo, M. (2016). Families first: The development of a new mentalization-based group intervention for first-time parents to promote
child development and family health. *Primary Health Care Research & Development, 17,* 3–17.

Kiel, E. J., Gratz, K. L., Moore, S. A., Latzman, R. D., & Tull, M. T. (2011). The impact
of borderline personality pathology on mothers' responses to infant distress. *Journal of
Family Psychology, 25*(6), 907.

Kiel, E. J., Viana, A. G., Tull, M. T., & Gratz, K. L. (2017). Emotion socialization strategies of mothers with borderline personality disorder symptoms: The role of maternal
emotion regulation and interactions with infant temperament. *Journal of Personality
Disorders, 31*(3), 399–416. https://doi.org/10.1521/pedi_2016_30_256

Klein, P. S. (1996). *Early intervention: Cross-cultural experiences with a mediational approach.*
New York: Routledge.

Kluczniok, D., Boedeker, K., Attar, C. H., Jaite, C., Bierbaum, A. L., Fuehrer, D., . . .
Winter, S. (2018). Emotional availability in mothers with borderline personality

disorder and mothers with remitted major depression is differently associated with psychopathology among school-aged children. *Journal of Affective Disorders, 231*, 63–73.

Linehan, M. (1993). *Cognitive-behavioral treatment of borderline personality disorder.* New York: Guilford Press.

Macfie, J., Kurdziel, G., Mahan, R. M., & Kors, S. (2017). A mother's borderline personality disorder and her sensitivity, autonomy support, hostility, fearful/disoriented behavior, and role reversal with her young child. *Journal of Personality Disorders, 31*(6), 721–737. https://doi.org/10.1521/pedi_2017_31_275

Mahan, R. M., Kors, S. B., Simmons, M. L., & Macfie, J. (2018). Maternal psychological control, maternal borderline personality disorder, and adolescent borderline features. *Personality Disorders: Theory, Research, and Treatment, 9*(4), 297–304. https://doi.org/10.1037/per0000269

Marcoux, A.-A., Bernier, A., Séguin, J. R., Boike Armerding, J., & Lyons-Ruth, K. (2017). How do mothers with borderline personality disorder mentalize when interacting with their infants? Mothers with borderline personality disorders. *Personality and Mental Health, 11*(1), 14–22. https://doi.org/10.1002/pmh.1362

McCarthy, K. L., Lewis, K. L., Bourke, M. E., & Grenyer, B. F. (2016). A new intervention for people with borderline personality disorder who are also parents: A pilot study of clinician acceptability. *Borderline Personality Disorder and Emotion Dysregulation, 3*(1), 10.

National Collaborating Centre for Methods and Tools. (2017). *Framework to adapt evidence-based interventions: ADAPT-ITT.* Hamilton, ON: McMaster University. (Updated 01 September 2017). Retrieved from www.nccmt.ca/resources/search/285

Newman, L. K., Stevenson, C. S., Bergman, L. R., & Boyce, P. (2007). Borderline personality disorder, mother-infant interaction and parenting perceptions: Preliminary findings. *Australian & New Zealand Journal of Psychiatry, 41*(7), 598–605. https://doi.org/10.1080/00048670701392833

Nijssens, L., Luyten, P., & Bales, D. L. (2012). Mentalization-based treatment for parents (MBT-P) with borderline personality disorder and their infants. In *Minding the child: Mentalization-based interventions with children, young people and their families* (pp. 79–97).

Preibler, S., Dziobek, I., Ritter, K., Heekeren, H. R., & Roepke, S. (2010). Social cognition in Borderline personality disorder: Evidence for disturbed recognition of the emotions, thoughts, and intentions of others. *Frontiers in Behavioral Neuroscience, 4*, 182. https://doi.org/10.3389/fnbeh.2010.00182.

Renneberg, B., & Rosenbach, C. (2016). "There is not much help for mothers like me": Parenting skills for mothers with borderline personality disorder—a newly developed group training program. *Borderline Personality Disorder and Emotion Dysregulation, 3*(1), 1–7.

Schacht, R., Hammond, L., Marks, M., Wood, B., & Conroy, S. (2013). The relation between mind-mindedness in mothers with borderline personality disorder and mental state understanding in their children: Mentalization and borderline personality disorder. *Infant and Child Development, 22*(1), 68–84. https://doi.org/10.1002/icd.1766

Shai, D., & Belsky, J. (2011). When words just won't do: Introducing parental embodied mentalizing. *Child Development Perspectives, 5*(3), 173–180.

Sharp, C. (2021). Enhancing the capacity for optimal social and personality function through the mediational intervention for sensitizing caregivers: A case illustration. *Journal of Clinical Psychology, 77*(5), 1162–1175.

Sharp, C., Shohet, C., Givon, D., Penner, F., Marais, L., & Fonagy, P. (2020). Learning to mentalize: A mediational approach for caregivers and therapists. *Clinical Psychology: Science and Practice, 27*(3), e12334. https://doi.org/10.1111/cpsp.12334

Sharp, C., & Vanwoerden, S. (2015). Hypermentalizing in borderline personality disorder: A model and data. *Journal of Infant, Child, and Adolescent Psychotherapy, 14*(1), 33–45. https://doi.org/10.1080/15289168.2015.1004890

Slade, A., Holland, M. L., Ordway, M. R., Carlson, E. A., Jeon, S., Close, N., . . . Sadler, L. S. (2020). Minding the baby®: Enhancing parental reflective functioning and infant attachment in an attachment-based, interdisciplinary home visiting program. *Development and Psychopathology, 32*, 123–137.

Sperber, D., Clement, F., Heintz, C., Mascaro, O., Mercier, H., Origgi, G., & Wilson, D. (2010). Epistemic vigilance. *Mind and Language, 25*(4), 359–393. https://doi.org/10.1111/j.1468-0017.2010.01394.x

Stepp, S. D., Whalen, D. J., Pilkonis, P. A., Hipwell, A. E., & Levine, M. D. (2012). Children of mothers with borderline personality disorder: Identifying parenting behaviors as potential targets for intervention. *Personality Disorders: Theory, Research, and Treatment, 3*(1), 76–91.

Suchman, N. E., DeCoste, C. L., McMahon, T. J., Dalton, R., Mayes, L. C., & Borelli, J. (2017). Mothering from the inside out: Results of a second randomized clinical trial testing a mentalization-based intervention for mothers in addiction treatment. *Development and Psychopathology, 29*, 617–636.

White, H., Flanagan, T. J., Martin, A., & Silvermann, D. (2011). Mother-infant interactions in women with borderline personality disorder, major depressive disorder, their co-occurrence, and healthy controls. *Journal of Reproductive and Infant Psychology, 29*(3), 223–235. https://doi.org/10.1080/02646838.2011.576425

Williams, A. E. S., Yelland, C., Hollamby, S., Wigley, M., & Aylward, P. (2018). A new therapeutic group to help women with borderline personality disorder and their infants. *Journal of Psychiatric Practice®, 24*(5), 331–340.

Wilson, S., & Durbin, C. E. (2012). Parental personality disorder symptoms are associated with dysfunctional parent-child interactions during early childhood: A multilevel modeling analysis. *Personality Disorders: Theory, Research, and Treatment, 3*(1), 55–65. https://doi.org/10.1037/a0024245

Wilson, R., Weaver, T., Michelson, D., & Day, C. (2018). Experiences of parenting and clinical intervention for mothers affected by personality disorder: A pilot qualitative study combining parent and clinician perspectives. *BMC Psychiatry, 18*(1), 1–7.

Wingood, G. M., & DiClemente, R. J. (2008). The ADAPT-ITT model: A novel method of adapting evidence-based HIV Interventions. *JAIDS Journal of Acquired Immune Deficiency Syndromes, 47*, S40–S46.

Winsper, C. (2020). Borderline personality disorder: Course and outcomes across the lifespan. *Current Opinion in Psychology, 37*, 94–97.

Winsper, C., Bilgin, A., Thompson, A., Marwaha, S., Chanen, A. M., Singh, S. P., . . . Furtado, V. (2020). The prevalence of personality disorders in the community: A global systematic review and meta-analysis. *The British Journal of Psychiatry, 216*(2), 69–78.

Zalewski, M., Stepp, S. D., Whalen, D. J., & Scott, L. N. (2015). A qualitative assessment of the parenting challenges and treatment needs of mothers with borderline personality disorder. *Journal of Psychotherapy Integration, 25*(2), 71–89.

11 Maternal Depression and MISC in Low- and Middle-Income Countries

Itziar Familiar

11.1 Maternal Depression and Anxiety and Young Children's Development

Maternal depression and anxiety are common in low-income countries (Fisher et al., 2012), with about 10% of pregnant women and 13% of those who have given birth experiencing some type of mental disorder, most commonly depression or anxiety (Hanlon, 2013). More generally and given the high rate of co-morbidity, the term "maternal psychological distress" is frequently used to include stress, depression, or anxiety symptoms and occurs in approximately 25% of women in the first three years after giving birth (Singer et al., 1999). Rates of maternal depression are higher among socio-economically disadvantaged women (Chaudron et al., 2005). Specifically, low-income women have higher rates (up to 50%) of post-partum depression (Boury, Larkin, & Krummel, 2004; Evans, Heron, Oke, & Golding, 2001; Hobfoll, Ritter, Lavin, Hulsizer, & Cameron, 1995; Price & Proctor, 2009) than do other income groups (Hobfoll et al., 1995; Scholle, Haskett, Hanusa, Pincus, & Kupfer, 2003), especially unrecognized and untreated depression (Chaudron et al., 2005). Low-income women are often exposed to chronic stress, and their high levels of perceived stress are strongly associated with increased risk for depression and/or anxiety (Scheyer, 2016). In addition, the consequences of depression are often more severe for low-income women when compared with high-income peers (Kessler et al., 2009).

Observational and longitudinal studies in low- and middle-income countries (LMIC) suggest that depression in mothers or primary caregivers can contribute to multiple early child growth and developmental problems, including nutritional status, health, and socio-emotional behavior problems (Bennett, Schott, Krutikova, & Behrman, 2016; Black et al., 2007; Grantham-McGregor et al., 2007; Surkan, Kennedy, Hurley, & Black, 2011). Maternal depressive symptoms double the likelihood of child behavioral and emotional disorders (Giallo et al., 2015) and lower school performance in young children (Augustine & Crosnoe, 2010). Maternal anxiety symptoms have been negatively associated with compromised parenting that in turn is negatively associated with child development and behavior, suggesting a

DOI: 10.4324/9781003145899-11

possible mechanism of action (Bass et al., 2016; Murray et al., 2017; Seffren et al., 2018) and has been associated with executive functioning problems (Familiar et al., 2019). The negative effects of untreated maternal psychological distress on mother-child interactions (Austin & Priest, 2005), maternal caregiving, child language development, executive functioning (Familiar et al., 2019), and other child outcomes (Moehler, Brunner, Wiebel, Reck, & Resch, 2006; Naicker, Wickham, & Colman, 2012) are substantial, and appear to be potentiated by the presence of socioeconomic adversity (Murray, Fiori-Cowley, & Hooper, 1996; Sohr-Preston, 2006; Stein, 2008). Among low-income women, the higher prevalence of depression, the reduced likelihood of treatment, and the impact of untreated depression on impaired development in children (Grace, Evindar, & Stewart, 2003; Murray, Halligan, & Cooper, 2009) lead to marked health disparities in children of these affected mothers (Federenko & Wadhwa, 2004).

In the context of interventions, maternal psychological distress may be a barrier to engage in or successfully complete child-focused programs, thereby limiting the opportunity for children to benefit from these programs (Rostad, Moreland, Valle, & Chaffin, 2018). Maternal psychological distress may also interact with other barriers (e.g. family sociodemographic characteristics, logistical and resource constraints, motivational barriers to treatment) (Kazdin, Holland, & Crowley, 1997) to intervention participation; psychological distress may make already-existing barriers more significant and may impact how a mother can manage other barriers.

A large body of literature shows that maternal depression responds positively to a range of psychological therapies (cognitive behavioral, interpersonal, supportive, and group therapy) and pharmacological therapies when delivered by specialists (Patel et al., 2016). Efforts to increase access to effective maternal depression treatment in LMIC, where the number of mental health specialists is limited, have been building. Several successful randomized controlled trials have been conducted, with lay health workers effectively delivering manualized, cognitive-based psychological therapies among adults (Singla et al., 2017) and specifically with mothers during the perinatal period (Rahman et al., 2013). Although few studies have directly assessed the effect of treatment of postpartum depression on child outcomes (Singla et al., 2017), taken together these results suggest that despite significant improvements in maternal mood, the only significant treatment effect in the parenting domain was related to parenting stress (Lynne Murray, Cooper, Wilson, & Romaniuk, 2003; Poobalan et al., 2007). This research suggests that approaches designed to target maternal depressive symptoms, regardless of the specific theoretical orientation, may not be sufficient to prevent negative child outcomes. An alternative approach put forth by Cramer (Cramer, 1993) suggests that maternal depression disrupts the mother-infant relationship and that this must receive attention for interventions to be effective on child outcomes. Hence, interventions designed to improve the mother-infant relationship (e.g. mother-infant parenting programs, home-based intervention programs) hold great potential for being an effective means of improving outcomes for children of depressed mothers.

11.2 Influence of Parental Care in Shaping Emotional Development, Stress Physiology, and Limbic Circuitry

Typical brain development manifests as dynamic changes that shape brain maturation and result in long-term behavioral outcomes. Sensitive periods in the developmental trajectory occur when the developing brain is especially susceptible to environmental restructuring (Andersen, 2003). A series of developmental cascades ensue, ultimately influencing behavioral phenotypes across the lifespan. This heightened capacity for change and remodeling of neuronal connections is referred to as neuroplasticity, and it can have both positive and negative impacts on brain development (Davidson & McEwen, 2012).

Brain development occurs in multiple stages, with each brain region having a unique course of ontogeny, setting the stage for differential periods of vulnerability in a regionally specific manner. The amygdala and frontoamygadala circuitry, brain regions involved in emotional processing, mature earlier than the prefrontal cortex, and sensitive periods correspond to the early structural development of the amygdala (Chareyron, Lavenex, Amaral, & Lavenex, 2012). In addition, the amygdala has a high density of glucocorticoid receptors linked to amygdala-mediated effects of stress (Han, Ding, & Shi, 2014). In normative development, children show robust amygdala reactivity to emotional stimuli, and reactivity is associated with the presence of normative childhood fears such as separation anxiety (Gee et al., 2013).

The parent-child relationship is critical to emotional wellbeing across development (Ainsworth, 1969; Bowlby, 1982), and strong evidence suggests that caregivers affect mental health and emotional behavior by influencing the neurobiology underlying emotion regulation. Research shows robust evidence for a sensitive period of parental buffering effects in which the developing brain is most open to parental shaping of frontoamygdala circuitry in early life. Parents can have strong buffering effects on children's emotional behavior and physiological reactivity by suppressing cortisol reactivity in children through physical presence and even facilitate the return of cortisol levels to baseline with verbal cues (Seltzer, Prososki, Ziegler, & Pollak, 2012). Parents are central to early emotion regulation patterns in childhood by modulating HPA and amygdala reactivity as they mature, shaping adult circuitry and associated phenotypes in typical rearing conditions. Thus, studies on how parental care modulates this development differently across the lifespan are essential to target critical developmental windows.

Children under 5 years of age are in a sensitive period of development with sustained dynamic capacity. Farah and colleagues (Farah et al., 2008) observed a relationship between parental nurturance and memory development consistent with the animal literature on maternal buffering of stress hormone effects on hippocampal development. Furthermore, Rao et al. (2010) noted that parental nurturance at age 4 predicts the volume of the left hippocampus in adolescence, with warmer and more loving nurturance associated with smaller hippocampal volume. In addition, the association between parental nurturance and hippocampal volume disappears at age 8 years. They concluded that this supports the existence of a sensitive developmental period for brain maturation, especially before the age of 4 years. Two of MISC core components, focusing and affecting, are directed to foster and strengthen secure and emotional attachments between caregiver and the child, thus nurturing environment in this early developmental window, creating learning experiences that allow a child's cognitive ability to blossom.

11.3 Nurturing Care Framework—Role of Caregiving for Very Young (< 5 Years) Children in Low- and Middle-Income Countries

One of the mechanisms linking maternal depression with poor child development is through family processes such as parenting behavior. In particular, studies from mostly high-income countries (HIC) have shown an association between maternal depression and suboptimal parenting practices, resulting in less secure mother-child attachments (Goodman et al., 2011; Santona et al., 2015). Depressed mothers are more likely to be inconsistent, withdrawn, or intrusive, increasing their children's risk for maladjustment (Goodman, 2007). These studies suggest a mediation mechanism that maternal depression impacts child outcomes through its negative influence on parenting. In studies from Sub-Saharan Africa, the relationship between maternal psychological distress and child behavior has also been explained by the negative impact of the child's behavior on family functioning and the perceived parental competence of the mother (Familiar et al., 2016, 2018; Murray et al., 2017), leading to increased maternal self-reported depressive symptoms, and a poorer sense of parental self-confidence (Augustinavicius et al., 2019). Although the underlying mechanisms associating maternal psychological wellbeing and child development might be similar in LMIC and HIC (Herba, Glover, Ramchandani, & Rondon, 2016), there is increased exposure to known risk factors for depression in LMIC, such as the high prevalence of HIV, war and trauma, low food security, child maltreatment, and low access to health care (Herba et al., 2016; Wekesa, 2000). In Uganda, contextual factors such as low educational attainment, food insecurity, low social support, and a high number of children were associated with higher depression levels among parents, and that in turn was associated with less optimal parenting (Huang, Abura, Theise, & Nakigudde, 2017).

The quality of parental care influences the socio-emotional and cognitive development in children. The attributes of this attachment are strongly associated with a child's cognitive, social, and emotional competence (Weinfield,

Sroufe, Egeland, & Carlson, 1999). However, the stress of poverty and illness can diminish a parent's ability to act as a "protective shield" (Bowlby, 1982) for the child. As a result, children raised in contexts of high adversity due to social, biological, and/or environmental insults are susceptible to a range of negative health and developmental outcomes. The main emphasis on the MISC approach is on improving this "protective shield" for the child and thus preventing negative developmental outcomes. Advantages of this approach include a strength-based focus. Carers are helped enhance their existing values and practices. A home training–based preventive approach enhances this model's feasibility and sustainability by bringing the services to the families themselves. Effective mediational behaviors taught as part of the MISC program to caregivers were found to be significantly related to children's social-emotional stability and the willingness to explore and learn about the world around them (Boivin et al., 2013; Sharp, 2021). This premise is foundational to the MISC method.

The MISC approach aligns with the nurturing care framework by placing on caregivers a central role, enhancing quality caregiving, in mitigating the negative effect of social, biological, and/or environmental stressors. In a US study, caregiving quality moderated the association between poverty and school readiness and language development in children, suggesting that caregiving practices can serve as a buffer (McCartney, Dearing, Taylor, & Bub, 2007). Findings from the US also suggest that improvements in caregiving quality can lead to positive cognitive development outcomes in young children already experiencing early signs of cognitive delay. Evidence from LMIC is slowly beginning to emerge, as the global under-5 mortality rates have decreased in the last 20 years, from an estimated 93 deaths per 1000 live births in 1990 to 39 deaths per 1000 live births in 2018 (Global Health Observatory. World Health Organization, 2018).

Another characteristic of the MISC approach emphasizing nurturing care of infants and children is expressing appropriate, intentional, and directed maternal responsiveness. This type of maternal sensitivity, defined as "timely and accurate responsivity to situationally dependent infant signals" (Pederson, Bailey, Tarabulsy, Bento, & Moran, 2014), is a critical influencer in the management of infant distress and a facilitator of autonomy. Maternal sensitivity and/or secure mother-child attachment predict social relationships (Pallini, Baiocco, Schneider, Madigan, & Atkinson, 2014) and enhanced cognitive abilities (Jacobsen, Huss, Fendrich, Kruesi, & Ziegenhain, 1997), and inversely relate to internalizing difficulties and externalizing problems (Garai et al., 2009).

At least two aspects of the caregiving environment enhanced by the MISC program may promote the development and cognitive function in at-risk children. First, cognitive stimulating environments may promote language development. For example, the quantity and diversity of language children hear at home (from the primary caregiver) is highly correlated with children's receptive vocabulary and cognitive development (Song,

Spier, & Tamis-Lemonda, 2014). Second, emotionally supportive environments may foster the emergence of behavioral control and emotion regulatory skills among at-risk children. Children's development of emotional self-regulation is important for many behavioral outcomes, including their ability to tolerate frustration, curb aggressive impulses, delay gratification, and express emotions in socially acceptable ways. A strong body of evidence supports that parents play an important role in children's development of self-regulation of emotions in the early years, offering comforting behaviors when infants express negative emotions and arouse positive emotions through praise and play (Morris, Criss, Silk, & Houltberg, 2017). In addition, positive parental behaviors (e.g. warmth, responsiveness, sensitivity) are associated with improved executive functioning in early childhood (Valcan, Davis, & Pino-Pasternak, 2018).

11.4 Promoting Early Child Development and Maternal Wellbeing With Parenting Interventions

A significant amount of evidence (Lanza, Rhoades, Greenberg, Cox, & Family Life Project Key, 2011) indicates that the child's early environment is associated with general cognitive development. Research has shown that a negative environment during the child's first three years is linked with developmental problems, including poor language development, behavior problems, and deficits in school readiness. Because children younger than 5 years tend to spend most of their time under their mother's care, interventions aimed at modifying the early environmental milieu are typically focused on the maternal-child relationship.

In general, parenting programs aim to support and strengthen existing parenting abilities and foster the development of new competencies so that parents promote children's cognitive, social, and emotional health. Many such programs intervene early in a child's life, reducing the harmful impact of detrimental prenatal parental health-related behaviors, poor infant caregiving practices, and stressful environmental conditions. Systematic reviews of home-based parenting programs in high- (Kendrick et al., 2000) (Nievar, Van Egeren, & Pollard, 2010) and low- and middle-income countries (Mejia, Calam, & Sanders, 2012) have found benefits, including enhanced cognitive and socio-emotional outcomes in the child, and improved parenting attitudes and behaviors in caregivers. Through numerous therapeutic approaches, parenting programs promote a secure attachment relationship between mother and infant through highlighting positive attachment behaviors when they occur, and focusing on maternal responsivity, sensitivity, and engagement (Murray et al., 2009). Home visits are commonly used with depressed mothers but especially with high-risk, low-socioeconomic samples.

Quality of caregiving and the home environment play an important role in optimizing child development and mitigating the negative effects of social and/or environmental disadvantage (Sarsour et al., 2011). Home-based child development programs aim to optimize children's developmental outcomes by educating, training, and supporting parents in their own homes to provide a nurturing and stimulating environment for their child. MISC is one such program designed to improve early childhood emotional and cognitive development among at-risk children in low-resource settings. The approach is family-oriented and provides training to the caregiver to improve sensitivity and responsiveness to her children's needs in the home context. Studies from Uganda (Bass et al., 2017; Boivin et al., 2013) and South Africa (Sharp, 2021) show that MISC is a culturally appropriate program in that it builds on existing caregiving norms and expectations of participants rather than through the introduction of Western concepts of appropriate caregiving. Targeting the home and caregiving environment is generally more feasible than attempting to reach youth in schools or other community contexts (Mejia et al., 2012).

The high-quality caregiver-child interactions (defined as the number of opportunities where mediated learning and praise occurs between caregiver and child) introduced as part of MISC can partially act as buffers in at-risk children, lessening negative environmental effects of poverty and adversity among Ugandan children (Bass et al., 2016; Familiar et al., 2018). In a Ugandan-based RTC of MISC, the quality and quantity of stimulation that the child was exposed to in their home resulted from MISC training as associated with a higher level of general neurocognitive development. These results support the view of program guidance for at-risk children (World Health Organization, 2018) that suggest family-oriented, home-based care with an emphasis on parent-child relationships and strengthening of caregiver's abilities to provide for the child as tenants for optimal child development. By focusing on the quality of caregiving, MISC is a program that reinforces specific positive influences within complex home environments in contexts of poverty and HIV that are highly prevalent in low-income settings, and that can impact a child's cognitive and neurodevelopment. In addition, parental use of positive parenting strategies (e.g. guidance and mediated learning) is associated with better child self-regulation. This critical cognitive process regulates behavior and emotional responses (Valcan et al., 2018).

Despite being a potentially modifiable component of child-development interventions aimed toward at-risk children in LMICs, the effect of maternal mental health interventions on child development has not been rigorously evaluated, with most studies focusing on measuring exclusive breastfeeding outcomes (Tol et al., 2020). Only a handful of randomized controlled trials in LMIC have evaluated the benefit of combining early childhood development curriculums with maternal psychotherapy or psychological support (Boivin et al., 2017; Rahman, Malik, Sikander, Roberts, & Creed, 2008; Singla, Kumbakumba, & Aboud, 2015) (Fuhr et al., 2019). In these studies, the focus has been mainly on the perinatal period and evaluating the impact of the intervention on growth infant outcomes (Fuhr et al., 2019; Rahman et al., 2008). Only Singla and colleagues (Boivin et al., 2017; Rahman et al., 2008; Singla et al., 2015) assessed infant neurodevelopment. Regardless, these recent studies provide evidence for the effects of interventions delivered by non-specialists for maternal depression and limited evidence on child development. More research is needed with trials designed to clarify the impact of mental health components on child cognitive development, including head-to-head comparisons of interventions with and without mental health components to estimate the additional contribution of these components in integrated interventions.

Similarly, scant research has addressed the potential benefits that parenting programs targeting children through early child development have on maternal psychological wellbeing. Evidence from the MISC RTC in Uganda indicated that depression and anxiety symptoms in participating women decreased after the one-year program (Bass et al., 2017; Boivin et al., 2013). Several explanations could account for these observed results. To internalize and understand the MISC approach, the program relies on 24 sessions spread over a year. This long-term format fosters the development of a bond between the caregiver and the MISC provider, both of whom are frequently women, with many of the characteristics of a therapeutic relationship. During MISC sessions, the interaction is confidential. There is a basic level of trust, frequent disclosure of difficult material (e.g. infidelity of a spouse, shameful affect), and an agreement about the program's goals. In addition, MISC focuses on enhancing verbal and non-verbal communication skills in the mother-child relationship to promote maternal sensitivity to the child's needs and attachment. As participants rehearse these communication skills with the MISC providers, they are communicating in a therapeutic manner, opening and creating a safe space where women can have a positive experience. Coupled with an increased sense of parent competency achieved through directed skill learning and practice (Augustinavicius et al., 2019), MISC may have indirect maternal psychological wellbeing effects, resulting in the observed reduction in maternal depression symptoms (Bass et al., 2017; Boivin et al., 2013). Hence, results provide evidence on the efficacy of MISC for reducing a primary source of risk for compromised development: maternal depression.

11.5 Conclusions

Overall, results from RCTs evaluating the psychological and developmental benefits of the MISC program are encouraging and should be evaluated further as interventions that can effectively and efficiently address mothers and infants' needs at risk for poor health and development outcomes are critically needed. There are several compelling reasons to integrate mental health services into routine maternal and child care, especially in low-resource settings. Dyadic approaches, such as the MISC program, are promising options for integrated services, with demonstrated efficacy in simultaneously providing relief for maternal depression and enhancing the infant's social and cognitive development.

References

Ainsworth, M. D. S. (1969). Object relations, dependency, and attachment: A theoretical review of the infant-mother relationship. *Child Development*, 969–1025.

Andersen, S. L. (2003). Trajectories of brain development: Point of vulnerability or window of opportunity? *Neuroscience & Biobehavioral Reviews, 27*(1–2), 3–18.

Augustinavicius, J. L., Familiar-Lopez, I., Winch, P. J., Murray, S. M., Ojuka, C., Boivin, M. J., & Bass, J. K. (2019). Parenting self-efficacy in the context of poverty and HIV in Eastern Uganda: A qualitative study. *Infant Mental Health Journal, 40*(3), 422–438. doi:10.1002/imhj.21774

Augustine, J. M., & Crosnoe, R. (2010). Mothers' depression and educational attainment and their children's academic trajectories. *Journal of Health and Social Behavior, 51*(3), 274–290.

Austin, M. P., & Priest, S. R. (2005). Clinical issues in perinatal mental health: New developments in the detection and treatment of perinatal mood and anxiety disorders. *Acta Psychiatrica Scandinavica, 112*(2), 97–104.

Bass, J. K., Nakasujja, N., Familiar-Lopez, I., Sikorskii, A., Murray, S. M., Opoka, R., . . . Boivin, M. J. (2016). Association of caregiver quality of care with neurocognitive outcomes in HIV-affected children aged 2–5 years in Uganda. *AIDS Care, 28* (Suppl 1), 76–83. doi:10.1080/09540121.2016.1146215

Bass, J. K., Opoka, R., Familiar, I., Nakasujja, N., Sikorskii, A., Awadu, J., . . . Boivin, M. (2017). Randomized controlled trial of caregiver training for HIV-infected child neurodevelopment and caregiver well being. *AIDS, 31*(13), 1877–1883. doi:10.1097/qad.0000000000001563

Bennett, I. M., Schott, W., Krutikova, S., & Behrman, J. R. (2016). Maternal mental health, and child growth and development, in four low-income and middle-income countries. *Journal of Epidemiology and Community Health, 70*(2), 168–173. doi:10.1136/jech-2014-205311

Black, M. M., Baqui, A. H., Zaman, K., McNary, S. W., Le, K., Arifeen, S. E., . . . Black, R. E. (2007). Depressive symptoms among rural Bangladeshi mothers: Implications for infant development. *Journal of Child Psychology and Psychiatry, 48*(8), 764–772. doi:10.1111/j.1469-7610.2007.01752.x

Boivin, M. J., Bangirana, P., Nakasujja, N., Page, C. F., Shohet, C., Givon, D., . . . Klein, P. S. (2013). A year-long caregiver training program to improve neurocognition in preschool Ugandan HIV-exposed children. *Journal of Developmental and Behavioral Pediatrics: JDBP, 34*(4), 269.

Boivin, M. J., Nakasujja, N., Familiar-Lopez, I., Murray, S. M., Sikorskii, A., Awadu, J., . . . Schut, E. E. (2017). Effect of caregiver training on the neurodevelopment of HIV-exposed uninfected children and caregiver mental health: A Ugandan cluster-randomized controlled trial. *Journal of Developmental & Behavioral Pediatrics, 38*(9), 753–764.

Boury, J., Larkin, K., & Krummel, D. (2004). Factors related to postpartum depressive symptoms in low-income women. *Women and Health, 39*(3), 19–34.

Bowlby, J. (1982). Attachment and loss: Retrospect and prospect. *American Journal of Orthopsychiatry, 52*(4), 664.

Chareyron, L. J., Lavenex, P. B., Amaral, D. G., & Lavenex, P. (2012). Postnatal development of the amygdala: A stereological study in macaque monkeys. *Journal of Comparative Neurology, 520*(9), 1965–1984.

Chaudron, L. H., Kitzman, H. J., Peifer, K. L., Morrow, S., Perez, L. M., & Newman, M. C. (2005). Self-recognition of and provider response to maternal depressive symptoms in low-income Hispanic women. *Journal of Women's Health, 14*(4), 331–338.

Cramer, B. (1993). Are postpartum depressions a mother-infant relationship disorder? *Infant Mental Health Journal, 14*(4), 283–297.

Davidson, R. J., & McEwen, B. S. (2012). Social influences on neuroplasticity: Stress and interventions to promote wellbeing. *Nature Neuroscience, 15*(5), 689–695.

Evans, J., Heron, J., H., F., Oke, S., & Golding, J. (2001). Cohort study of depressed mood during pregnancy and after childbirth. *British Medical Journal, 323*, 257–260.

Familiar, I., Collins, S. M., Sikorskii, A., Ruisenor-Escudero, H., Natamba, B., Bangirana, P., . . . Young, S. L. (2018). Quality of caregiving is positively associated with neurodevelopment during the first year of life among HIV-exposed uninfected children in Uganda. *Journal of Acquired Immune Deficiency Syndromes, 77*(3), 235–242.

Familiar, I., Nakasujja, N., Bass, J., Sikorskii, A., Murray, S., Ruisenor-Escudero, H., . . . Boivin, M. J. (2016). Caregivers' depressive symptoms and parent-report of child executive function among young children in Uganda. *Learning and Individual Differences, 46*, 17–24.

Familiar, I., Sikorskii, A., Murray, S., Ruisenor-Escudero, H., Nakasujja, N., Korneffel, C., . . . Bass, J. (2019). Depression symptom trajectories among mothers living with HIV in rural Uganda. A*IDS and Behaviour, 23*, 3411–3418.

Farah, M. J., Betancourt, L., Shera, D. M., Savage, J. H., Giannetta, J. M., Brodsky, N. L., . . . Hurt, H. (2008). Environmental stimulation, parental nurturance and cognitive development in humans. *Developmental Science, 11*(5), 793–801.

Federenko, I. S., & Wadhwa, P. D. (2004). Women's mental health during pregnancy influences fetal and infant developmental and health outcomes. *CNS Spectrums, 9*, 198–206.

Fisher, J., Cabral de Mello, M., Patel, V., Rahman, A., Tran, T., Holton, S., & Holmes, W. (2012). Prevalence and determinants of common perinatal mental disorders in women in low- and lower-middle-income countries: A systematic review. *Bulletin of the World Health Organization, 90*(2), 139g–149g.

Fuhr, D. C., Weobong, B., Lazarus, A., Vanobberghen, F., Weiss, H. A., Singla, D. R., . . . D'Souza, E. (2019). Delivering the thinking healthy programme for perinatal depression through peers: An individually randomised controlled trial in India. *The Lancet Psychiatry, 6*(2), 115–127.

Garai, E. P., Forehand, R. L., Colletti, C. J. M., Reeslund, K., Potts, J., & Compas, B. (2009). The relation of maternal sensitivity to children's internalizing and externalizing problems within the context of maternal depressive symptoms. *Behavior Modification, 33*(5), 559–582.

Gee, D. G., Humphreys, K. L., Flannery, J., Goff, B., Telzer, E. H., Shapiro, M., . . . Tottenham, N. (2013). A developmental shift from positive to negative connectivity in human amygdala—prefrontal circuitry. *Journal of Neuroscience, 33*(10), 4584–4593.

Giallo, R., Bahreinian, S., Brown, S., Cooklin, A., Kingston, D., & Kozyrskyj, A. (2015). Maternal depressive symptoms across early childhood and asthma in school children: Findings from a longitudinal Australian population based study. *PLoS One, 10*(3), e0121459. doi:10.1371/journal.pone.0121459

Global Health Observatory. World Health, O. (2018). *Under-five mortality.* Retrieved from www.who.int/gho/child_health/mortality/mortality_under_five_text/en/#:~:text= Globally%2C%20under%2Dfive%20mortality%20rate,1%20in%2026%20in%202018.

Goodman, S. H. (2007). Depression in mothers. *Annual Review Clinical Psychology, 3*, 107–135. doi:10.1146/annurev.clinpsy.3.022806.091401

Goodman, S. H., Rouse, M. H., Connell, A. M., Broth, M. R., Hall, C. M., & Heyward, D. (2011). Maternal depression and child psychopathology: A meta-analytic review. *Clinical Child and Family Psychology Review, 14*(1), 1–27.

Grace, S. L., Evindar, A., & Stewart, D. E. (2003). The effect of postpartum depression on child cognitive development and behavior: A review and critical analysis of the literature. *Archives of Women's Mental Health, 6*(4), 263–274.

Grantham-McGregor, S., Cheung, Y. B., Cueto, S., Glewwe, P., Richter, L., & Strupp, B. (2007). Developmental potential in the first 5 years for children in developing countries. *Lancet, 369*(9555), 60–70. doi:10.1016/s0140-6736(07)60032-4

Han, F., Ding, J., & Shi, Y. (2014). Expression of amygdala mineralocorticoid receptor and glucocorticoid receptor in the single-prolonged stress rats. *BMC Neuroscience, 15*(1), 77.

Hanlon, C. (2013). Maternal depression in low-and middle-income countries. *International Health, 5*(1), 4–5.

Herba, C. M., Glover, V., Ramchandani, P. G., & Rondon, M. B. (2016). Maternal depression and mental health in early childhood: An examination of underlying mechanisms in low-income and middle-income countries. *The Lancet Psychiatry, 3*(10), 983–992.

Hobfoll, S. E., Ritter, C., Lavin, J., Hulsizer, M., & Cameron, R. (1995). Depression prevalence and incidence among inner-city pregnant and postpartum women. *Journal of Consulting and Clinical Psychology, 63*(3), 445–453.

Huang, K.-Y., Abura, G., Theise, R., & Nakigudde, J. (2017). Parental depression and associations with parenting and children's physical and mental health in a sub-Saharan African setting. *Child Psychiatry & Human Development, 48*(4), 517–527.

Jacobsen, T., Huss, M., Fendrich, M., Kruesi, M. J. P., & Ziegenhain, U. (1997). Children's ability to delay gratification: Longitudinal relations to mother-child attachment. *The Journal of Genetic Psychology, 158*(4), 411–426.

Kazdin, A. E., Holland, L., & Crowley, M. (1997). Family experience of barriers to treatment and premature termination from child therapy. *Journal of Consulting and Clinical Psychology, 65*(3), 453.

Kendrick, D., Elkan, R., Hewitt, M., Dewey, M., Blair, M., Robinson, J., . . . Brummell, K. (2000). Does home visiting improve parenting and the quality of the home environment? A systematic review and meta analysis. *Archives of Disease in Childhood, 82*(6), 443–451.

Kessler, R. C., Aguilar-Gaxiola, S., Alonso, J., Chatterji, S., Lee, S., Ormel, J., . . . Wang, P. (2009). The global burden of mental disorders: An update from the WHO World Mental Health (WMH) Surveys. *Epidemiology Psychiatric Sciences, 18*(1), 23–33.

Lanza, S. T., Rhoades, B. L., Greenberg, M. T., Cox, M., & Family Life Project Key, I. (2011). Modeling multiple risks during infancy to predict quality of the caregiving environment: Contributions of a person-centered approach. *Infant Behavior and Development, 34*(3), 390–406.

McCartney, K., Dearing, E., Taylor, B. A., & Bub, K. L. (2007). Quality child care supports the achievement of low-income children: Direct and indirect pathways through caregiving and the home environment. *Journal of Applied Developmental Psychology, 28*(5–6), 411–426.

Mejia, A., Calam, R., & Sanders, M. R. (2012). A review of parenting programs in developing countries: Opportunities and challenges for preventing emotional and behavioral difficulties in children. *Clinical Child and Family Psychology Review, 15*(2), 163–175.

Moehler, E., Brunner, R., Wiebel, A., Reck, C., & Resch, F. (2006). Maternal depressive symptoms in the postnatal period are associated with long-term impairment of mother—child bonding. *Archives of Women's Mental Health, 9*(5), 273–278.

Morris, A. S., Criss, M. M., Silk, J. S., & Houltberg, B. J. (2017). The impact of parenting on emotion regulation during childhood and adolescence. *Child Development Perspectives, 11*(4), 233–238.

Murray, L., Cooper, P. J., Wilson, A., & Romaniuk, H. (2003). Controlled trial of the short-and long-term effect of psychological treatment of post-partum depression: 2. Impact on the mother-child relationship and child outcome. *The British Journal of Psychiatry, 182*(5), 420–427.

Murray, L., Fiori-Cowley, A., & Hooper, R. (1996). The impact of postnatal depression and associated adversity on early mother-infant interactions and later infant outcome. *Child Development, 67*, 2512–2526.

Murray, L., Halligan, S. L., & Cooper, P. J. (2009). *Effects of postnatal depression on mother-infant interactions, and child development.* Oxford: Wiley-Blackwell.

Murray, S. M., Familiar, I., Nakasujja, N., Winch, P. J., Gallo, J. J., Opoka, R., . . . Bass, J. K. (2017). Caregiver mental health and HIV-infected child wellness: Perspectives from Ugandan caregivers. *AIDS Care, 29*(6), 793–799.

Naicker, K., Wickham, M., & Colman, I. (2012). Timing of first exposure to maternal depression and adolescent emotional disorder in a national Canadian cohort. *PLoS One, 7*(3), e33422.

Nievar, M. A., Van Egeren, L. A., & Pollard, S. (2010). A meta-analysis of home visiting programs: Moderators of improvements in maternal behavior. *Infant Mental Health Journal, 31*(5), 499–520.

Pallini, S., Baiocco, R., Schneider, B. H., Madigan, S., & Atkinson, L. (2014). Early child—parent attachment and peer relations: A meta-analysis of recent research. *Journal of Family Psychology, 28*(1), 118.

Patel, V., Chisholm, D., Parikh, R., Charlson, F. J., Degenhardt, L., Dua, T., . . . Levin, C. (2016). Addressing the burden of mental, neurological, and substance use disorders: Key messages from disease control priorities. *The Lancet, 387*(10028), 1672–168.

Pederson, D. R., Bailey, H. N., Tarabulsy, G. M., Bento, S., & Moran, G. (2014). Understanding sensitivity: Lessons learned from the legacy of Mary Ainsworth. *Attachment & Human Development, 16*(3), 261–270.

Poobalan, A. S., Aucott, L. S., Ross, L., Smith, W. C. S., Helms, P. J., & Williams, J. H. G. (2007). Effects of treating postnatal depression on mother-infant interaction and child development: Systematic review. *The British Journal of Psychiatry, 191*(5), 378–386.

Price, S., & Proctor, E. (2009). A rural perspective on perinatal depression: Prevalence, correlates, and implications for help-seeking among low-income women. *The Journal or Rural Health, 25*(2), 158–166.

Rahman, A., Fisher, J., Bower, P., Luchters, S., Tran, T., Yasamy, M. T., . . . Waheed, W. (2013). Interventions for common perinatal mental disorders in women in low- and middle-income countries: A systematic review and meta-analysis. *Bulletin of the World Health Organization, 91*(8), 593–601.

Rahman, A., Malik, A., Sikander, S., Roberts, C., & Creed, F. (2008). Cognitive behaviour therapy-based intervention by community health workers for mothers with depression and their infants in rural Pakistan: A cluster-randomised controlled trial. *The Lancet, 372*(9642), 902–909.

Rao, H., Betancourt, L., Giannetta, J. M., Brodsky, N. L., Korczykowski, M., Avants, B. B., . . . Detre, J. A. (2010). Early parental care is important for hippocampal maturation: Evidence from brain morphology in humans. *Neuroimage, 49*(1), 1144–1150.

Rostad, W. L., Moreland, A. D., Valle, L. A., & Chaffin, M. J. (2018). Barriers to participation in parenting programs: The relationship between parenting stress, perceived barriers, and program completion. *Journal of Child and Family Studies, 27*(4), 1264–1274.

Santona, A., Tagini, A., Sarracino, D., De Carli, P., Pace, C. S., Parolin, L., & Terrone, G. (2015). Maternal depression and attachment: The evaluation of mother-child interactions during feeding practice. *Frontier in Psychology, 6*, 1235.

Sarsour, K., Sheridan, M., Jutte, D., Nuru-Jeter, A., Hinshaw, S., & Boyce, W. T. (2011). Family socioeconomic status and child executive functions: The roles of language, home environment, and single parenthood. *Journal of the International Neuropsychological Society: JINS, 17*(1), 120.

Scheyer, K., & Urizar, G. G. (2016). Altered stress patterns and increased risk for postpartum depression among low-income pregnant women. *Archives of Women's Mental Health, 19*, 317–328.

Scholle, S. H., Haskett, R. F., Hanusa, B. H., Pincus, H. A., & Kupfer, D. J. (2003). Addressing depression in obstetrics/gynecology practice. *General Hospital Psychiatry, 25*(2), 83–90.

Seffren, V., Familiar, I., Murray, S. M., Augustinavicius, J., Boivin, M. J., Nakasujja, N., . . . Bass, J. (2018). Association between coping strategies, social support, and depression and anxiety symptoms among rural Ugandan women living with HIV/AIDS. *AIDS Care, 30*(7), 888–895.

Seltzer, L. J., Prososki, A. R., Ziegler, T. E., & Pollak, S. D. (2012). Instant messages vs. speech: Hormones and why we still need to hear each other. *Evolution and Human Behavior, 33*(1), 42–45.

Sharp, C. K. P., Marais, L., Shoet, C., Rani, K., Lenka, M., Cloete, J., Vanwoerden, S., Givon, D., & Boivin, M. (2021). Mediational intervention for sensitizing caregivers to improve mental health outcomes in orphaned and vulnerable children. *Journal of Clinical Child and Adolescent Psychology.* https://doi.org/10.1080/15374416.2021.1881903.

Singer, L. T., Salvator, A., Guo, S., Collin, M., Lilien, L., & Baley, J. (1999). Maternal psychological distress and parenting stress after the birth of a very low-birth-weight infant. *Jama, 281*(9), 799–805.

Singla, D. R., Kohrt, B. A., Murray, L. K., Anand, A., Chorpita, B. F., & Patel, V. (2017). Psychological treatments for the world: Lessons from low- and middle-income countries. *Annual Review Clinical Psychology, 13*, 149–181.

Singla, D. R., Kumbakumba, E., & Aboud, F. E. (2015). Effects of a parenting intervention to address both maternal psychological wellbeing and child development and growth in rural Uganda: A community-based, cluster randomised trial. *Lancet Global Health, 3*(8), e458–469.

Sohr-Preston, S., & Scaramella, L. (2006). Implications of timing of maternal depressive symptoms for early cognitive and language development. *Clinical Child and Family Psychology Review, 9*, 65–83.

Song, L., Spier, E. T., & Tamis-Lemonda, C. S. (2014). Reciprocal influences between maternal language and children's language and cognitive development in low-income families. *Journal of Child Language, 41*(2), 305–326.

Stein, A., Malberg, L. E., Sylva, K., Barnes, J., Leach, P., FCCC Team. (2008). The influence of maternal depression, caregiving, and socioeconomic status in the postnatal year on children's language development. *Child: Care, Health and Development, 34*(5), 603–612.

Surkan, P. J., Kennedy, C. E., Hurley, K. M., & Black, M. M. (2011). Maternal depression and early childhood growth in developing countries: Systematic review and meta-analysis. *Bulletin of the World Health Organization, 89*(8), 608–615.

Tol, W. A., Greene, M. C., Lasater, M. E., Le Roch, K., Bizouerne, C., Purgato, M., . . . Barbui, C. (2020). Impact of maternal mental health interventions on child-related outcomes in low-and middle-income countries: A systematic review and meta-analysis. *Epidemiology and Psychiatric Sciences*, *29*, e174.

Valcan, D. S., Davis, H., & Pino-Pasternak, D. X. (2018). Parental behaviours predicting early childhood executive functions: A meta-analysis. *Educational Psychology Review*, *30*, 307–349.

Weinfield, N. S., Sroufe, L. A., Egeland, B., & Carlson, E. A. (1999). The nature of individual differences in infant–caregiver attachment. In J. Cassidy & P. R. Shaver (Eds.), *Handbook of attachment: Theory, research, and clinical applications* (pp. 68–88). New York: The Guilford Press.

Wekesa, E. (2000). The impact of HIV/AIDS on child survival and development in Kenya. *AIDS Anal Afr*, *10*(4), 12–14.

World Health Organization, U. N. C. s. F., World Bank Group. (2018). Nurturing care for early childhood development: A framework for helping children survive and thrive to transform health and human potential. Retrieved from https://apps.who.int/iris/bitstream/handle/10665/272603/9789241514064-eng.pdf

12 MISC Applied to Families Reunited After Migration-Related Separation

Amanda Venta, Kalina Brabeck, Jodi Berger Cardoso, Arlene Bjugstad, Jessica Hernandez Ortiz, Natasha Prosperi, and Carla Sharp

12.1 Migration-Related Family Separation

Family and youth migration from Central America has rapidly grown in recent years, drawing attention to the already-large numbers of parents (without children), families, and youth (without parents) migrating from Central America and Mexico to the U.S. (U.S. Customs & Border Patrol, 2019). Likewise, recent outrage regarding the forced separation of migrant parents from their children at the U.S. and Mexico border shone a spotlight on the process of migration as a threat to family relationships, safety, and mental health. While U.S. policies of separation are certainly reprehensible from a mental health standpoint (APA, 2018), Mexican and Central American families have been experiencing migration-related separation for decades. Indeed, parents will travel to the U.S. alone to seek employment or security before coordinating migration for their children (Gindling & Poggio, 2012).

Estimates from a Latin American college sample indicate that approximately 10% of young adults who continue to reside in Latin America have experienced at least one parent's migration (and subsequent separation), whereas the rate is much higher—exceeding 60%—in a U.S. sample of Central American immigrant youth (Venta, Bailey, Mercado & Colunga-Rodríguez, 2021; Venta et al., 2020). These figures suggest that for Latinx immigrants to the U.S. in particular, caregiver separations due to migration are likely an important feature of their psychosocial history.

In-depth interview data from a small sample of Central American high school students who had experienced parental migration in their home countries and subsequently migrated to the U.S. demonstrated that these family separations could last up to 14 years and, on average, separations lasted 5–6 years (Venta et al., 2020). Disruption in the youth-caregiver relationship was associated with caregiver migration in that study. Though more than 85% of youth ultimately felt that their parent made the right decision in migrating, reunifications with caregivers were complex, characterized by previous feelings of loss and ongoing mistrust. Interview narratives in that study indicated variety in the substitute caregivers available after parental migration,

DOI: 10.4324/9781003145899-12

with respondents often indicating that even when they remained with a close family member (e.g., grandparent), parental migration, particularly concerning mothers, was a source of ongoing sadness. Indeed, quantitative research conducted with Latin American young adults who previously experienced family separation due to parental migration confirms that the child's closeness with subsequent caregivers varies considerably and affects their relationship with their caregiver into young adulthood, as does frequency of contact with the parent after migration (Venta et al., 2021). As these studies suggest, youth who ultimately migrate to the U.S. following a migrant parent are likely to be reunified and live with that parent, and doing so is associated with reduced emotional and behavioral symptoms with moderate to large effect sizes (Walker, Venta & Galicia, 2020). Still, reunified families struggle with the emotional and relational difficulties previously noted (Venta et al., 2020), exacerbated by pragmatic challenges like lack of documentation status (Walker et al., 2020). Currently, there are no available interventions that target the parent-child relationships during and following reunification.

The need for interventions targeting parent-child relationships is further justified by the implications of separation for attachment security. As aforementioned, migration-related separations from caregivers are associated with reduced attachment security in adolescence (Venta et al., 2020) and young adulthood (Venta et al., 2021). Attachment security—characterized by generalized views of the self as worthy of care and others as reliable caregivers—is often cited as a transdiagnostic protective factor for youth mental health, and, indeed, in Latinx immigrant youth, attachment security is associated with reduced emotional and behavioral symptoms as well as increased resilience (Venta et al., 2019). Importantly, secure attachment relationships have also been shown, in this population, to buffer the effects of childhood trauma on acculturation, or cultural adaptation, in the year following migration (Venta, 2020). As such, intervening to nurture and maintain attachment relationships that have been threatened due to long-term separations has significant clinical implications. Indeed, recent waves of Central American and Mexican migrants are demonstrating startling levels of trauma exposure and posttraumatic distress. Among Latinx children and adolescent migrants, most have been exposed to three to four traumatic events with significant exposure to community violence (39% among children and 64% among adolescents), and 60% exhibit clinically significant symptoms of posttraumatic stress disorder (Venta & Mercado, 2019). Further, trauma symptoms among Latinx migrant parents and children have profound, cross-cutting effects. Indeed, in parents, trauma symptoms are significantly associated with reduced physical functioning; role limitations in work, family, and social life; emotional and social functioning; pain; and energy/fatigue (Mercado, Venta, Henderson & Pimentel, 2019). Similarly, in migrant children, trauma symptoms are associated with mental and physical health, broadly, and role limitations in schooling, family, social life, self-esteem, behavior problems, and family activities (Mercado et al., 2019). Against this background, it is no surprise that immigrant youth face long-term challenges relating to mental health, community functioning, school attachment and engagement, and family cohesion, though, relevant to MISC, relational interventions have shown promise in mitigating challenges related to schooling (Suárez-Orozco, Pimentel, & Martin, 2009; Suárez-Orozco, Onaga, & de Lardemelle, 2010).

12.2 Potential Relevance of MISC to Immigrant Families

The previously described attachment trauma associated with separation and the ensuing attachment stress involved in reunification necessitates attachment-informed intervention programs that can scaffold repairing attachment relations. As discussed in other chapters in this volume, the Mediational Intervention for Sensitizing Caregivers (MISC; Klein, 1996) has been successfully used in Uganda and South Africa to train laypersons (mothers infected by HIV/AIDS and community-based caregivers working with HIV orphans) to increase sensitive caregiving with direct effects on child outcomes (Bass et al., 2017; Boivin et al., 2013a, 2013b; Boivin et al., 2017; Sharp et al., 2021). MISC is a semi-structured, manualized, and evidence-based treatment that combines attachment principles with principles of learning (Shohet & Jaegermann, 2012). The acronym, MISC, stands for both the *objective* of the intervention (to help children become **M**ore **I**ntelligent and **S**ensitive (**S**ocially **C**ompetent) **C**hildren) and the *process* through which this objective is achieved (i.e. the mediating role of adult caregivers to become sensitized to their child—a **M**ediational **I**ntervention for **S**ensitizing **C**aregivers). MISC trains caregivers how to maximize psychosocial and cognitive development in children and is designed specifically for low-resource settings affected by trauma (P. S. Klein, 1996). Its evidence base is, therefore, most established in poor communities in Africa, Asia, and the United Kingdom and Europe (P. S. Klein, 1996), which share many similar health disparities (trauma, poverty, limited access to health care, minority stress, discrimination) as communities affected by immigration in the United States (Weinstein, Geller, Negussie, & Baciu, 2017).

The theoretical foundation of MISC is grounded in Bowlby's attachment theory (Bowlby, 1973, 1980a, 1980b) and Feuerstein's theory of Cognitive Modifiability and Mediated Learning Experience (MLE) (Feuerstein, 1979). The first of these, attachment, provides the basis for a set of "emotional components" in MISC, including eye contact, smiles, vocalization, touch, physical closeness, turn-taking, sharing of joy, expression of positive affect, synchrony, length of communication chains, and excitement expressed toward things, people, and experiences in the environment. When these components are present in the everyday interactions between caregiver and child, the child receives messages that communicate "I love you," "I'm with you," and "It's worthwhile to act." However, these messages are not enough to optimize cognitive and socio-emotional development in children. To do so, a set of cognitive (mediational) components needs to characterize an interaction. To constitute an MLE, the following components need to be present: focusing, affecting (providing meaning), expanding, regulating, and rewarding. These components provide caregivers with the step-by-step know-how of how to interact with their child to slow down the interaction and mediate a child's subjective experience. In MISC, these components are observed through video-based coding and feedback to the caregiver using the Observing Mediational Interaction (OMI) (P. S. Klein, 2014) tool. By influencing these mediational processes, children's need system is positively affected, including the capacity to focus, seek meaning, regulate behavior, plan before doing, seek success or approval, and inquire about and associate past, present, and future experiences.

While a mediated learning environment is accessible for most children, children exposed to traumatic separation due to migration experience attachment disruption and toxic levels of trauma and stress. Their mothers similarly undergo immense stress in navigating migration that involves separation from their children, homelessness, violence, and the rupture of their own attachment relationships. Vulnerability and stress are further compounded if mothers and children are victims of social determinants of ill health, which is often the case for migrants. Therefore, these caregivers may be depleted in the emotional resources needed to mediate their child's social and emotional needs, as suggested by MISC. The MISC intervention addresses this depletion and builds resilience by teaching caregivers' aforementioned emotional and cognitive components through video-based feedback.

There are several advantages to MISC specifically for caregivers and children affected by migration. MISC trainers are laypersons—MISC scale-up, therefore, does not rely on master-level or Ph.D-level mental health professionals. Moreover, MISC does not require a mother to do any new activities with children but changes the nature of everyday interactions with children ("the serve and return"). In the same way that we invest in math literacy, reading literacy, or nutrition literacy, MISC provides a vehicle for investing in the "literacy of interaction", thereby providing a much needed "mental diet" for children most in need. MISC is highly suitable for cross-cultural adaptation, because it does not depend on importing the dominant culture's methods, ideas, and tools and operationalizing existing cultural caregiving practices (P.S. Klein, Wieder, & Greenspan, 1987). It is also highly adaptable developmentally, because MISC is not highly structured, and instils the basic components of high-quality interactions regardless of age or interaction partner (Sharp et al., 2020). We would like to point out, however, that the MISC takes time. Consistent with other attachment-based interventions (Fonagy, 2006), and prior experience with MISC (Bass et al., 2017; Boivin et al., 2013a, 2013b; Boivin et al., 2017; Sharp et al., 2021), one year is required, because human caregiving behavior is difficult to influence all at once. In contrast to short-term, highly structured interventions that use instructional formats and materials, MISC requires internalization of basic concepts rather than short-term skills-building. It is designed to affect the child's needs system, to create a new, more differentiated caregiving context. The time-cost is balanced by the fact that no additional tools or materials are purchased. Moreover, the Cognitive-Behavior Therapy (CBT) framework of short-term, intense program sessions most often used in parenting interventions (Weisz et al., 2017) may be considered culturally intrusive. Indeed, imposing structured programs based on the dominant culture's values produces three negative effects: dependency, alienation, and feelings of inferiority in caregivers (P. S. Klein & Rye, 2004).

Taken together, MISC is ideal for resource-poor environments like those often seen in communities affected by intimate partner violence (IPV) and the social determinants of ill health but needs to be systematically adapted for Spanish-speaking caregivers and children affected by migration separation. This requires a rigorous, evidence-based, and iterative adaptation approach until "fit" with the context is achieved.

12.3 Adaptation of MISC: Wingwood and DiClemente's ADAPT-ITT Model

In the following, we document the stage 1a process (Onken, Carroll, Shoham, Cuthbert, & Riddle, 2014) of adapting MISC for mothers and youth separated by migration. Wingwood and DiClemente's ADAPT-ITT model guides MISC adaptation for immigrant youth and mothers experiencing migration-related separation and reunification. The ADAPT-ITT model consists of eight sequential phases, including assessment, decision, administration, production, topical experts, training, and testing. ADAPT-ITT is one of the few frameworks for adaptation of evidence-based interventions (Wingood & DiClemente, 2008). This framework has been applied to adolescents in various U.S. and international settings and has been widely utilized in adapting HIV treatment and prevention interventions for different populations. Three of the eight phases of the ADAPT-ITT model have been completed to facilitate a practical and cultural adaptation of the MISC intervention (the final phases will be completed in a larger study). In the following, we describe how the 8 phases of the ADAPT-ITT framework are applied to adapt MISC for youth and mothers separated by migration.

Phase 1: Assessment involved conducting a needs assessment to determine the unique needs of the target population. To inform the needs assessment, researchers formed a community advisory board (CAB) that comprised of community-based organizations in Houston that work to create opportunities for refugees, immigrants, and other underserved and vulnerable residents in Houston. The CAB consisted of 17 organizations that included mental health providers, case managers, school counsellors, school administrators, and social service providers in the Houston area. CAB members were recruited from immigrant-serving organizations that include federally qualified health care centers, non-profit organizations that serve immigrants, post-release programs that serve unaccompanied minors, two large school districts, non-profit legal organizations, and university academics whose research focuses on Latinx families, migration, and/or attachment in youth. Four CAB meetings during the two-year project period were planned. Additionally, to examine how MISC would fit within the structure of community-based organizations (CBOs), we held a 2.5-day workshop on MISC and led discussion sessions following the MISC training about the content, delivery, and proposed cultural adaptations.

The main task of the assessment phase was to conduct semi-structured individual interviews with immigrant youth and their mothers ($n = 16$ mothers and 16 children) to better understand their experiences with reunification and needs related to the parent-child relationship. Mothers and youth were included if they: (a) immigrated to the U.S. from Mexico and/or Central America and (b) were separated by migration. Individual interviews sought to understand the factors that challenge parent-child reunification and strategies that families have used to resolve these challenges.

Phase 2: Decision involved (a) reviewing the evidence on culturally relevant evidenced-based interventions and determining how MISC should be adapted to include key cultural values critical to Latinx cultures (i.e., familismo, confianza, and respeto); and (b) determine how MISC fits within the structure of the Alliance, a Houston-based CBO.

Phase 3: Administration involved the use of a theater-testing approach with stakeholders. This included five Latinx immigrant families and five mental health professionals ($n = 10$). During the theater testing, facilitators implement critical components of MISC. Using this methodology, participants provide feedback via discussion meant to elicit their reactions regarding the appropriateness of the new content. In the administration phase, we included mental health professionals to probe about the feasibility and acceptability of MISC within their organizational structure. We then held discussions with mothers and youth to solicit their reaction about MISC, including the concepts, use of videos, messages, materials, etc.

Phase 4: Production involves drafting an adapted version of MISC. A careful assessment of balancing the fidelity, underlying theory, and core elements and logic of the original MISC will occur under a MISC-approved trainer's supervision.

Phase 5: Topical experts assist with the production and integration of the adapted MISC. We will engage our CAB members; five youth and their mothers who have lived experiences of separation and reunification; and researchers and trainers who have MISC expertise. This phase's primary goal is to solicit input on all aspects of adaptation, including cultural and language adaptation of MISC.

Phase 6: Integration will involve having the same experts give feedback on MISC materials, videos, and other content. MISC will be translated into Spanish using a translation-back/translation method by bilingual/bicultural language translators. Following the translation, the readability and acceptability of MISC will be assessed via formal, individual, qualitative interviews that will be analyzed as described next. Changes will be implemented before dissemination. Two sets of interviews will be conducted. The first set will be with the community-based organization (CBO) members. Researchers will use a modified interview guide that has been used in previous studies to assess the feasibility and acceptability of MISC within the CBO context. The second set of interviews will be conducted with Latinx parents and youth to obtain feedback on the final MISC guide and delivery process. This final feedback will be integrated into the MISC manual and used in phases 7 and 8.

Phase 7: Training will involve training in MISC. Here we intend to pull from the members of the CBO. The CBO members have invested time and expertise in learning about MISC. Now, they will receive formal training and supervision.

Phase 8: Testing will occur using a quasi-experimental or experimental design. Researchers will analyze the pilot study results and build evidence for a phase 2 study. Following a phase 2 study, researchers will need to determine the efficacy of MISC for mothers and youth separated by migration.

12.4 Progress in MISC Adaptation

12.4.1 Results of Phase 1 Assessment

Thus far, Phase 1 of the MISC adaptation process has been completed, and we present preliminary results here. The goal of Phase 1: Assessment was to understand how mothers and youth perceived the migration-related separation and the reunification. The research team conducted 16 semi-structured dyadic interviews with immigrant youth and their mothers (see Berger Cardoso et al., 2020, for a full description of methodology). Dyadic interviews were analyzed via a process of collaborative, multi-phase, and iterative coding (see Berger Cardoso et al., 2020 for details on analysis).

Participating families were from Honduras ($n = 7$), El Salvador ($n = 4$), Mexico ($n = 3$), and Guatemala ($n = 2$). They lived in the U.S. on average, six years. About half of the youth lived with maternal grandparents during separation ($n = 9$, 56.3%). Youths' average age at the time of separation was 4 and at the time of youth migration was 8. Mothers and youth were separated between 1–10 years (average five years). About half of the youth participants were female ($n = 9$, 56.3%). Youths' current age ranged from 10–18.

Disruption during separation. For mothers, the multiple uncertainties surrounding the separation created anxiety. In addition to primary emotions (e.g., sadness and fear), mothers internalized blame for leaving their children, creating secondary emotions (e.g., guilt). Mothers assumed blame even though their decisions to migrate occurred within contexts of systems of oppression and historical and ongoing inequity. Such self-blame is also reflective of responses to traumatic events.

I wouldn't stop crying, and I would tell her how much I loved her and everything, but it was painful for me to live without my daughter and think that I had been partially to blame . . . because to me, it was my fault.

(6A)

Youths' recollections of the separation period depended on their age at the time of separation. Those who remembered recalled the fear that they would never see their mothers again. Notably, the separation from the mother for most youth occurred on top of a previous separation from their father due to separation, death, or migration. Youth recalled having to navigate essential milestones, like first menstruation, without their mother. They recalled jealously comparing themselves to peers whose mothers were present, and some described symptoms of posttraumatic stress disorder (PTSD).

<u>Coping during separation.</u> Although it varied based on the child's age, many mothers communicated a rationale for the separation—that they migrated for a better life, opportunity, or safety. Mothers thereby provided a counter-narrative to a child's tendency to personalize negative events: to assume they are to blame or caused the separation. When they left their children, mothers emphasized hope for a reunion and promises for the material and physical benefits that would result from their sacrifice:

I didn't have the courage to see her, to turn around. When I started to walk, I didn't have the courage. I just hugged her, I told her I loved her a lot and promised her that I was going to . . . that she was going to be here someday with me and that I was going to buy her the prettiest doll that I could find.

(11A)

During separation, mothers coped by working, which allowed them to send gifts, support education, secure housing, and contribute to their children's future. The ability to translate the pain of separation into meaning and purpose was instrumental in their ability to cope. Work and caretaking roles in the U.S. also provided an important distraction.

Youth also articulate mothers' reasons for the migration; this was protective in that it allowed youth to externalize the reason for migration—i.e., it was not their fault. Moreover, this framing helped preserve an internal representation of their mother as prioritizing their wellbeing, and themselves as deserving of such care. There was also evidence of how youth managed their own emotional reactions to protect their mothers. This compartmentalization of emotion is in the short-term protective. In the long term, the foreclosure of emotional processing may contribute to psychological challenges.

When I said goodbye . . . she told me, "You don't have to cry because if I'm leaving, it is in search of a better future. Here we barely have anything and I don't want you to cry because I need to leave to make things better for you." So I promised her that I wasn't going to cry, and the next day, when it was time for her to leave and she left, I made her the promise that I wasn't going to cry, and I didn't cry.

(15B)

Daily activities and routines, such as school, visiting a certain *tienda* (store) each day, and playing soccer, helped distract youth and establish a sense of normalcy and predictability: "That's why church was my escape and school, too. To take a break from everything and just have fun" (6B). Siblings played essential roles, providing companionship and shared understanding of the experience of separation.

Alternative caregivers: experiences of protection and maltreatment. Participating mothers came from small, close-knit communities where extended families lived in the same or close-by households. For most, choosing an alternative caregiver during the mother's absence was fairly straightforward. Mothers who trusted the alternative caregiver psychologically fared better during the separation. However, the cost was that some youth formed stronger bonds with the alternative caregiver, which complicated the later reunion with the mother. The youth who reported positive relationships with their caregiver(s) developed strong attachments with them, referring to them as "mom", and longing for them when they later migrated to the U.S.

One-quarter of mothers did not have a trusted family member to care for their children. These alternative arrangements were more likely to expose the children to maltreatment. Seven youth (44%) experienced abuse from alternative caregivers; this included experiences of emotional abuse; being exploited for work; neglect; physical abuse; and sexual abuse from family members. When mothers understood the alternative caregiving situations to be unsupportive, neglectful, or dangerous, their own anxiety, sadness, and guilt intensified. Children who were maltreated during separation also had more psychological difficulty after reunification. They were affected by both the attachment disruption and the chronic exposure to traumatic events perpetrated by those meant to protect them.

Protecting relationships through communication: Most mothers reported communicating with their children daily, often multiple times per day, primarily via phone videoconferencing. Communication was complicated by lack of access to technology, caregivers acting as gatekeepers, mothers' busy work schedules, and youths' anger and resentment. Despite this, mothers tried their best to mother from a distance. They instructed youth on how to behave and how to protect themselves, tell them to take their medication, and monitor school attendance. They also reiterate the reasons for separation, again providing a counter-narrative to youth assuming rejection or blame and searching for meaning in their loss.

In their recollections, youth focused on gifts or necessities sent and viewed these as proof of their mother's love and commitment to care for them. This reinforced the internal representation of mothers as caring and of themselves as worthy. Yet youth also express their ambivalence about communicating with mothers. They repeatedly ask why they were left behind, and they resist and sometimes resent mothers' efforts to assert authority over the phone.

> Because we wouldn't talk before, even though I had a phone and she had a phone, we didn't talk and it was largely my fault because first I would say I didn't have a phone as an excuse. . .
>
> (15B)

Thus there is the erosion of cultural norms, like *respeto* (respect) for elders, being *bien educado/a* (well behaved), and traditional parent/child hierarchies.

Office of Refugee Resettlement (ORR) detention. The majority of the families decided to bring the child to the U.S. based on fears for safety. At the border, youth described horrible conditions, which included cold rooms and harsh treatment: "I behaved well there because I knew it was really bad. They would wake us up early. I always liked to wake up early because they would throw really ice cold water on anyone who doesn't wake up." (9B). After several days, most youths were transferred to ORR shelters. This represented an additional separation and event in which they lacked control and power.

Complicated reunifications. Upon finally being reunited with their mother, most youth struggled with grief, trauma symptoms, and sometimes mental health disorders, like PTSD. Some mothers struggle with their youth's mood, rebellion, disrespect and/or resentment, and were unsure how to effectively parent youth through these challenges.

> She would lock herself up in her room and didn't want to come out. She wanted to be in her own world, locked up, and I didn't know what to do anymore as much as we tried. I would buy her things. She had it all. I would go to the stores. I tried to give her the best, but no, she didn't want it.
>
> (14A)

Similarly, youth reported feeling angry, isolated, and sad. Many were conflicted; on the one hand, they were happy to be reunited, but on the other, they were trying to make sense of the separation, experiencing memories of maltreatment, and grieving relationships in the country of origin: "Sometimes my emotions change. Sometimes I'm good. Sometimes I'm bad. Sometimes I'm sad" (4B). In addition, youth are trying to adjust to new families, norms, culture, and language. Moreover, their insecure legal status put them at risk for another separation through deportation. Mothers similarly described reunification as a "double-sided coin" that involved, on the one hand, relief and joy, and on the other hand, stress and unfamiliarity.

The psychological toll of separation and reunification affected the mother-child relationships. Mother and child had to become reacquainted, and often expectations did not match reality:

> But unfortunately, he's not the boy I left anymore. Because he was a quiet child, humble even . . . and now, I wasn't expecting his reactions, his behavior. . . . I wish I could turn back time, but it's not possible.
>
> (9A)

Because separation occurred during critical periods of development, developing trust was a significant source of stress. Initially, all youth described feeling guarded and mistrustful of their mothers. While acknowledging that mothers typically have authority over children, the felt deference and respect were not earned: "It wasn't that I didn't call her 'mom', but I just didn't have that trust between mother and son" (3B).

Integrating into new families and communities. In addition to navigating complicated reunifications with their mothers, many youth were joining stepparents and new siblings. While this was a positive experience for many, for others resentment and jealousy toward stepparents and U.S.-born siblings complicated their reunification with their mother. Additionally, youth were challenged to integrate into schools with new languages, norms, and expectations. Psychological struggles, academic gaps, language challenges, parental engagement, and bullying all complicated school experiences. Additionally, because many families lived in unsafe communities in the U.S., mothers limited youths' mobility outside of the home, leaving the youth to feel "trapped". At the same time, engagement in the community, e.g., via sports or church, was a protective experience: "And when I got to do track and skateboarding, it's like a new thing, and it opened me up a lot" (6B).

12.4.2 Results of Phase 2: Decision

Our review of the literature suggests that MISC is likely consistent with Latinx cultural values. Values, such as familismo (family orientation), personalismo (friendliness), simpatía (niceness), confianza (trust), and respeto (respect) are essential in Latinx cultures. These cultural values have emerged as critically important protective factors reducing internalizing and externalizing symptoms in Latinx youth. Because these cultural values are communicated in the context of family relationships, psychotherapeutic interventions that are focused solely on the individual can be less effective in treating mental health symptoms (Suarez-Morales, Mena, Schlaudt, & Santisteban, 2017). Based on this premise, MISC likely builds resilience by scaffolding parental capacity to protect children against the negative effects of trauma. Although we have not yet tested the effectiveness of MISC with this population, we hypothesize that sensitized caregiving (learned in MISC) will be the primary mechanism of change between MISC and mental health outcomes and parent-child relational satisfaction in Latinx mothers and children who experienced migration-related separation.

12.5 Summary and Future Directions

The work for Phases 3–8 is underway. In summary, preliminary findings from our formative work thus far, based on qualitative research with 16 immigrant mother-child dyads that will inform subsequences of cultural adaptation, are (a) separations in the context of migration negatively impact mothers and youth psychologically and negatively impact their relationship. This is particularly true when youth experience maltreatment from alternative caregivers. The separation from the mother is compounded by additional separations the child endures, including from their father, while in ORR custody, and threatened separation due to insecure legal status. The negative consequences of separation, combined with additional stressors such as integrating into new families/communities/schools and grieving the loss of relationships in the country of origin, make reunification a "double-sided coin", at once relieving and joyful, but also stressful and tenuous. Culturally situated norms, such as respect for elders, and essential qualities of attachment, such as trust, are eroded and take time to rebuild. (b) Mothers and youth demonstrate resiliency and adaptation through finding meaning in their sacrifices; framing mothers as prioritizing youths' care and youth as deserving of such care; daily virtual communication; stable alternative caregiving during the separation; distraction through work, school, and activities; and connecting to faith and supportive others. Thus far, our findings speak to both the vulnerability and resilience of immigrant communities, highlighting the critical need for MISC to address mother, child, and relational difficulties and the potential of MISC to capitalize and build upon strengths already evident in the dyads.

Refereces

American Psychological Association (APA). (2018). *Statement of APA president regarding the traumatic effects of separating immigrant families.* Retrieved from www.apa.org/news/press/releases/2018/05/separating-immigrant-families

Bass, J. K., Opoka, R., Familiar, I., Nakasujja, N., Sikorskii, A., Awadu, J., . . . Boivin, M. (2017). Randomized controlled trial of caregiver training for HIV-infected child neurodevelopment and caregiver well being. *Aids, 31*(13), 1877–1883. doi:10.1097/QAD.0000000000001563

Berger Cardoso, J., & Brabeck, K. (2020, October 26-27). "*Una Moneda De Dos Caras:" Central American and Mexican Immigrant Mothers and Youths' Experiences of Separation and Reunification.*" [Symposium presentation]. University Park, PA: Penn State's National Symposium on Family Issues.

Boivin, M. J., Bangirana, P., Nakasujja, N., Page, C. F., Shohet, C., Givon, D., . . . Klein, P. S. (2013a). A year-long caregiver training program improves cognition in preschool Ugandan children with human immunodeficiency virus. *Journal of Pediatrics, 163*(5), 1409–1416, e1401–1405. doi:10.1016/j.jpeds.2013.06.055

Boivin, M. J., Bangirana, P., Nakasujja, N., Page, C. F., Shohet, C., Givon, D., . . . Klein, P. S. (2013b). A year-long caregiver training program to improve neurocognition in preschool Ugandan HIV-exposed children. *Journal of Developmental and Behavioral Pediatrics, 34*(4), 269–278. doi:10.1097/Dbp.0b013e318285fba9

Boivin, M. J., Nakasujja, N., Familiar-Lopez, I., Murray, S. M., Sikorskii, A., Awadu, J., . . . Bass, J. K. (2017). Effect of caregiver training on the neurodevelopment of HIV-exposed uninfected children and caregiver mental health: A Ugandan cluster-randomized controlled trial. *Journal of Developmental and Behavioral Pediatrics, 38*(9), 753–764. doi:10.1097/DBP.0000000000000510

Bowlby, J. (1973). *Attachment and loss: Separation.* New York: Basic Books.

Bowlby, J. (1980a). *Attachment and loss: Loss, sadness and depression.* New York: Basic Books.

Bowlby, J. (1980b). *Attachment and loss (vol 3). Loss, sadness and depression.* London: Hogarth Press.

Feuerstein, R. (1979). The ontogeny of learning in man. In M. A. B. Brazier (Ed.), *Brain mechanisms in memory and learning* (pp. 361–371). New York: Raven Press.

Fonagy, P. (2006). The Mentalization-focused approach to social development. In G. Allen & P. Fonagy (Eds.), *Handbook of mentalization-based treatment* (pp. 53–99). London: John Wiley & Sons Inc.

Gindling, T. H., & Poggio, S. (2012). Family separation and reunification as a factor in the educational success of immigrant children. *Journal of Ethnic and Migration Studies, 38*(7), 1155–1173.

Klein, P. S. (1996). *Early intervention: Cross-cultural experiences with a mediational approach.* Oxford: Routledge.

Klein, P. S. (2014). *OMI—observing mediational interaction manual.* Israel: Bar-Ilan University.

Klein, P. S., & Rye, H. (2004). Interaction-oriented early intervention in Ethiopia. The MISC approach. *Infants and Young Children, 17*(4), 340–354.

Klein, P. S., Wieder, S., & Greenspan, S. I. (1987). A theoretical overview and empirical study of mediated learning experience: Prediction of preschool performance from mother-infant interactions patterns. *Infant Mental Health Journal, 8*(2), 110–129.

Mercado, A., Venta, A., Henderson, C., & Pimentel, N. (2019, April). Trauma and cultural values in the health of recently immigrated families. *Journal of Health Psychology,* 1–13. doi:1359105319842935.

Onken, L., Carroll, L., Shoham, V., Cuthbert, B., & Riddle, M. (2014). Reenvisioning clinical science: Unifying the discipline to improve public health. *Clinical Psychological Science, 2,* 22–34.

Sharp, C., Kulesz, P., Marais, L., Shohet, C., Rani, K., Lenka, M., Cloete, J., Vanwoerden, S., Givon, D., & Boivin, M. (2021). Mediational Intervention for Sensitizing Caregivers to improve mental health outcomes in orphaned and vulnerable children. *Journal of Clinical Child and Adolescent Psychology, 49*(4), 545–557.

Sharp, C., Shohet, C., Givon, D., Penner, F., Marais, L., & Fonagy, P. (2020). Learning to mentalize: A mediational approach. *Clinical Psychology: Science and Practice, 27*(3), e12334.

Shohet, C., & Jaegermann, N. (2012). Integrating infant mental health into primary health care and early childhood education settings in Israel. *Zero to Three, 33*(2), 55–58.

Suarez-Morales, M., Schlaudt, V. A., & Santisteban, D. (2017). Trauma in Hispanic youth with psychiatric symptoms: Investigating gender and family effects. *Psychological Trauma, 9*(3), 334–343.

Suárez-Orozco, C., Onaga, M., & de Lardemelle, C. (2010). Promoting academic engagement among immigrant adolescents through school-family-community collaboration. *Professional School Counseling, 14*(1), 15–26. doi:2156759X1001400103.

Suárez-Orozco, C., Pimentel, A., & Martin, M. (2009). The significance of relationships: Academic engagement and achievement among newcomer immigrant youth. *Teachers College Record, 111*(3), 712–749.

U.S. Customs and Border Patrol. *Southwest border apprehensions (FY2020).* (2019). www. cbp.gov/newsroom/stats/sw-border-migration/usbp-sw-border-apprehensions

Venta, A. C. (2020). Attachment facilitates acculturative learning and adversity moderates: Validating the theory of epistemic trust in a natural experiment. *Child Psychiatry & Human Development, 51,* 471–477.

Venta, A., Bailey, C., Mercado, A., & Colunga-Rodríguez, C. (2021). Family separation and attachment in young adults who were once left behind by caregiver migration. *Psychiatry Research,* 114039.

Venta, A. C., Bailey, C., Muñoz, C., Godinez, E., Colin, Y., Arreola, A., . . . Lawlace, S. (2019). Contribution of schools to mental health and resilience in recently immigrated youth. *School Psychology, 34*(2), 138.

Venta, A. C., Galicia, B., Bailey, C., Abate, A., Marshall, K., & Long, T. (2020). Attachment and loss in the context of U.S. immigration: Caregiver separation and characteristics of internal working models of attachment in high school students. *Attachment & Human Development, 22*(4), 474–489.

Venta, A. C., & Mercado, A. (2019). Trauma screening in recently immigrated youth: Data from two Spanish-speaking samples. *Journal of Child and Family Studies, 28*(1), 84–90.

Walker, J., Venta, A., & Galicia, B. (2020, May). Who is taking care of central American immigrant youth? Preliminary data on caregiving arrangements and emotional-behavioral symptoms post-migration. *Child Psychiatry and Human Development,* 1–8. doi:10. 1007%2Fs10578-020-01002-8.

Weinstein, J. N., Geller, A., Negussie, Y., & Baciu, A. (Eds.). (2017). *Communities in action: Pathways to health equity.* Washington, DC: The National Academic Press.

Weisz, J. R., Kuppens, S., Ng, M. Y., Eckshtain, D., Ugueto, A. M., Vaughn-Coaxum, R., . . . Fordwood, S. R. (2017). What five decades of research tells us about the effects of youth psychological therapy: A multilevel meta-analysis and implications for science and practice. *American Psychologist, 72*(2), 79–117. doi:10.1037/a0040360

Wingood, G. M., & DiClemente, R. J. (2008). The ADAPT-ITT model: A novel method of adapting evidence-based HIV interventions. *JAIDS Journal of Acquired Immune Deficiency Syndromes, 47,* S40–S46.

Acronyms

ADAPT-ITT = Assessment, Decision, Adaptation, Production, Topical Experts, Integration, Training, Testing
AIDS = Acquired immunodeficiency syndrome
CAB = Community advisory board
CBO = Community-based organization
CBT = Cognitive-Behavior Therapy
HIV = Human immunodeficiency virus
IPV = intimate partner violence
MISC = Mediational Intervention for Sensitizing Caregivers
MLE = Mediated Learning Experience
OMI = Observing Mediational Interaction
ORR = Office of Refugee Resettlement

13 The Mediational Intervention for Sensitizing Caregivers for Mothers and Children Exposed to Intimate Partner Violence

Barbie Brashear, John Bickel, Veronica McLaren, Quenette Walton, Judith McFarlane, and Carla Sharp

13.1 Intimate Partner Violence and Its Intergenerational Transmission

13.1.1 What Is Intimate Partner Violence

There are many terms used to label a pattern of assault and coercive behaviors and control tactics that are often used in intimate relationships. These terms include domestic violence, family violence, battering, wife-beating, and intimate partner violence. The Centers for Disease Control defines intimate partner violence as physical, sexual, or psychological violence by a current or former partner (Centers for Disease Control and Prevention, 2020). The National Coalition Against Domestic Violence describes domestic violence as "the willful intimidation, physical assault, battery, sexual assault, and/or other abusive behavior as part of a systematic pattern of power and control perpetrated by one intimate partner against another" (National Coalition Against Domestic Violence, n.d.). Intimate Partner Violence (IPV) is a life-altering trauma that has devastating effects on all those exposed to and harmed by it. It includes physical, emotional, financial, social, and psychological abuse that occurs over time and varies in intensity and duration. It is not a limited, one-time event. It occurs in every culture, in every country, in every community. Women are often on the receiving end of the violence, experiencing higher rates of victimization and increased risk of serious injury (Walby & Towers, 2017; Walby & Allen, 2004). Much of the time, children are nearby or present in homes when violence occurs.

Coercive control is important to understand in the context of IPV. We having worked with hundreds of survivors over the past 20 years and hearing their survival stories, many women describe the most difficult times of the relationship as not including the physical violence, but rather the terrorism of the emotional and psychological abuse they endured from their partner. Ellen Pence was a co-creator of the Domestic Violence Power and Control

DOI: 10.4324/9781003145899-13

Wheel (Gondolf, 2010). The wheel came directly from asking women what it was like to live with a batterer and recording hundreds of answers. The answers to that question were the basis for categorizing control into eight core tactics. These tactics include Using Coercion and Threats, Using Intimidation, Using Emotional Abuse, Using Isolation, Minimizing Denying and Blaming, Using Children, Using Male Privilege, and Using Economic Abuse. These tactics do not occur in isolation; often many are used within the intimate relationship, and all can severely traumatize the family system.

Coercive control describes the controlling violence used as a systemic pattern of behavior one partner uses to dominate and control the other person. This includes intimidation, isolation, and the threat of violence (Dichter, Thomas, Crits-Christoph, Ogden, & Rhodes, 2018). This coercive control is a dynamic that has also been found to influence child adjustment (Jouriles & McDonald, 2015). When violence is present in a family, all members are affected; it does not occur in isolation or without long-term consequences for all in the family system.

13.1.2 Prevalence

The National Intimate Partner Violence Survey of 2015 found that one in every four women and one in every ten men experience sexual violence, physical violence, and/or stalking by an intimate partner during their lifetime (Centers for Disease Control, Violence Prevention Data Brief, 2020). Every day in the United States, domestic violence hotlines receive over 19,000 calls (National Network to End Domestic Violence, 2020). IPV is most common against women between the ages of 18 and 24 (Morgan & Oudekerk, 2019). Women are most the victims of IPV. They also experience higher rates of IPV and are more often the primary caregivers for children. Therefore, exposure and risk of harm for children increases when IPV is present. The National Coalition Against Domestic Violence reports that 1 in 15 children are exposed to intimate partner violence each year, and 90% of these children are eyewitnesses to this violence (National Coalition Against Domestic Violence, n.d.).

13.1.3 Intersectionality

IPV does not occur in a vacuum. Human beings are complex and dynamic. The oppressions that permeate our world are causes and the effects of the trauma that so many are forced to endure. Kimberlé Crenshaw introduced the term intersectionality to address the marginalization of Black women at the individual level to reflect macro-level systems of oppression within domestic violence and anti-discrimination law (Bowleg, 2012; Carbado, Crenshaw, Mays, & Tomlinson, 2013; Crenshaw, 1991; Mehrotra, 2010). For Black women, intersectionality sees their identity holistically, highlighting "that one is neither Black or a woman, nor is one Black plus woman, but rather a Black woman" (Walton & Oyewuwo-Gassikia, 2017, p. 4). Thus, this term describes how social problems and challenges are interconnected and how those that suffer from one problem or one oppression are not singularly oppressed. Race, religion, gender, sexuality, identity, age, socioeconomic status, or lack thereof are all part of the dynamics and ingredients at play when the trauma of IPV is present. These ingredients make the development of interventions for achieving physical, emotional, social, financial, and spiritual safety even more complex.

13.1.4 Intergenerational Patterns of IPV

There are many schools of thought about how IPV is learned and passed to the next generation. Feminist theories suggest that gender inequalities and patriarchal attitudes perpetuate and insulate IPV as part of the dominate culture (Dobash & Dobash, 1979). Many have heard the saying "children see, children do" and some parents have a philosophy of "do as I say, not as I do." For children growing up in homes where there is violence, seeing the violence, hearing the violence, witnessing the violence are all forms of exposure that harm the development of children (Wathen & Macmillan, 2013).

For children, exposure can also mean never directly observing the violence. Anecdotal clinical evidence derived from working in a long-term housing program that had an onsite childcare program offers an example of the lasting effects of IPV exposure on children. One afternoon while observing the toddler room (ages 18–24 months), one non-verbal 22-month-old played out a scene he must have heard. This young one pretended to knock on a door and babbled loudly and angrily over and over until redirected by another child in the playroom. This observation was described to the mother when she picked him up that afternoon. The mother winced, saying she had no idea that "Joey" could hear any of the goings on from the night before. She stated his father showed up at the door and yelled at her until she threatened to call the police and the father left. Children are at greater risk for repeating the cycle as adults by entering into abusive relationships or becoming abusers themselves. Boys who see their mother being abused can be 10 times more likely to abuse their own partners as adults, and girls who grow up in homes exposed to fathers abusing their mothers can be six times more likely to be sexually abused than is a girl who grows up in non-abusive homes (Vargas, Cataldo, & Dickson, 2005).

There is evidence that mothers who experience maltreatment in their own childhoods may show up in later life during their own parenting behaviors as mothers. For example, Thompson-Booth et al. (2019) suggested that mothers may be less likely to show curiosity about a baby's distress when a mother experienced her own maltreatment in childhood. For many mothers who are working hard to employ safety strategies from the violence in their intimate relationship, parenting is not the priority; survival is. Early development and attachment are critical for a child's wellbeing. The mother's attachment to her own mother, or its disruption, also affects how she may have learned to attach to her own children. When this is added to the extra stress of a mother now living through the trauma of adult intimate partner violence, parenting becomes even more challenging and difficult.

13.2 The Effects of IPV on Mothers and Children

> "The boys had always been her reason to stay, but now for the first time they were her reason to leave. She'd allowed violence to become a normal part of their life."
>
> —**Liane Moriarty** (Author, *Big Little Lies*)

13.2.1 Survivor

Women who suffer the trauma of intimate partner violence are impacted physically, mentally, sexually, cognitively, and financially. The physical impact can include bruising, broken bones, strangulation, lacerations, burns, and the ultimate—death. However, the longer the exposure, the greater the physical costs to women. This can extend to long-term health problems, poor health status, and chronic pain syndromes, as well as higher rates of depression, anxiety, post-traumatic stress disorder, sleeping and eating disorders, self-harm and suicide attempts, and poor self-esteem (World Health Organization, Understanding and addressing violence against women, 2010).

Women are killed by husbands, boyfriends, or ex-partners at nine times the rate of women killed by strangers. IPV is the seventh-leading cause of death to women and the second-leading cause of death to African American women (Campbell, Webster, & Glass, 2009). Women are at the highest risk when they decide to leave the relationship. In approximately 19% of IPV homicides, children are also killed (Campbell et al., 2009).

Exposure and victimization of IPV can have significant effects on the mental wellbeing of women. IPV can precipitate a mental health crisis and make it more difficult to access resources (Warshaw, Brashler, & Gil, 2009). Women who are abused are at an increased risk for depression and post-traumatic stress disorder that can function intergenerationally to impact the child (McFarlane et al., 2017). Long-term exposure to ongoing abuse relates to increased physical and psychological health problems, with the mother's mental health problems frequently displayed in behavioral disorders and poor academic functioning of the children (Symes, McFarlane, Maddoux, & Fredland, 2020).

Coping mechanisms for women who experience IPV can include healthy and unhealthy behaviors ranging from drug and alcohol use and abuse to engaging in risky and unprotected sexual relationships. Women who are frequently abused experience PTSD and, if a parent, face many challenges of protecting their children physically and emotionally as they strive to survive (Symes et al., 2020). The focus on survival, safety, and prevention of children becoming physically assaulted by the partner require a great deal of energy both physically and emotionally. Focusing on a child's education and learning is not one of the highest priorities when daily survival is at stake.

Women who suffer from IPV trauma are more likely to suffer from severe financial distress (Gilroy et al., 2018). Women lose over 8 million days of paid work each year due to IPV (World Health Organization, The economic dimensions of intimate partner violence, 2004). Women also suffer higher rates of homelessness due to IPV (Gilroy, McFarlane, Maddoux, & Sullivan, 2016). The National Network to End Domestic Violence (2020) reports that over 90% of homeless women have experienced severe physical or sexual abuse at some point in their lives and 63% have been victims of domestic violence (www.nnedv.org). Often, interventions for those seeking services for IPV are organized in ways that focus on women leaving the abusive relationship to gain access to resources and help. This includes leaving and going to shelter. There are very few financial resources that women can access to stay safely in their own place, there are even fewer interventions that seek to remove and rehabilitate the person using the violence in the relationship, while affording adequate financial support to women and children to prevent losing safe and stable housing.

A lack of social support networks keeps women isolated and reliant upon the intimate partner. Along with the fear of increased violence, financial insecurity, lack of resources, and lack of social support systems are the very things that women often cite as the reasons for not leaving the relationship. Fear of not having money to support children, fear of not finding a job and childcare, and fear of being alone are all fears that can cause women to remain or return to violent relationships. The use of power and control tactics to isolate a partner from friends and families means that the survivor is often left with little access to significant relationships that can be a helpful resource. Women have described being moved across the county by an abusive partner and left with no friends or family to reach out to for support. Isolation is an extremely powerful tool to maintain control over another. Living in constant fear of so many things, including fearing for physical safety, means less energy and resources to focus on the wellbeing of self and children. Basic survival needs are prioritized above many other things—the tank is truly empty.

13.2.2 Children

Children who are exposed to IPV have many long-lasting effects (Wathen & Macmillan, 2013). Children living in homes where IPV is present are at increased risk for personal injuries. They can be caught by the crossfire of arguments and injured unintentionally, or they can be injured intentionally as a pawn by the abusive parent to maintain power and control in the relationship. As discussed earlier, using children as a tactic for power and control can include physically harming children to control the mother. A mother's fear of harm to her children is used against her as a means to keep her in the relationship, and many children become the victims of physical assault (Modi, Palmer, & Armstrong, 2014).

Furthermore, children whom IPV impacts are at an increased risk for other types of abuse, neglect, and other stressors. Eighty-six percent of adults who had been exposed to IPV in childhood (including mother being treated violently) had also been exposed to at least one of the other six types of Adverse Childhood Experiences (ACEs), and 62% to at least two other ACEs (Felitti et al., 1998). They also found that the more types of ACE exposure that occurred resulted in higher likelihoods of risky health behavior such as smoking, severe obesity, and so forth. This led to increases in ischemic heart disease, some cancers, and other disease processes. They also examined the relationship to mental illness and found that these individuals were more likely to suffer from mental illness. Those with four or more ACE categories had a statistically significant 4.9 times increased risk of having had an episode of depression, and attempting suicide of over 12.2 times when the effects of age, gender, race, and educational attainment are controlled for (Felitti et al., 1998).

Numerous additional studies have looked at the relationship between exposure to ACEs, and IPV in particular, and mental health challenges in children and adults. Pelcovitz, Kaplan, DeRosa, Mandel, and Salzinger (2000) found increases in both anxiety and depression among this group. Weissman et al. (2020) showed that violence (child maltreatment and domestic violence) corresponded to a general decrease in activation of the dorsal anterior cingulate cortex and frontal pole when shown fearful or neutral faces. This decreased activation was associated with lowered general psychopathology scores two years later. These studies may indicate a general mechanism for how these early traumas lead to mental health challenges in the short and long term.

13.2.3 *Effects on Parent–Child Relationships*

In the context of IPV, the parent-child relationship cannot escape being affected. The types of harm are quite diverse. Mothers in abusive relationships often cite fear of causing harm to children as a primary reason they stay in abusive relationships (Kelly, 2009; Cravens, Whiting, & Aamar, 2015). This places the mother at ongoing risk of harm (Jack, Petrosky, & Lyons, 2018; Smith et al., 2018), and also for the children who witness a primary attachment figure being battered and mistreated (Geffner, Igelman, Zellner, & Doyle, 2014; Niolon et al., 2017). This is linked to various internalizing (depression, anxiety, and poor self-concept) and externalizing (aggression, oppositionality, and ultimately abusive romantic relationships). When this occurs early, it may be that it also interferes with the child's ability to learn how to "read" and infer the internal states (emotions, thoughts, intentions, and so forth) of others based on behavior (Asen & Fonagy, 2017).

If previously learned, it may also be associated with an inability to efficiently and effectively use this very basic skill (Asen & Fonagy, 2017; Fonagy & Bateman, 2016). The consequences of this are associated with an increased risk of lifelong mental health challenges (Felitti et al., 1998).

These consequences collide in the parent-child relationship. For instance, mothers may be more frustrated with oppositional children and make poor parenting choices either overly authoritarian to control behaviors or overly permissive to protect children from the often controlling and abusiveness of the battering partner.

13.3 Current Approaches to Addressing IPV in Domestic Violence Organizations

13.3.1 Domestic Violence Agency-Based Approach

Before 1970, there were very little to no formal services for those suffering from intimate partner violence. The Battered Women's Movement, specifically the shelter movement, brought the emergence of domestic violence shelters to cities across the United States in the early to mid-1970s. Advocates were "sheltering" women fleeing from an abusive partner in their homes or within churches for temporary or "cooling off" periods before the development of shelters. Formal shelters created safe spaces for women to flee and bring their children. Service delivery was organized around providing the person fleeing from the violence with a safe place to stay. This was and remained almost always a woman with her children. With the creation of shelters came the need for funding and formalization of those interventions and services. What started as small shelters with two or three rooms for families, has grown today to large complexes in some urban areas with rooms for 100–200 families and various services for the families. These services range from short-term emergency housing assistance to long-term housing programs for two or more years. Many shelter programs now include individual and group counseling, legal assistance, employment assistance, onsite childcare and schools, children's counseling and therapy programs, and financial assistance. These comprehensive centers are focused on increasing safety for families and providing for basic needs until families can do so independently. Advocacy work is organized to address the immediate crisis needs by assessing the level of dangerousness of the relationship and crisis intervention and safety planning for the whole family. Interventions also include accessing other systems for safety such as law enforcement, civil and criminal legal systems, and immigration assistance when needed.

Emergency shelter beds are often in great demand and can be difficult to access due to being full. They typically provide short-term stays, and caseworkers and advocates assess needs and create access to resources to meet those needs so that families can move from the shelter into safe housing solutions. Many communities have short-term housing programs that provide rental assistance and case management services for families that needed longer-term support. A family is provided with up to two years of rental assistance, and the goal is to find the financial resources to sustain rent independently at the end of two years. Long-term and permanent housing programs are in lesser supply, and when available, they provide case management and support for adults who have greater needs resulting from mental or physical health conditions that warrant a more intense level of housing support. All the interventions for short, medium, and long-term housing are in great demand, often have waiting lists, and often are prioritized based on the greatest safety and vulnerability needs for families fleeing IPV. These interventions are also centered around the adult or head of household. Children's services are a part of the array of offerings specific to the child's needs. Much of the focus is on the principle of caseworkers for the adults and separate services for the child/children.

13.3.2 Evidence-Supported Interventions (California Evidence-Based Clearinghouse)

According to the California Evidence-Based Clearinghouse for Child Welfare (CEBC), there are no programs that currently meet the highest standard for being well supported by research evidence for children affected by IPV. Two programs meet the second highest level of "Supported by Research Evidence", Child-Parent Psychotherapy (CPC) and the Community Advocacy Project (CAP) (CEBC, 2021a).

CPC is designed for children ages 0–5 and their caregivers. The non-offending caregiver and the child are treated together weekly over about one year by a trained mental health professional. The goal of the treatment is to foster the parent-child relationship to build support systems for the child's mental health. The program is cognizant of the parent-child social environment context, and this is considered in treatment. The therapist helps the parent and child create a narrative of the violence together and address triggers that lead to behavioral problems (CEBC, 2021b). Special attention is paid to safety, affect regulation, reciprocity in relationships, focus on traumatic events, continuity of daily living, and reflective supervision (CEBC, 2021b).

Several studies have demonstrated support for improved parental empathic response (Lieberman, Weston, & Pawl, 1991), improved emotional regulation (Lieberman et al., 1991), higher levels of secure attachment (Cicchetti, Toth, & Rogosch, 1999; Cicchetti, Rogosh & Toth, 2006; Stronach, Toth, Rogosch, & Cicchetti, 2013), reductions in negative self-representations (Toth, Maughan, Manly, Spagnola, & Cicchetti, 2002), decrease in PTSD symptoms (Lieberman, Van Horn, & Ghosh Ippen, 2005), and a decrease in parental stress (Toth, Sturge-Apple, Rogosch, & Cicchetti, 2015). Additionally, Guild, Toth, Handley, Fogosch, and Cicchetti (2017) found that not only was there a lasting decrease in insecure attachment, but this was also associated with better peer relationships seven to eight years later.

CAP is a home- and community-based program that seeks to link women and their children with appropriate services which seek to increase women's quality of life and decrease the likelihood of future violence (CEBC, 2021c). The program is designed to be provided to women and children affected by IPV over 10 weeks of four to six hours per week. It seeks to increase child self-competence and decrease women's depression while increasing women's quality of life, access to resources, social support, and safety (CEBC, 2021c). The services are tailored to the community setting and are home-based. The provider, often an extensively trained paraprofessional, seeks to demonstrate empathy while letting the client drive the process by dictating what services are provided (CEBC, 2021c). Several studies have demonstrated that the women participating in these programs experience less violence for years after their participation (Allen, Bybee, & Sullivan, 2004; Bybee & Sullivan, 2002, 2005; Sullivan & Bybee, 1999). Less evidence supports this as an intervention that directly benefits children. However, Sullivan and Bybee (1999), when used in combination with another program (the Learning Club), found there was a significant increase in the self-competence of children compared to a treatment as usual control group.

Other programs show promising research evidence, such as child-centered play therapy (Kot, Landreth, & Giordano, 1998; Ray, Schottelkorb, & Tsai, 2007) and Kids Club and Moms Empowerment (Graham-Bermann, Lynch, Banyard, DeVoe, & Halabu, 2007). However, the programs discussed, except CPC, generally do not focus on the child-parent relationship, and thus there seems to be a desire for programs like MISC to address the needs of children and their mothers.

13.4 MISC for IPV-Exposed Mothers and Children

"Trauma creates change you don't choose. Healing is about creating change you do choose."

—Michelle Rosenthall

Systematic reviews (Anderson & Van Ee, 2018; Austin, Shanahan, Barrios, & Macy, 2019) identify 19 parenting intervention studies (1992–2016) for IPV-exposed women. While these studies signal significant advancement, several limitations remain. These interventions are costly, require highly skilled mental health professionals trained in delivering the specific form of treatment, are often culturally insensitive, are not relational, and are delivered on an outpatient basis that is not accessible to homeless mothers. Interventions are typically also limited to specific age ranges. While this is developmentally appropriate, an alternative approach is to consider developmentally transportable interventions where a set of cross-developmental principles are instilled in caregivers that can generalize to other developmental periods as children mature. Notably, most interventions take a deficit-approach to the parenting of IPV-exposed mothers and children, aiming to teach mothers skills instead of leveraging existing strengths.

For all of these reasons, particularly for scalability, what is needed are community-based interventions utilizing care systems already in place. That is, the intervention must live in the community. This can be achieved by training those already in contact with families (e.g., caseworkers) to foster higher-quality caregiving, ultimately affecting both the mental health outcomes of children and their mothers. Because IPV exposure is now defined as a form of child maltreatment (Hamby, Finkelhor, Turner, & Ormrod, 2011), CPS case plans direct women to complete parent training to end CPS involvement and maintain child custody (Child Welfare Information Gateway, 2016). However, due to the expense and level of training required by the evidence-based interventions reviewed earlier, such services rarely use these interventions (Austin, Shanahan, Barrios, & Macy, 2019). Moreover, within IPV rehousing programs (which is a common IPV intervention), the focus is on housing stability, increasing income, and connection to other resources through case management. This means that caseworkers do not focus on the mother-child relationship. Consistent with extant research (Holt, Buckley, & Whelan, 2008), caseworkers do not routinely assess the effects of IPV on children and struggle to understand the dynamics of children's experiences and respond appropriately to their individual needs. Reasons for this include a knowledge, training, and skills base deficit and the seemingly incompatible theoretical approaches and dichotomous agendas of the child-focused social services mandate and the woman-focused ethos of rehousing and shelter work. It follows that there is an urgent need for training of caseworkers delivering woman-focused IPV services in how to address the needs of IPV-exposed children simultaneously. Community-based mental health can be addressed through community development (Christens, 2012), an emphasis on human care (Jordans & Tol, 2013), and task shifting ("task sharing"), where caseworkers learn new skills directly addressing shortages in human resources for mental health.

In addition, what is needed is a strengths-based intervention that plays to the existing assets in mother-child relationships. A strengths-based approach emphasizes that a positive relationship with a caring and responsive adult, usually the mother, serves as a protective buffer against the traumatizing effects of IPV exposure (*Centers for Disease Control and Prevention, I. P. C. Preventing Child Abuse and Neglect*, 2021; Holt et al., 2008). Many abused women internalize a model of healthy parenting that predates their abuse, and can locate their caregiving from this earlier experience with appropriate help. Children themselves cite mothers as "their most important source of help than anyone else in their lives" (Mullender et al., 2002). Indeed, among IPV-exposed children, those who had mothers with better parenting skills were more resilient against negative outcomes (Graham-Bermann, Gruber, Howell, & Girz, 2009). We propose here that the Mediational Intervention for Sensitizing Caregivers (MISC; Klein, 1996) can scaffold mothers' capacity to act as a buffer against the adverse effects of IPV trauma on children, harnessing the expressed desire of mothers to protect and care for children as they navigate the adverse effects of IPV trauma on themselves and their children (Levendosky & Graham-Bermann, 2000).

MISC is an evidence-based, semi-structured intervention that was developed to restore disrupted caregiving practices and, in turn, enhance mental health and cognitive outcomes for youth. In MISC, socio-emotional and cognitive learning opportunities arise in the course of natural everyday caregiver/child interactions. MISC is highly suitable for cross-cultural adaptation because it does not depend on importing Western-based methods, ideas, and tools and operates inside existing cultural caregiving practices. It is also highly adaptable across developmental periods because MISC was developed to flexibly adapt to different contexts. As outlined in Chapter 1 of this volume, MISC is theoretically grounded in Bowlby's theory of attachment and Feuerstein's theory of cognitive modifiability. We will not reiterate the MISC model here, but will highlight that IPV-exposed children experience attachment disruption and toxic trauma and stress levels. Their mothers similarly undergo immense stress in navigating homelessness and the rupture of their own attachment relationships. Vulnerability and stress are further compounded if mothers and children are victims of social determinants of ill health. MISC builds resilience by scaffolding the caregiving capacity of IPV-exposed mothers to protect their children against trauma's negative effects. MISC does not require a mother to do any new activities with children but changes the nature of everyday interactions with children ("serve and return"). In the same way that we invest in math literacy, reading literacy, or nutrition literacy, MISC provides a vehicle for investing in the "literacy of interaction", thereby providing a much-needed "mental diet" for children, interrupting the intergenerational transmission of IPV.

Our group has begun to adapt MISC for the IPV context. In 2018, a partnership was forged between the University of Houston and the Harris County Domestic Violence Care Collaborative (HCDVCC) to lay the groundwork for a randomized control trial to assess the effectiveness of MISC in a population of IPV exposed mothers and children. Four HCDVCC caseworkers underwent the three-day MISC training. Questionnaires and interviews assessed attitudes, initial feasibility, and acceptability of MISC. This small-scale investigation revealed that caseworkers feel frustrated by their sole function of rehousing/employment when the effects of IPV exposure on parenting were so visible. They expressed appreciation of the MISC approach to combine the needs of children alongside the family's material needs.

Additionally, eight interviews were conducted with mothers who had experienced IPV. Fifty percent of those interviewed were Black, 25% White, and 12.5% Hispanic, and 12.5% wished not to report their race/ethnicity. All of the mothers interviewed had a child between the ages of 7 and 11. In these interviews, MISC was presented to the mothers, and feedback was solicited. Comprehensive qualitative analysis of these interviews is currently in progress, but preliminary results reveal that these mothers noticed changes in their relationships and interactions with their children due to their abuse. According to one mother, "it changes how you view the world. And obviously, it's going to change how you parent your children." According to another mother, mothers expressed a desire to improve these interactions that are often based on "negativity and worry", according to another mother. Mothers reported that they worried about their children's future and felt that a program like MISC would help "break the cycle" and allow their children to "raise their children better when they're parents". Mothers felt that receiving support from not only their caseworker, but also other mothers who had experienced abuse, would be valuable for their relationships with their children, as well as their own mental health. Another mother reported feeling "isolated, alone, like I'm the only one going through this". This mother also expressed that to "hear that there are other women out there who are going through the same thing and seeing them flourishing and getting better and parenting their kids better" would encourage and empower her to do the same.

13.5 Conclusion

"Alone we can do so little, together we can do so much."

—Helen Keller

Relationships have the power to create positive change. When interventions are focused on building relationships, and time, energy, and resources are dedicated to building relationships, might there be great promise for increased learning and family healing? Domestic violence organizations are tasked with meeting the crisis needs of families fleeing IPV. Much of the focus of the interventions is centered on immediate access to increasing safety through housing, civil legal remedies, and criminal justice advocacy. There is a great opportunity to apply interventions that work with the parent-child relationship to improve long-term outcomes for children. MISC is a promising program that gives much hope to practitioners and parents. It shifts the focus to what mothers have great concern about, their sense and need to be good parents to their children, and their need to ensure healthy environments for their children to grow physically, mentally, socially, and cognitively. When mothers living with the trauma of IPV cannot access their internal assets to support their children, the trauma of violence intensifies and deepens, and what mothers feared most—harm to their children—happens. MISC is a program that has the potential to restore hope.

References

Allen, N. E., Bybee, D. I., & Sullivan, C. M. (2004). Battered women's multitude of needs: Evidence supporting the need for comprehensive advocacy. *Violence Against Women, 10*(9), 1015–1035.

Anderson, K., & Van Ee, E. (2018). Mothers and children exposed to intimate partner violence: A review of treatment interventions. *International Journal of Environmental Research and Public Health, 15*(9), 1955.

Asen, F., & Fonagy, P. (2017). Mentalizing family violence part 1: Conceptual framework. *Family Process, 56*(1), 6–21.

Austin, A. E., Shanahan, M. E., Barrios, Y. V., & Macy, R. J. (2019). A systematic review of interventions for women parenting in the context of intimate partner violence. *Trauma, Violence, & Abuse, 20*(4), 498–519.

Bowleg, L. (2012). The problem with the phrase women and minorities: Intersectionality—an important theoretical framework for public health. *American Journal of Public Health, 102*(7), 1267–1273.

Bybee, D. I., & Sullivan, C. M. (2002). The process through which an advocacy intervention resulted in positive changes for women over time. *American Journal of Community Psychology, 30*(1), 103–132.

Bybee, D., & Sullivan, C. M. (2005). Predicting re-victimization of battered women 3 years after exiting a shelter program. *American Journal of Community Psychology, 36*(1–2), 85–96.

California Evidence Based Clearinghouse. (2021a). *Domestic/intimate partner violence: Services for victims and their children.* Retrieved January 10, 2021, from www.cebc4cw.org/topic/domestic-intimate-partner-violence-services-for-women-and-their-children.

California Evidence Based Clearinghouse. (2021b). *Child-parent psychotherapy.* Retrieved January 18, 2021, from www.cebc4cw.org/program/child-parent-psychotherapy/

California Evidence Based Clearinghouse. (2021c). *The community action project (CAP).* Retrieved January 18, 2021, from www.cebc4cw.org/program/the-community-advocacy-project/

Campbell, J., Webster, D., & Glass, N. (2009). The danger assessment: Validation of a lethality risk assessment instrument for intimate partner femicide. *Journal of Interpersonal Violence, 24*(4), 653–674.

Carbado, D., Crenshaw, K., Mays, V., & Tomlinson, B. (2013). Intersectionality: Mapping the movements of a theory. *Du Bois Review: Social Science Research on Race, 10*(2), 303–312.

Center for Disease Control and Prevention, I. P. C. (2020, October 9). *Intimate partner violence.* www.cdc.gov/violenceprevention/intimatepartnerviolence/index.html

Centers for Disease Control and Prevention, I. P. C. (2021, March 15). *Preventing child abuse and neglect.* www.cdc.gov/violenceprevention/childabuseandneglect/fastfact.html

Child Welfare Information Gateway. (2016). *Child witnesses to domestic violence.* Washington, DC: U.S. Department of Health and Human Services, Children's Bureau.

Christens, B. D. (2012). Targeting empowerment in community development: A community psychology approach to enhancing local power and wellbeing. *Community Development Journal, 47*(4), 538–554.

Cicchetti, D., Rogosh, F. A., & Toth, S. L. (2006). Fostering secure attachment in infants in maltreating families through preventive interventions. *Development and Psychopathology, 18*, 623–649.

Cicchetti, D., Toth, S. L., & Rogosch, F. A. (1999). The efficacy of toddler-parent psychotherapy to increase attachment security in off-spring of depressed mothers. *Attachment & Human Development, 1*(1), 34–66.

Cravens, W., Whiting, J. B., & Aamar, R. O. (2015). Why I stayed/left: An analysis of voices of intimate partner violence on social media. *Contemporary Family Therapy, 37*(4), 372–385. https://doi.org/10.1007/s10591-015-9360-8

Crenshaw, K. (1991). Mapping the margins: Intersectionality, identity politics, and violence against women of color. *Stanford Law Review, 43*, 1241–1299.

Dichter, M. E., Thomas, K. A., Crits-Christoph, P., Ogden, S. N., & Rhodes, K. V. (2018). Coercive control in intimate partner violence: Relationship with women's experience of violence, use of violence, and danger. *Psychology of Violence, 8*(5), 596–604.

Dobash, R. E., & Dobash, R. (1979). *Violence against wives: A case against the patriarchy.* New York: Free Press.

Felitti, V. J., Anda, R. F., Nordenberg, D., Williamson, D. F., Spitz, A. M., Edwards, V., . . . Marks, J. S. (1998). Relationship of childhood abuse and household dysfunction to many of the leading causes of death in Adults: The adverse childhood experiences (ACE) study. *American Journal of Preventive Medicine, 14*(4), 245–258.

Fonagy, P., & Bateman, A. W. (2016). Adversity, attachment, and mentalizing. *Comprehensive Psychiatry, 64*, 59–66.

Geffner, R., Igelman, R., Zellner, J., & Doyle, M. (2014). *The effects of intimate partner violence on children.* London: Routledge.

Gilroy, H., McFarlane, J., Fredland, N., Cesario, S., Nava, A., & Maddoux, J. (2018). Using a model of economic solvency to understand the connection between economic factors and intimate partner violence. *Journal of International Women's Studies, 19*(6), 305–325.

Gilroy, H., McFarlane, J., Maddoux, J., & Sullivan, C. (2016). Homelessness, housing instability, intimate partner violence, mental health, and functioning: A multi-year cohort study of IPV survivors and their children. *Journal of Social Distress and the Homeless, 25*(2), 86–94.

Gondolf, E. W. (2010). The contributions of Ellen Pence to batterer programming. *Violence Against Women, 16*(9), 992–1006.

Graham-Bermann, S. A., Gruber, G., Howell, K. H., & Girz, L. (2009). Factors discriminating among profiles of resilience and psychopathology in children exposed to intimate partner violence (IPV). *Child Abuse & Neglect, 33*(9), 648–660.

Graham-Bermann, S. A., Lynch, D., Banyard, V., DeVoe, E. R., & Halabu, H. (2007). Community-based intervention for children exposed to intimate partner violence: An efficacy trial. *Journal of Consulting and Clinical Psychology, 75*(2), 199–209.

Guild, D., Toth, S., Handley, E. D., Fogosch, F. A., & Cicchetti, D. (2017). Attachment security mediates the longitudinal association between child-parent psychotherapy and peer relations for toddlers of depressed mothers. *Development and Psychopathology, 29*(2), 587–600.

Hamby, S., Finkelhor, D., Turner, H., & Ormrod, R. (2011). *Children's exposure to intimate partner violence and other family violence: (725322011–001)* [Data set]. American Psychological Association. https://doi.org/10.1037/e725322011-001

Holt, S., Buckley, H., & Whelan, S. (2008). The impact of exposure to domestic violence on children and young people: A review of the literature. *Child Abuse & Neglect, 32*(8), 797–810.

Jack, S. P., Petrosky, E., & Lyons, B. H. (2018). Surveillance for violent deaths—national violent death reporting system, 27 states, 2015. *MMWR Surveillance Summaries, 67*(SS–11), 1–32. http://dx.doi.org/10.15585/mmwr.ss6711a1external

Jordans, M. J., & Tol, W. A. (2013). Mental health in humanitarian settings: Shifting focus to care systems. *International Health, 5*(1), 9–10.

Jouriles, E. N., & McDonald, R. (2015). Intimate partner violence, coercive control, and child adjustment problems. *Journal of Interpersonal Violence, 30*(3), 459–474.

Kelly, U. A. (2009). "I'm a mother first": The influence of mothering in the decision-making processes of battered immigrant Latino women. *Research in Nursing & Health, 32*(3), 286–297.

Klein, P. S. (1996). *Early intervention: Cross-cultural experiences with a mediational approach.* New York: Garland Publishing.

Kot, S., Landreth, G. L., & Giordano, M. (1998). Intensive child-centered play therapy with child witnesses of domestic violence. *International Journal of Play Therapy, 7*(2), 17–36.

Levendosky, A. A., & Graham-Bermann, S. A. (2000). Behavioral observations of parenting in battered women. *Journal of Family Psychology, 14*(1), 80.

Lieberman, A. F., Van Horn, P., & Ghosh Ippen, C. (2005). Toward evidence-based treatment: Child-parent psychotherapy with preschoolers exposed to marital violence. *Journal of the American Academy of Child and Adolescent Psychiatry, 44*(12), 1241–1448.

Lieberman, A. F., Weston, D. R., & Pawl, J. H. (1991). Preventive interaction and outcome with anxiously attached dyads. *Child Development, 62*, 199–209.

McFarlane, J., Fredland, N. M., Symes, L., Zhou, W., Jouriles, E. N., Dutton, M. A., & Greeley, C. S. (2017). The intergenerational impact of intimate partner violence against mothers on child functioning over four years. *Journal of Family Violence, 32*(7), 645–655.

Mehrotra, G. (2010). Toward a continuum of intersectionality theorizing for feminist social work scholarship. *Affilia, 25*(4), 417–430.

Modi, M. N., Palmer, S., & Armstrong, A. (2014). The role of violence against women act in addressing intimate partner violence: A public health issue. *Journal of Women's Health, 23*(3), 253–259.

Morgan, R. E., & Oudekerk, B. A. (2019). *Criminal victimization, 2018*. Bureau of Justice Statistics. Retrieved from www.bjs.gov/content/pub/pdf/cv18.pdf

Mullender, A., Hague, G., Imam, U. F., Kelly, L., Malos, E., & Regan, L. (2002). *Children's perspectives on domestic violence*. London: Sage.

National Coalition Against Domestic Violence. (n.d.). *Statistics.* https://ncadv.org/STATISTICS#:~:text=1%20in%2015%20children%20are,are,%20eyewitnesses%20to%20this%20violence

National Network to End Domestic Violence. (2020). *14th annual domestic violence counts report*. Retrieved from www.NNEDV.org/DVCounts.org

Niolon, P. H., Kearns, M., Dills, J., Rambo, K., Irving, S., Armstead, T., & Gilbert, L. (2017). *Preventing intimate partner violence across the lifespan: A technical package of programs, policies and practices*. Atlanta, GA: National Center for Injury Prevention and Control, Centers for Disease Control and Prevention.

Pelcovitz, D., Kaplan, S. J., DeRosa, R. R., Mandel, F. S., & Salzinger, S. (2000). Psychiatric disorders in adolescents exposed to domestic violence and physical abuse. *American Journal of Orthopsychiatry, 70*(3), 360–369.

Ray, D. C., Schottelkorb, A., & Tsai, M. H. (2007). Play therapy with children exhibiting symptoms of attention deficit hyperactivity disorder. *International Journal of Play Therapy, 16*(2), 95–111.

Smith, S. G., Zhang, X., Basile, K. C., Merrick, M. T., Wang, J., Kresnow, M., & Chen, J. (2018). *The national intimate partner and sexual violence Survey (NISVS): 2015 data brief—updated release*. Atlanta, GA: National Center for Injury Prevention and Control, Centers for Disease Control and Prevention.

Stronach, E. P., Toth, S. L., Rogosch, F., & Cicchetti, D. (2013). Preventive interventions and sustained attachment security in maltreated children. *Development and Psychopathology, 25*(4), 919–930.

Sullivan, C. M., & Bybee, D. I. (1999). Reducing violence using community-based advocacy for women with abusive partners. *Journal of Consulting and Clinical Psychology, 67*(1), 43–53.

Symes, L., McFarlane, J., Maddoux, J., & Fredland, N. (2020). Evaluating an intergenerational model to explain the path from violence against mothers to child behavior and academic outcomes. *Violence Against Women, 26*(6–7), 730–749.

Thompson-Booth, C., Viding, E., Puetz, V., Rutherford, H., Mayes, L., & McCrory, C. (2019). Ghosts in the nursery: An experimental investigation of a parent's own maltreatment experience, attention to infant faces, and dyadic reciprocity. *Emotion, 19*(6), 1093–1102.

Toth, S. L., Maughan, A., Manly, J. T., Spagnola, M., & Cicchetti, D. (2002). The relative efficacy of two interventions in altering maltreated preschool children's representational models: Implications for attachment theory. *Development and Psychopathology, 14*, 877–908.

Toth, S. L., Sturge-Apple, M. L., Rogosch, F. A., & Cicchetti, D. (2015). Mechanisms of change: Testing how preventative interventions impact psychological and physiological stress functioning in mothers in neglectful families. *Development and Psychopathology, 27*(4pt2), 1661–1674.

Vargas, L. Cataldo, J., & Dickson, S. (2005). Domestic violence and children. In G. R. Walz & R. K. Yep (Eds.), *VISTAS: Compelling perspectives on counseling* (pp. 67–69). Alexandria, VA: American Counseling Association.

Walby, S., & Allen, J. (2004). *Domestic violence, sexual assault and stalking: Findings from the British crime survey.* Home Office Research Study 276. London: Home Office.

Walby, S., & Towers, J. (2017, May). Measuring violence to end violence: Mainstreaming gender. *Journal of Gender-Based Violence, 1*(1), 11–31.

Walton, Q. L., & Oyewuwo-Gassikia, O. (2017). The case for #BlackGirlMagic: Application of a strengths-based intersectional practice framework for working with Black women with depression. *Affilia, 32*(4), 461–475.

Warshaw, C., Brashler, P., & Gil, J. (2009). Mental health consequences of intimate partner violence. In C. Mitchell & D. Anglin (Eds.), *Intimate partner violence: A health-based perspective* (pp. 147–171). Oxford: Oxford University Press.

Wathen, C. N., & Macmillan, H. L. (2013). Children's exposure to intimate partner violence: Impacts and interventions. *Paediatric Child Health, 18*(8), 419–422.

Weissman, D. G., Jenness, J. L., Colich, N. L., Miller, A. B., Sambrook, K. A., Sheridan, M. A., & McLaughlin, K. A. (2020). Altered neural processing of threat-related information in children and adolescents exposed to violence: A transdiagnostic mechanism contributing to the emergence of psychopathology. *Journal of the American Academy of Child & Adolescent Psychiatry, 59*(11), 1274–1284.

World Health Organization. (2002). *World report on violence and health* (Krug, E. G., et al., Eds.). Geneva: WHO.

World Health Organization. (2004). *The economic dimensions of intimate partner violence.* Retrieved from http://apps.who.int/iris/bitstream/10665/42944/1/9241591609.pdf

World Health Organization, Understanding and Addressing Violence Against Women. (2010). Retrieved from https://apps.who.int/iris/bitstream/handle/10665/77431/WHO_RHR_12.43_eng.pdf;jsessionid=7FEA31070227FF35E6DE9DF0FCEFBB02?sequence=1

14 Considerations for Implementing MISC as Part of Asset-Based Community Development

Lochner Marais, Kholisa Rani and Molefi Lenka

14.1 Introduction

There is substantial agreement that investing in children has life-long benefits for society. The emphasis on the first 1000 days has now become conventional wisdom, but the argument for investing in children goes beyond the first 1000 days. Consequently, programmes have been developed to improve parenting skills and thus the developmental outcomes and socio-emotional health of children. However, in the Global South many children grow up in dysfunctional households and without their parents. The HIV&AIDS pandemic and poverty have been the leading disrupters. To some degree, looking after orphans and vulnerable children has become a community responsibility.

The South African government funds a range of community-based organisations (CBOs) that provide additional services to families and children. One such funding stream is for CBOs that provide after-school care for orphans and vulnerable children. Most of these CBOs give the children an afternoon meal. Some provide social services, such as identifying abuse, helping children obtain a birth certificate or assisting with homework. The question is whether these qualify as services or whether they should be seen as community development work (Marais et al., 2018). As a concept, community development has been debated in the literature and has changed in context and approach in recent years. The notion of asset-based community development (ABCD) has risen to prominence over the past two decades. The overall aim of ABCD is to build on existing assets rather than emphasise needs.

This chapter discusses the potential of MISC (Mediational Intervention for Sensitising Caregivers) as a candidate for ABCD. We argue that some of the basic principles of ABCD make it possible to view MISC as an asset-based intervention. To discuss this, we use evidence from a three-year-long MISC programme in a low-resource setting in South Africa and conducted with children who attend a typical after-school care facility.

14.2 Community Development and Assets

Community development has a long history which has been discussed extensively elsewhere. Here we focus on the history and development of

DOI: 10.4324/9781003145899-14

ABCD and explain how it differs from needs-based approaches. Many needs-based approaches originate from government and non-governmental approaches to community development in the 1970s and 1980s. For Mathie and Cunningham (2003, p. 474), the value of ABCD as opposed to needs-based community development "lies in its premise that people in communities can organise to drive the development process themselves by identifying and mobilising existing (but often unrecognised) assets, thereby responding to and creating local economic opportunity". In ABCD, the emphasis is on the skills, associations and networks that communities already have, on which community development workers can build.

ABCD is an alternative to needs-based approaches. Needs-based approaches are based on a needs analysis, which determines the gap between reality and what people need. These approaches often characterise communities in negative and deficit-oriented terms (McKnight & Kretzmann, 2012).

A focus on needs could disempower communities and increase the need for welfare services. It can create the impression that government, business or society can fix societal problems. The assumption that external agents can fix problems can weaken local organisations and encourage external organisations to maintain the dependency to maintain their roles (Mathie & Cunningham, 2005). Other concerns include an expectation that local leadership should attract funding from external sources. This requirement has two unintended consequences: to attract the funding, communities and their leadership are obliged to portray themselves as needy, and often a transactional relationship develops between the communities and the funders (Mathie & Cunningham, 2003). All of this helps to create the impression that change is only possible through outside agents. Funding organisations also often develop their funding criteria according to levels of need. The more needy a community can make itself appear, the more funding it is likely to receive. Although very few practitioners will acknowledge that they take a needs-based approach, the assumption that such an approach is necessary remains inherent in many community development programmes. Mathie and Cunningham (2003, p. 475) argue that ABCD is "more likely to inspire positive action for change in a community" because it is based on recognizing strengths and assets rather than focusing exclusively on needs and problems.

What are community assets? Forrester, Kurth, Vincent, and Oliver (2020, p. 444) define them as typically "physical, tangible resources or spaces in communities (such as schools, parks and recreational areas, religious places of worship, sports facilities, community centres, etc.) as well as the more intangible personal and social qualities". Kretzman and McKnight (1993) note that ABCD focuses on relationships, strengths, dialogue and partnerships. ABCD theory begins by mapping the positive capabilities of communities and emphasising "where communities are at", rather than being idealistic about how development should take place (Forrester et al., 2020). Proponents of ABCD all emphasise the existing capacities (assets). Mathie and Cunningham (2003) list four important points for implementing ABCD: constructing shared meaning, emphasising social capital, developing and recognising community economic capacity, and managing the distribution of power.

The ABCD approach has been widely applied since the early 1990s, particularly in the US but more recently in the UK. Public health interventions have used it extensively (Friedli, 2013; Stuteley & Cohen, 2014), for three reasons: to bring about behaviour change, to save costs (community-based approaches can reduce the load on the hospitals) and to promote good health and well-being rather than just prevent disease. The ABCD approach is attractive for achieving these goals and long-term change, but it does require community consent. Table 14.1 provides a comparison of needs-based community development and ABCD.

ABCD has not escaped criticism. Three points of criticism dominate. It has been accused of neoliberalism in its emphasis on individualism and privatisation (Macleod & Emejulu, 2014). Seen as a way to reduce the role of the state by overemphasising the community's role, it has attracted this criticism particularly in the US, where government programmes do not always receive acknowledgement. It has been accused of underplaying the structural reasons for poverty and inequality (Missingham, 2017). And because of its inherent inward-looking focus, it has been accused of being vulnerable to outside control (Owen & Kemp, 2012). Among other criticisms, it has also been accused of lacking an evidence base and theoretical depth (Ennis & West, 2010). In response, some researchers have argued that the problem is not ABCD per se, but the way it gets applied (Garven, MacLean, & Pattoni,

Table 14.1 Comparing needs-based community development and ABCD

Needs-Based Community Development and Typical International Development	*ABCD*
Focusing on community deficiencies	Focus on community assets
Problem response/Technical solutions	Opportunity identification/Assets are a springboard
Charity in favour of orientation	Investment and right orientation
Experts provide solutions in a one-way exchange	Solutions devised in mutual exchange/ technical ally
Grants to agencies/government/ overseer	Grants, investments, volunteer support to associations
Service needs to be determined outside the community	Service needs to be determined inside the community
High emphasis on government's role	High emphasis on community role
People as beneficiaries	People as citizens, co-creators in control
The aim is to "fix people"	It aims to develop potential in people
Root concerns are developing territories	The root concern is developing people
Programmes as the answer	People as the answer
The main concern at project conclusion: maintenance	The main concern at project conclusion: what is next?

Source: CatCom, 2021

2016). Often, application means a fall back into a needs-based approach or the development workers not doing enough the listen and create dialogue.

ABCD has also faced implementation difficulties (Mathie & Cunningham, 2003). The focus on community-driven processes prompts questions about what the role of external organisations is. Most external organisations find it difficult to play a facilitative role and not create dependencies. It can be difficult to create inclusive partnerships, because unequal power relationships can be hard to manage. Sustained community leadership is often not available. And creating institutional environments and trust is not easy.

14.3 MISC and ABCD

We do not repeat here the detailed conceptual framework for MISC (see Chapter 2), but we emphasise two points: that MISC deals with not only children's cognitive development but also their socio-emotional development and mental health, and that MISC can be applied by community workers, teachers and parents. Our application of MISC with CBOs gave us the idea of merging MISC with ABCD. Here we identify and discuss five critical aspects of MISC that we believe make the merger a good idea: its sensitivity to culture, the way it can be integrated into existing programmes, the possibility of in-service training, the mediation between child and caregiver, and the focus on relating directly to the child.

Sensitivity to the existing culture has advantages in community development. It reduces the risk of making value judgements, and is thus in line with the ABCD emphasis on dialogue and respect for the existing situation. Being sensitive to culture also minimises the need for MISC practitioners to aim for an ideal state of development or culture. A typical MISC engagement will start with a dialogue with parents (or teachers and community workers) about what *they* view as an ideal child and *their* dreams for the children. In contrast, a programme based on a needs-based approach would start by explaining to parents the development deficit of their children and the importance of filling this gap. The focus on understanding, dialogue and building on assets in ABCD could easily be transferred to MISC, where such an approach is central, particularly not judging culture or behaviour.

Having no strict prescribed implementation plan with pre-set times and activities, MISC can be integrated into existing programmes. Caregivers (parents, guardians, careworkers or teachers) must use normal day-to-day activities to apply the principles of MISC. Teachers need not teach differently or set aside time for MISC, but can integrate it into their daily interactions with children. Parents need not allocate specific times to MISC, and CBOs need not adjust their programmes or activities to make room for MISC. The initial dialogue about the ideal child also includes discussion about the existing interactions between children and the caregiver. An understanding of these interactions provides the foundation on which to build. Effectively, MISC builds on existing interactions, while ABCD builds on assets—the principle is the same (focusing on strengths rather than needs or weaknesses).

To apply MISC requires training, but participants learn through in-service training and applying MISC in everyday interactions with children. No separate course takes them away from home or out of the classroom. This means that whoever takes on MISC can determine when and where such training can take place. Participants can integrate MISC training sessions into household duties or into field and garden work in rural communities. Once again, MISC builds on existing activities, similar to ABCD's building on strengths and assets.

For the children, learning takes place through mediation, a two-way process between them and the caregiver. This emphasis on process as opposed to just outcome is also central to ABCD. Like community agency, learning agency can develop not through direction but through facilitation or mediation. Mediating experiences are at the heart of MISC and are similar to facilitation in community development. This focus on process and medication in MISC is similar to the principle of dialogue and understanding in ABCD.

To improve children's mental health, MISC emphasises the need for the caregiver to relate to the child by, for example, making eye contact and smiling. To some degree, it is about building an appropriate partnership between child and caregiver. MISC teaches caregivers to convey three essential messages (see Chapter 2):

- That it is worthwhile to act and the child experiences that "I can do".
- That the caregiver is with the child and the child experiences that "I am safe".
- That the caregiver loves the child and the child experiences that "I am loved".

Partnerships are also central to ABCD, though at the community level.

14.4 Methods

We implemented a MISC programme with two CBOs in a low-resource setting, the former black township of Bloemfontein, Mangaung, in the Mangaung Metropolitan Municipality, from 2016 to 2018. The project created the opportunity to work with existing community structures and their existing programmes. The overall study was part of a quasi-experimental trial implemented by the University of the Free State and the University of Houston in partnership (Sharp et al., 2021). The two CBOs provided eight careworkers for the programme, all of them from the surrounding communities and speaking the local languages. These careworkers worked without a salary. Among other services, they usually provided the children with a meal (mostly funded by the Department of Social Development) in the afternoon after school. The project provided the two CBOs with R2800[1] a month each (in addition to any other funding they received, for example from the government). We required the CBOs to provide the children with food in the afternoon. They used our funds if they did not have an allocation from the Department of Social Development.

The project management employed two trainers who spoke the local language to teach MISC to the careworkers. The trainers themselves underwent an in-service training session between April 2016 and March 2017, run by well-established MISC experts. The careworkers received in-service training, in the form of one-on-one sessions, from the trainers during years two and three of the programme and did not have to attend any formal training. We measured progress with the implementation of MISC by videoing careworkers with individual children at baseline, six months and one year.

14.5 Results and Discussion

The results of the intervention for children's mental health outcomes are discussed elsewhere in this volume (Chapter 8.). Here, we discuss the results in terms of community developmental outcomes. The project was essentially an intervention. It was developed outside the community and applied with the consent of the two CBOs. We thus did not start with extensive dialogue and discussions with the broader community. However, our initial workshop with CBOs and establishing a Community Advisory Board (CAB) have been attempts to create initial dialogue. There were other ways in which we used a contractual rather than relational arrangements. For example, the small financial contribution to the CBOs ensured that the CBOs provided food and constituted a contract with the CBOs. Despite these elements that reflect the contractual arrangements like the provision of meals and services, we argue that the evidence from the programme shows that MISC lends itself to ABCD. Although we implemented the project from the outside, we argue that it nevertheless proved suitable for being implemented through more appropriate community development processes, and we consulted extensively with the CAB during the adaptation of MISC for the local context. We list next seven factors from our experience to support this claim.

First, in implementing MISC, we did not require the community to set up a new structure to apply MISC. We used existing CBOs (assets) that provide services in the community. The community already trusted these CBOs and valued their work, especially in providing food to children after school. A meeting with legal guardians, arranged by the CBOs, to discuss the implementation of MISC, did not raise any significant concerns. The main issue we had to explain to legal guardians had to do with whether their children would benefit from the money we paid the CBOs to provide meals in the afternoon. They asked whether their children would benefit from the food if they were not formally part of the study. We assured legal guardians that the project money paid to the CBOs was for all children attending the afternoon care.

Second, we did start with dialogue with the CBOs and instituted a CAB to understand the current situation and services at the CBOs. The small financial incentive that we provided did appear to play a role in persuading the CBOs to participate. However, our central contractual arrangement was for the provision of food (something we did monitor). Once the CBOs had agreed to participate, we were able to have open discussions about what they did, why they did it, what they view as their ideal child and what their ultimate goals for the children were. We used two methods to elicit this information: we interviewed each careworker before the implementation, and the trainers held discussions with the careworkers to discover how the careworkers view the children and what the daily programme at the CBOs is. These conversations were part of the continued dialogue to understand and build on existing assets, as opposed to merely applying a programme for the CBOs. During these interviews, we found that the careworkers tried very hard to convince us of the levels of deprivation in the community. In their minds, they had to showcase high levels of poverty to ensure that we would see deprivation. They were also swift to point out the limitations of their kitchens. Although our trainers did listen to these needs assessments, they tried rather to see how they could work with the existing arrangements. We never invested in any new kitchen equipment despite some of the needs being legitimate. Our initial conversations showed that much effort goes into making the meals. This was understandable as the Department of Social Development and our programme required it from the CBOs. The careworkers also listed many services they provided on behalf of government departments. Examples included obtaining birth certificates or dealing with and reporting child abuse. They also said they helped children with their homework and sometimes played with the children. Providing care was central to their existing programmes and MISC fitted into this. In applying MISC, our trainers did not require the CBO careworkers to develop a new daily programme. Instead, they used making meals (dishing up and cleaning up afterwards), doing homework and playing with children as activities into which MISC had to be integrated—a good example of building on assets.

Third, as mentioned in the literature review, health interventions tend to find common ground with ABCD. The literature points to the cost savings in healthcare and the importance of obtaining consent for behaviour change during health interventions. However, this focus on cost savings could also quickly change the emphasis to providing services rather than concentrating on community development. Although we did not manage to escape this danger entirely, our overall focus was on getting the careworkers to apply MISC appropriately irrespective of the outcomes for the children.

Fourth, we focused on developing a partnership with CBOs and the careworkers. Although we could not avoid the formal contract for the food which ensured that the careworkers carried out the terms of the contract, our trainers developed an excellent relationship with the careworkers. These relationships were built on a one-on-one basis, and in the post-programme interviews some of the careworkers referred to the trainers as their "sisters". These good relationships were achieved through the initial dialogue and making an effort to understand the existing context and culture.

Fifth, many needs-based programmes tend to overwhelm community workers and take up a large amount of their time. In our programme, every two weeks the MISC trainers required one hour from each of the careworkers individually and one hour of group work. Thus, although the careworkers had to integrate aspects of MISC from day one, they spent only two hours every two weeks formally learning the approach. Although they were initially afraid of these sessions, our post-evaluation interviews suggest that towards the end of the programme they were eagerly anticipating them. Our trainers kept a low profile by listening rather than leading and by supporting rather than instructing.

Sixth, as we have already argued, the focus in MISC on cultural sensitivity links well with ABCD. For example, although we knew that corporal punishment is a feature of the society we worked in (despite being unlawful), we did not discuss this with the careworkers. We did not make any normative judgements. However, there was one issue that did spark a debate. Because of the authoritative nature of the community we worked in, children are taught not to look adults in the eye when they talk to them. In contrast, MISC requires eye contact. Although our trainers did not force it at the beginning, we slowly managed to get the careworkers to encourage the children to look them in the eye. We could see this in the videos. In the end, the careworkers thought that it elicited much better responses from the children.

Finally, we think the programme was well accepted, for several reasons, such as the overall training approach described earlier, the valuable role the trainers played, and the non-intrusive nature of MISC (using existing programmes, taking only two hours of careworkers' time every second week, not challenging cultural practices). Further feasibility and acceptability results are presented in Rani et al. (under review) and Sharp et al. (2021). Table 14.2 next compares ABCD with our application of MISC.

The previous points emphasise the possibility of fit between MISC and ABCD. Despite our mostly positive findings, we do recognize some limitations. Despite the MISC principle to avoid interfering with culture, there were lengthy discussions at the community advisory meetings[2] about cultural issues. Two pertinent issues received attention: eye contact and corporal punishment. As we explained earlier, we slowly made progress in convincing the careworkers that eye contact is important. As regards corporal punishment, we did not find ourselves having to make any value judgement during the project.

14.6 Conclusion

ABCD has become a common approach to community development. Despite criticism, it is slowly replacing needs-based approaches. In contrast

Table 14.2 Comparing ABCD and the application of MISC

ABCD	ABCD Application
Focus on community assets	We used existing CBO. There was no need to create new institutions
Opportunity identification/ Assets are a springboard	The existing caregiving practices provided a base to build on. We devoted much time to understand existing programmes
Investment and right orientation	We invested in the food programme for the children. Ensuring that everybody has a meal
Solutions devised in mutual exchange/technical ally	We fostered mutual exchange through our trainers that tried to mediate interactions and the CAB that provided feedback on our existing processes
Grants, investments, volunteer support to associations	Our grants provided the CBOs to expand the volunteer support in the community
Service needs to be determined inside the community	We did not predetermine the needs and the training programme. Identifying and developing service needs were part of a process
High emphasis on community role	Throughout the programme, we valued the contribution of the CBOs and careworkers
People as citizens, co-creators in control	We placed much emphasis on listening in CAB meetings and the training process
It aims to develop potential in people	This was one of our main objectives as we tried to develop the potential of the careworkers
The root concern is developing people	This was one of our main objectives as we tried to develop the potential of the careworkers
People as the answer	This was one of our main objectives as we tried to develop the potential of the careworkers
The main concern at project conclusion: what is next?	We are in the process to expand the project, and we think the skill that careworkers developed are practised daily

to such approaches, ABCD does not start with the level of deprivation or need or make a normative judgement about the community. Instead, it starts by focusing on existing strengths and assets in communities. Despite this shift, many community development programmes still contain elements of needs-based approaches. In this chapter, we investigated the possible alignment of MISC with ABCD.

We think MISC does have a set of characteristics that align well with ABCD: being sensitive to the existing culture, not being prescriptive in implementation, using an in-service training approach, mediating and not teaching, and building appropriate relationships. Of course, all of these are not enough to ensure the adequate application of ABCD. But they do lay the foundation for ABCD. From our programme in Mangaung, we believed it was possible to implement MISC within an ABCD approach. For example, the implementation of MISC did not require the establishment of new organisations but used the existing CBOs. It was not very difficult to persuade them to take part, since we did not have to change their daily programmes or take up too much of their time. Ultimately, the programme supported their existing aim of providing care to the children. Furthermore, we started with conversations and dialogue and never judged community culture. We admit that the MISC focus on mental health (in addition to cognitive outcomes) makes it, like many other health-related programmes, comparatively easy to apply. We think we did develop a good partnership with the CBOs and MISC did not place too much pressure on their time commitments. MISC's inherent cultural sensitivity prevented a normative approach to issues like eye contact and corporal punishment. We accepted the slow change concerning eye contact. Consequently, programme acceptability was high. We believe that because MISC is about what the careworkers do anyway (care for children), and because the trainers maintain contact with the careworkers after the project and help to answer their questions, there is hope for continuity. As happens with many projects like this, the funding runs out. We were transparent about this and helped the CBOs to submit applications to other possible funders. Two years after the project conclusion, they are still functioning, which is a hopeful sign. We are not precisely clear, however, to what extent the careworkers are applying MISC. Figure 14.1 provides a conceptual framework for the application of ABCD through MISC.

Despite these achievements, we were aware of remaining elements of a needs-based approach. At an individual level, the project and its implementation still represent a form of contract requiring participants to perform specific tasks. The programme was not initially developed from within, despite building on existing strengths in the community.

In conclusion, our implementation of MISC through CBOs in Mangaung was a first attempt to think about MISC within the context of

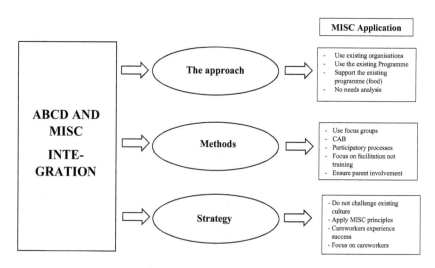

Figure 14.1 Conceptual framework for integrating ABCD and MISC

community development. Although there is much room for improvement, we believe that MISC has several inherent characteristics that make its application within ABCD possible. Of course, that approach would require less of a contractual arrangement and more of local ownership. We plan to work harder to make this possible in follow-up programmes.

Notes

1 At the time of the intervention (2017 and 2018 when the community project was implemented), the exchange rate was approximately 13.2 ZAR to 1 USD.
2 The project required the establishment of a community advisory board.

References

Catcom. (2021). *Asset-based community development*. Retrieved from https://catcomm. org/abcd/

Ennis, G., & West, D. (2010). Exploring the potential of social network analysis in ABCD practice and research. *Australian Social Work, 63*(4), 404–417.

Forrester, G., Kurth, J., Vincent, P., & Oliver, M. (2020). Schools as community assets: An exploration of the merits of an asset-based community development (ABCD) approach. *Educational Review, 72*(4), 443–458.

Friedli, L. (2013). "What we've tried, hasn't worked": The politics of assets based public health. *Critical Public Health, 23*(2), 131–145.

Garven, F., MacLean., J., & Pattoni, L. (2016). *Asset-based approaches: Their rise, role and reality*. Edinburgh: Dunedin Academic Press.

Kretzman, J., & McKnight, J. (1993). *Building communities from the inside out: A path toward finding and mobilising a community's assets*. Chicago: ACTA Publications.

Macleod, M., & Emejulu, E. (2014). Neoliberalism with a community face? A critical analysis of ABCD in Scotland. *Journal of Community Practice, 22*, 430–450.

Marais, L., Rani, K., Sharp, C., Skinner, D., Serekoane, J., Cloete, J., . . . Lenka, M. (2018). What role for community? Critical reflections on state-driven support for vulnerable children and orphans in South Africa. In L. Shevellar & P. Westoby (Eds.), *The Routledge handbook of community development* (pp. 71–83). London: Routledge.

Mathie, A., & Cunningham, G. (2003). From clients to citizens: ABCD as a strategy for community-driven development. *Development in Practice, 13*(5), 474–486.

Mathie, A., & Cunningham, G. (2005). Who is driving development? Reflections on the transformative potential of ABCD. *Canadian Journal of Development Studies, 26*(1), 175–186.

McKnight, J., & Kretzmann, J. (2012). Mapping community capacity. In M. Minkler (Ed.), *Community organising and community building for health and welfare* (pp. 171–186). New Brunswick: Rutgers University Press.

Missingham, B. (2017). Asset-based learning and the pedagogy of community development. *Community Development, 48*(3), 339–350.

Owen, J., & Kemp, D. (2012). Assets, capitals, and resources: Frameworks for corporate community development in mining. *Business & Society, 51*(3), 382–408.

Rani, K., Marais, L., Sharp, C., Cloete, J., Serekoane, M., Lenka, M., . . . Phakisi, T. (under review). The acceptability and feasibility of MISC in a low resource setting in South Africa. *International Journal of Child Care and Educational Policy*.

Sharp, C., Kulesz, P., Marais, L., Shohet, C., Rani, K., Lenka, M., . . . Boivin, M. (2021). Mediational Intervention for Sensitizing Caregivers to improve mental health outcomes in orphaned and vulnerable children. *Journal of Clinical Child and Adolescent Psychology, 49*(4), 545–557.

Stuteley, H., & Cohen, C. (2014). Community partnership for health and well-being: The Falmouth beacon project. *Journal of Integrated Care, 12*(4), 19–27.

15 Negotiating With and Situating MISC Within Context-Specific Nuances for Sustainable Use

Motsaathebe Serekoane

15.1 Introduction

Child vulnerability and the need for early childhood intervention in resource-limited settings remain a challenge (Sharp et al., 2018). Given the increase of orphanhood due to, among other things, parents dying of HIV and AIDS-related diseases, the child-rearing challenges facing communities in general—but especially those in resources-limited settings—have increased exponentially (Cluver & Gardner, 2007; Cluver, Fincham, & Seedat, 2009). We can accept that all community members recognize changing family needs to raise children in an environment that provides optimal health, safety, and learning conditions. Subsequently, the need to empower parents and community workers with skills critical to all aspects of child-care, wellbeing, learning, and development is a pressing one. Furthermore, community-based care centers cannot meet all the educational needs of young children, given their often limited resources (Jeynes, 2005). As Davis and Meltzer (2007, p. 2) state:

> When thinking about how to help parents or needy communities, it is easy to assume implicitly that helping is simply about doing something for them, providing them with the correct solution, the right answer, or appropriate advice to remove the problem.

This idea, underpinned by the so-called Expert Model (Davis, Day, & Bidmead, 2002), which is essentially normative and effectively top-down, permeates most piloting and implementation of intervention programs. Butin (2015) expressed concern that many intervention programs assume that community outreach (also phrased as community work, community engagement, community development, service-learning) is possible through, in the interest of time and efficiency, doing it for them. These efficiencies involve powerful actors (like universities or funded projects) assisting vulnerable and needy communities. It is not necessarily the result of actors with ill intention. However, the approach neglects the person with the need and effectively results in disempowerment.

DOI: 10.4324/9781003145899-15

This chapter argues against the one-size-fits-all approach and rather advances a careful and negotiated process to integrate tools to aid local after-care child practices. Unfortunately, many partnerships have little stakeholder input. Instead, people are told to "just do it", which can be a predictor for project failure and compromises sustainability. This chapter aims to present valuable discernment emerging from the consideration of "context" and "culture", aided by forging partnerships with community advisory boards. In this chapter, I propose a conceptual model to illustrate the numerous factors and processes that intervene and influence each other in such a collective enterprise to develop partnerships.

Often research teams do not have the firsthand information and experience of community-based aftercare centers or contextual and culturally underscored child-rearing practices. Accordingly, piloting intervention tools require a negotiated and situated conceptual practice model that is responsive to contextual nuances in enhancing acceptability and sustainable use. Ultimately, contextual barriers can significantly inhibit the effectiveness of promising interventions. An intervention exerts its influence within a specific context by changing relationships, reappropriating existing child-rearing or aftercare child practices, and redistributing and transforming resources. In our prior work in the Mangaung township in South Africa (see also Chapters 8 and 14, this volume), the MISC project's context is that of a community-based care center with many actors, including caregivers and other stakeholders such as households, schools, and communities. I argue that although this project took place in community-based care centers, contextual factors, directly and indirectly, influence the acceptability of MISC. Subsequently, incorporating the community advisory board as a partner to the MISC project was deemed critical in representing the community's interest.

15.2 Situating MISC in the South African Low-Resource Community Context

The complexity and peculiarity of child-rearing practices depend on the particular context and needs rooted in situational understanding. Understanding whether the need exists for child-development intervention requires a context-specific approach (Nduna, 2007). The critical pragmatism review process rejects the notion of generalized analysis removed from the historical, cultural, or lived experience in which the challenge or need is located (Mitchell, 2008; Forester, 2013). My understanding of community is that it is inclusive to all affected by implementing MISC and subsequent research results. This definition includes children, lay-residents of a local area, community practitioners, and service agencies (Green & Mercer, 2001, p. 1926). I use the construct "culture" to denote the set of distinctive beliefs and behaviors shared by a group of people and regulating their daily living (Eriksen, 2001; Bornstein, 2012). These beliefs and behaviors shape how parents care for their children. Therefore, embedded in the concept of culture is the expectation that different cultural groups possess distinct worldviews (loosely translates to beliefs that informs everyday actions) and behave in unique ways concerning their parenting (Bornstein, 2012). These differences can act as a baseline for childcare and caregiver practice. It is the immediate, if not the only, source to draw lessons from establishing caring practices.

Many intervention programs, usually with good intent, are less effective than anticipated in real-life settings (Robertson, Jepson, Macvean, & Gray, 2016). The deficit response to this outcome is that the beneficiaries lack interest in and ownership of the intervention program. In South Africa, dependency and a sense of entitlement are often the main reasons for failed intervention programs. Understanding the role of context in aiding effectiveness (or lack thereof) is useful in assessing the intervention program's outcome. On the one hand, the unique culture (including ethnic and language aspects) of each community, as well as its township nature, offer both opportunities and challenges for establishing responsive partnerships and sustainable program implementation outcomes (Bornstein, 2012). On the other hand, context is beneficial in decisions about the nature of the mediational intervention. Furthermore, context appropriation considers whether the program's outcomes are socially, ethically, and culturally feasible and acceptable.

The MISC intervention was implemented in Mangaung, in South Africa (see also Chapters 8 and 14 for details). The geographic site was historically known as a township to denote an area predominantly occupied by black people. The area includes formal and informal settlement and forms part of the City of Bloemfontein and the Mangaung Metropolitan. It is a typical extension, growing from surrounding areas, and the spoken languages are SeSotho and SeTswana (dominant) and pockets of IsiXhosa.

The context of this project is one of limited resources. Poverty and high levels of unemployment are endemic. Furthermore, poor health and schooling systems and infrastructure are pervasive. However, communal capital embedded in the principle of Ubuntu, loosely translating to "I am because you are", provides a necessary resource (in particular indigenous knowledge content) to harness from, for the implementation of MISC. The existing community-based centers, although under-resourced, also provide an ideal site for the program's piloting and implementation. Acknowledging the existing cultural capital, the project adopted cumulative integrative and strength-based approaches in which forging a partnership with the local community was crucial.

15.3 Forging Partnerships for the Effective Implementation of MISC

Suppose we accept that child-rearing is contextual and culturally rooted. We also need to acknowledge that community members' involvement in the piloting and implementing any form of child development is essential. It is then inevitable to engage community partners who can bring their perspectives and understandings of community child-rearing practices and development issues, especially emotional and cognitive aspects, into the project.

This assertion emanates from the theoretical conversation on universities' institutionalization of community engagement (see also Center for Disease Control and Prevention [CDC], 1997) and sustainable project outcomes (Matthews et al., 2018). For this chapter, community engagement speaks to the process of working collaboratively with and through community-based organizations affiliated by geographic proximity and particular interest to address issues affecting the wellbeing of the people (CDC, 1997). It often involves partnerships and coalitions that help mobilize resources, influence systems and serve as the catalyst to add value and improve existing practices (CDC, 1997). Recognizing overlapping expertise and interest emanating from the nuances of the implementation context and culture, we forged a partnership with local welfare organizations, community-based care centers, and members of faith-based non-profit organizations.

By collaborating with both welfare and community organizations, we combined resources to lower cost and increase impact. All those involved in the project had an interest in the children's developmental needs. These partners shared strengths and expertise to empower frontline workers (careworkers at aftercare day centers) to develop and provide holistic care amidst the continuous demand for care and caregiving in resource-limited communities. Whereas the traditional approach to community intervention programs tends to focus on doing it *for* the community, it was critical for the MISC project to first foreground the needs of the community concerned (Marais et al., 2014) and doing it *with* them (see Mitchell, 2008; Nduna, 2007; Oldfield, 2008). Israel, Schulz, Parker, and Becker (1998) discuss principles to guide the partnerships between academic researchers and communities.

Similarly, Hoekstra et al. (2020) review principles, strategies, outcomes, and impacts of research partnerships approaches. For the MISC project, we recognized the community as a unit of identity and built on strengths and resources within that community. Fostering co-learning and capacity-building among all partners, and espousing a collaborative, equitable partnership in all phases of the research was crucial (Israel et al., 1998). Accordingly, we integrated a balance between knowledge capital (particularly indigenous knowledge content) and MISC for all parties' mutual benefit focused on the local relevance.

Three basic principles underscored the South African MISC project partnership: we advanced the principles of *reciprocity, democratic process,* and openness for various *learning opportunities* (Flinders, Nicholson, Carlascio, & Gilb, 2013). Reciprocity in the partnership depends on the spirit of shared and collective learning. It is not only the community that benefits from the partnership; the implementation team also draws valuable lessons from the process. Inherent in partnership is often both overlapping and competing interests due to differences in worldviews. Effectively, participants in the partnership should resolve conflicts through the democratic processes of mediation, negotiation, and compromise. To illustrate, the MISC project was developed in Israel by Klein, Shohet, and Givon. Its evidence base in Africa started in Uganda by Boivin (an American—see Chapter 6, this volume), transported to South Africa by Sharp (a South African citizen living in the United States), and led on the ground by Marais (a South African community development researcher). Our team, therefore, included those that worked with Klein in Israel, Boivin with some of his team members from Uganda, Sharp with team members from the United States, and Marais, with team members from the local community. The team intersect with the local community, which constituted a very complex system for negotiating meaning.

For effective partnership, each member must have equal opportunities to participate in the planning, decision-making, and strategies that will facilitate the implementation process, as this advances sustainable use. The community partners can also contribute knowledge and understanding of the specific community the project team is working with to optimize its service. Elsewhere, we argued for the successful implementation of the mediational community intervention to rest on the appropriateness and acceptability of the strategies and methods (Rani et al., under review). Stith et al. (2006) found that community coalitions and program fidelity aided the program's successful implementation. Ultimately, the effectiveness, acceptability, sustainability, and public impact of an intervention program depend on the partnership and level of consultation, involvement, collaboration, and empowerment within the target community (Oldfield, 2008; Davies, 1991).

The community-partnership approach adopted for the MISC project used theoretical lessons discerned from publications on the community advisory board in community-based participatory research, health and well-being research, and implementation of an intervention program (Minkler, Vásquez, Warner, Steussey, & Facente, 2006; Shalowitz et al., 2009; Quinn, 2004; Newman et al., 2011; Cramer, Lazoritz, Shaffer, Palm, & Ford, 2018). Child-rearing necessities should be considered in their socio-cultural context. A firm understanding of cultural lenses and local worldview provides the conditions necessary to inform the implementation process. Subsequently, through the community advisory board, the project team formalized the academic-community partnership.

15.4 The Role of a Community Advisory Board in the Implementation of MISC

The community advisory board (CAB) effectively builds mutually beneficial partnerships between academic researchers and communities (Mott, Crawford, & NIMH, 2008; Reddy, Buchanan, Sifunda, James, & Naidoo, 2010; Ortega, McAlvain, Briant, Hohl, & Thompson, 2018). Although most CABs share similar principles, their variations in how they function respond to context particularities and the nature of the research or intervention program. For the MISC-SA project, the CAB served as the liaison between researchers and the community, expressing community concerns and clarifying cultural bottlenecks. The CAB provided assistance and suggestions in the refinement of the tools to enhance acceptability. Their participation in the MISC-SA project's planning stages contributed to the project's sustainability.

Their continuous participation served to improve research through ongoing dialogue between the researchers and the community (Strauss et al., 2001). CAB members provided firsthand knowledge that the project team used in project planning and implementation decision-making. Furthermore, the added value that CAB members bring to a community-academic partnership was the interrogation and validation of baseline research findings.

To eliminate competing child-rearing ideological practices, we espoused an open and ongoing consultation with the partners through face-to-face meetings and technology-mediated techniques (e.g. email) to solicit inputs from all affected and interested groups to establish a pragmatic MISC implementation nexus. At these meetings, we interrogated MISC concepts[1] (as discussed in Chapter 2; see also Sharp et al., 2018) associated with socio-emotional and cognitive development against the local cultural understandings and caregivers' own established child-rearing knowledge capital and beliefs. Communication was ongoing in line with the reflection by Kimme-Hea and Wendler-Shah's (2016). The project team committed to establishing channels for ongoing communication during the MISC-SA project implementation (see Chapter 14; Rani et al., under review).

15.5 MISC as to Aid Local Cultural Child-Rearing Practices

Advancing best practices and facilitating acceptability and sustainable use of an intervention program entails that we free ourselves from the arrogance of the Expert Model and align ourselves with establishing context-responsive practices. It compels professional bodies to regularly revisit the validity and applicability of mainstream knowledge and assertions and requires reflective questions (see Copple & Bredekamp, 2009). For example, does existing content need modification in light of working in a different context? Are there other forms of knowledge or practices to inform the planning and implementation process? Are there aspects of the existing content that have given rise to misunderstandings and misconceptions that need correcting? These reflective questions, especially in cross-cultural interaction, also serve as a checklist against an ethnocentric[2] undertone in MISC. The inability to anticipate, understand, and manage cultural bottlenecks can lead to the failure of cross-cultural MISC implementation.

The importance of recognizing the expertise and insights of the people we work with is highlighted (Knox, Mok, & Parmenter, 2000) and is vital for project ownership and sustainability. Speaking in the context of community development. Ife (2013, p. 139) argues:

> Community workers [including community researchers] face the temptation common to all human-service workers: to assume that somehow they are the experts, with specialist knowledge to be brought to the community and used to help in some way. . . . There is no doubt

that community workers do often have specialist knowledge, but to privilege this knowledge, and thereby devalue the local knowledge (see Briggs, 2005; Nel, 2005 reflections on Indigenous Knowledge System) of the community itself, is the antithesis of community development. The valuing of local knowledge is an essential component of any community development work, and this can best be summed up by the phrase "the community knows best".

Acknowledging that the community knows best does not loosely translate to advancing a strong anthropological form of cultural relativism[3] (Donnelly, 1984) in implementing community mediational programs. Mindful of existing assets and strengths (including the community's indigenous knowledge capital), we must create opportunities for uncomfortable conversations that encourage people to rethink their customary behavior or long-held beliefs about child-rearing practices. These conversations should take place in ways that do not devalue lived experiences. In the following, I present a conceptual model to guide the piloting and implementation of an intervention or mediational program.

15.6 Conceptual Model Towards Aiding Acceptability and Sustainable Use

It is essential to tailor services or mediational intervention programs to the unique community needs by building upon existing strengths (NTAECSC, 2008). Figure 15.1 illustrates a schematic representation of the MISC-SA project implementation process to facilitate acceptability and sustainable use. It especially challenges the expert model, which is essentially top-down and advances the strength–based partnership approach (Bryan & Henry, 2008).

The MISC research team must situate the mediation intervention in both context and culture through collaboration (to foster strength–based partnership) with stakeholders from the target community. This collaboration will enable them to implement a mediational intervention that supports frontline

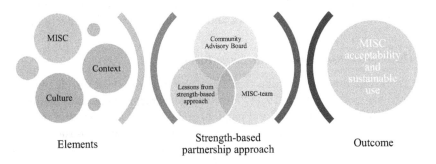

Figure 15.1 A conceptual model for best practice

workers to deliver culturally relevant and contextual responsive childcare. The CAB represents the community as more than their needs and what they lack. They bring to the partnership a body of local knowledge to share based on direct experience and firsthand observations, and CABs are arguably important gatekeepers in accessing such knowledge.

The strength-based partnership adopted for the MISC-SA project is sensitive to cross-cultural matters. It utilizes assets in the community, such as indigenous knowledge capital, to add value and broaden local caring practices for holistic child development. From this approach, the research team can discover that there is much to be gained from the lived experiences and indigenous knowledge of different communities. Although it is crucial to understand the context and acknowledge the community's socio-cultural and economic challenges, one must guard against "deficit perspectives" (Harry, Klingner, & Hart, 2005). The assumptions and narratives of deficit discredit the community partner as a valuable member of the partnership. After all, they are experts within their context, in charge of their own lives.

Additional to the conceptual model justification is the ability to move from individual units of the partnership, harness each other's expertise to establish a pragmatic, context-specific, and responsive program implementation nexus. The operational nexus will demonstrate interdependency and the interaction with one another towards a common outcome. In the advocacy for community empowerment, I discourage the top-down strategies and call for a project implementation process that honors and creates a space for the community's voice (through, for example, a CAB) and underpinned by lessons from a strength-based approach. If we can understand these processes properly, we will be more able to meet the communities' needs. This process begs to understand how people function as individuals and how they relate to each other since communication is intimately related to interventions' outcomes (see Davis & Meltzer, 2007).

15.7 Emerging Themes or Patterns From the MISC-SA Project Implementation

As the project's cultural consultant, I discerned from the CBO's meetings the following themes, bottlenecks, and patterns as critical for reflection.

The Individualism-Versus-Collectivism Binary

I think that research on collectivism and individualism entrench the either-or binary (see Hofstede, 1980). However, recognizing differences within a culture (including ethnicity and religion) and connection to another context (local, national, and international), and acknowledging the construct of culture as dynamic and continuously changing, expanded this view. Although the research provides a good baseline for a differentiated approach, voluntary subscription (cf. diffusion) through direct, stimulus and intermediate contact collapses the binary (particularity often used to rationalize essentialism and cultural racism) for a complementary approach, underscored by the convergence of various knowledge systems (Ember & Ember, 2014). The contribution of and access to new technologies and the international media facilitates disseminating values, beliefs, and perceptions about different cultural child-rearing practices (Costin, 2015). Effectively, it is safe to say critical features of what was considered dominant for individualism and collectivism context practices are not mutually exclusive (see Parker, Haytko, & Hermans, 2009). Local child-rearing practices can reflect universal principles of the global culture. Although the concept of "global culture" is gaining traction, in understanding this phenomenon, two opposite tendencies should be considered: homogenization versus heterogenization. It is essential to consider the homogenization of child-rearing practices through denouncing local practices in favor of an internationally dominant culture (cultural imperialism). Within this frame, only some cultures found their place and legitimize representatives of the international culture (Costin, 2015). Heterogeneity supports the principle of cultural pluralism and the doctrine of multiplicity (Haviland, Prins, & McBride, 2013). If we accept local practices as legitimate practice globally, child-rearing practices can form part of the "glocal" culture (see Eriksen, 2015). Global practices interface with the local to establish best practices. In practice, then, the global messages (or intervention) will be adapted, integrated, and transmitted through local perspectives. In other words, an intervention developed by global knowledge should use a local lens for implementation.

MISC-SA project was a semi-structured intervention program that combines socio-emotional health and cognitive development (Klein, 1996; Shohet & Jaegermann, 2012). Successful MISC implementation has taken place in Ethiopia (Klein & Rye, 2004) and Uganda (Boivin et al., 2013). MISC situates every activity within the cultural framework that the careworkers use to interact with the children. Klein (1996) recommends the use of everyday caregiving interaction. This application of a cross-cultural approach should mitigate concerns that MISC-caregiving depends on western cultural norms (Klein, Wieder, & Greenspan, 1987; Klein, Shohet, & Givon, 2017).

A complementary approach guided the MISC-implementation in South Africa. This complementary approach involved interaction and collaboration with partners as a connected group, resulting in a significant implementation experience. Experiences, ranging from the acceptability and feasibility of MISC implementation, are reported by Rani et al. (under review).

Eye Contact: Clearly and Visibly Looking Each Other in the Eye

Empirical studies have demonstrated that eye contact has a fundamental role in human social interaction. However, cross-cultural studies suggest that cultural norms affect eye contact behaviors (Akechi et al., 2013). Socialization processes are central to infant behavioral development. Although there are many spheres of influences, parents remain highly effective in scaffolding and regulating infant behavior (Neale & Whitebread, 2019; Rosanbalm & Murray, 2017). Assertions by human development theorists of newborns' vocal and facial recognition abilities are a good baseline to accept that eye contact is innate to humans. However, the meaning of eye contact varies across different cultural contexts (Akechi et al., 2013). In some cultural contexts, wary of generalization (especially Asia, Latin America, and Africa), this inborn reflex is discouraged, and children are taught to look away when conversing with an older person. This form of non-verbal social behavior is sign of respect. In the United States and Western Europe, looking away will be interpreted as being distracted and disinterested (and as such is discouraged). For Vygotsky (1978), signs lead humans to a specific behavior structure that breaks away from biological development and creates new forms of what is understood as culturally based acceptable values and norms. My view is that children adapt this kind of behavior and respond with eye contact (or averting the eyes) as required by the particular context.[4] MISC's emphasis on eye contact is not a disregard for the local context of normative behavior.

A Cultural Expectation Blind-Spot: The Female-Versus-Male Socialization Script

Given the gender (male versus female) socialization script, the MISC attributes of physical closeness, touching, emotional expression, and synchrony present interesting cultural distinctions and overlaps. Culture-specific influences shape fundamental decisions about which behavior caregivers or parents should promote concerning specific genders (Bornstein, 2012). We can expect these attributes to find expression discrepancy within cultural-specific patterns of child-rearing gender role norms, expectations, and needs attributes. For instance, emotional expression and touching tend to be promoted in the rearing of a female child but discouraged in a male child, especially in countries with an over-emphasis on masculinity (a practice that leans towards toxic masculinity). Although the stereotypical differences between boys and girls are considered invalid, given their traditional context, some do appear significant in the present. General observations are that socialization institutions (like schools, churches, traditional initiation schools, boys' and girls' clubs) will reinforce the male image of dominance and independence. In contrast, girls receive rewards for passive and submissive behavior. The most frequent traits used to define the two roles are that boys are socialized to be assertive and competitive (often leading to aggressive behavior) and girls for modesty and servitude. From Hewlett, Lamb, Shannon, Leyendecker, and Schölmerich's (1998) research on child-parent proximity among Aka foragers and Ngandu farmers, they discern that parents from Aka communities hold their children close when they feed them. In contrast, Ngandu children are left to feed themselves. Two decades since this study, we can accept that this pattern has shifted and mostly changed. However, this observation's key lesson supports Bornstein's (2012) assertion that caregivers normally organize and distribute their caregiving faithful to indigenous cultural belief systems and behavior patterns.

Beyond MISC's immediate outcomes, in South Africa as a country engulfed by gender-based violence, it may be even more critical for male children to be raised within a caring environment. For example, Child Welfare South Africa (https://childwelfaresa.org.za/boy-child/) has an intervention program aiming to help boys make life choices. The program should lead to improved skills in relating to women and girls through planned self-care and positive interaction with girls and increased community participation. This demonstrates the earnest need for mediational intervention. I think that MISC principles can add value to the development of boys in contributing to a safe, healthier, and happier society.

- **From talking *to* children to talking *with* them**
  Care-workers probably grew up with the adage that children should be seen and not heard (see Nel, 2016), and to some extent, they have internalized and considered it a baseline for child-rearing practices. This form of silencing serves the authoritarian parenting style to disadvantage the child's emotional and cognitive development. In this context, individual agency is discouraged, and children are taught to internalize without questioning or asking for clarification and understanding. MISC encourages the real interaction between careworker and child that creates opportunities for taking turns, initiation and response.
- **From doing it for the child to doing it with them**
  There is a growing literature on careworker/parent-child scaffolding in the preschool years (Conner & Cross, 2003). Parental or careworker's responsiveness has been identified as necessary for certain aspects of child regulatory development (Kochanska & Aksan, 2004). Adult-child interaction for scaffolding and the modelling of regulatory strategies and behaviors are critical for implementing MISC. In the long term, this interaction leads to the child's self-regulation. This interaction is underscored by:

  - mutual engagement, as both the child and the careworker, collaborate on a task or activity; and
  - mutual attention, as both the child and the careworker focus on the same task or activity.

This advancement challenges the cultural authority inherent in parenting (atypical of an authoritarian parenting style). Careworkers must relinquish their position of power as one who sees the child as a clean slate that needs imprinting (through instruction or commands) to creating opportunities for scaffolding (through suggestions, akin to the MISC principle of expanding). Bornstein (2012) asserts that children are comprehending partners. Through scaffolding, the careworker guides the child's learning during a goal-oriented MISC-task by offering and withdrawing support at different levels (Neale & Whitebread, 2019).

- **Closing the gap for cumulative and integrated best practice**
  Careworkers are socilaized in a particular cultural context. They grew in the same context, observing and caring for their younger siblings. Some of them are mothers, so effectively, they have a body of caregiving knowledge that is underscored by lived experience. These culturally constructed childcare practices are internalized, often dictate compliance in the face of new realities and experiences, and silence individual agency. Therefore, having experienced unique caregiving patterns is a principal reason that individuals in different cultures are who they are and often differ from one another (Bornstein, 2012). Given an opportunity to provide care, Bornstein (2012) is of the view that they would "normally organize and distribute their caregiving faithful to indigenous cultural belief systems and behavior patterns". Subsequently, exposure to new ways of doing or opportunities for learning new skills creates cognitive dissonance and can disrupt the spontaneous response to childcare practices. Often new experiences require individual adjustment or practice modification. Lessons from the MISC-SA project is that careworkers had to:

- close the gap between own socialization and rearing script through the incorporation of MISC-principles in their current practice; and
- situate MISC into the center's daily activities.

15.8 Conclusion

This chapter presents valuable discernment emerging from the consideration of "culture" and "context" aided by forging a partnership with the CAB. As the project's cultural consultant, a discursive approach was followed, and I acknowledge my role being part of the context and process from which arguments are made. The descriptive reflections in this piece speak to the South African context of limited resources—the intention is not to prescribe its assertion as a baseline approach for mediational intervention program implementation.

I have argued against a one-size-fits-all approach. It should effectively be read and understood as a piece that sensitizes and advocates a context-specific and responsive approach. In line with the latter, the establishment of the partnership underscored by a strength-based approach is inevitable. The strengths-based practice involves shifting from a deficit approach, which emphasizes problems, to a positive partnership with the community. A strength-based approach is highly resonant with mediational intervention acceptability and sustainable use. The CAB helped the research team to understand the local particularities to advance a context responsive mediational program. In such practice, CABs should be active partners in the planning, appropriation, and implementation of MISC. Subsequently, the MISC-SA project has transformed the community-based organization climate by cultivating a strengths-enhancing environment that supports and empowers community-based care workers to deliver holistic childcare practices, including providing food and socio-emotional care.

Notes

1 Focusing, exciting/affecting, expanding, encouraging/rewarding, regulating.
2 The point of view that one's own way of life is to be preferred to all others.
3 Akin to "anything goes", which may compromise the protection of human rights.
4 The SeSotho proverb "taba di mahlong" ("the face is the index of the mind") emphasizes eye contact in social interaction, but it is common practice to discourage eye contact between children and adults. Is this not a contradiction?

References

Akechi, H., Senju, A., Uibo, H., Kikuchi, Y., Hasegawa, T., & Hietanen, J. K. (2013). Attention to eye contact in the West and East: Autonomic responses and evaluative ratings. *PloS One, 8*(3), e59312.

Boivin, M., Bangirana, P., Nakasujja, N., Page, C., Shohet, C., Givon, D., & Klein, P. (2013). A year-long caregiver training program to improve neurocognition in preschool Ugandan HIV-exposed children. *Journal of Developmental and Behavioral Pediatrics, 34*(4), 269–278.

Bornstein, M. H. (2012). Cultural approaches to parenting. *Parenting, 2*(2–3), 212–221.

Briggs, J. (2005). The use of indigenous knowledge in development: Problems and challenges. *Progress in Development Studies, 5*(2), 99–114.

Bryan, J., & Henry, L. (2008). Strengths-based partnerships: A school-family-community partnership approach to empowering students. *Professional School Counseling, 12*(2), 149–156.

Butin, D. W. (2015). Dreaming of justice: Critical service-learning and the need to wake up. *Theory into Practice, 54*(1), 5–10.

Centers for Disease Control and Prevention (CDC). (1997). *Principles of community engagement* (1st ed.). Atlanta, GA: CDC/ATSDR Committee on Community Engagement.

Cluver, L., Fincham, D., & Seedat, S. (2009). Posttraumatic stress in AIDS-orphaned children exposed to high levels of trauma: The protective role of perceived social support. *Journal of Traumatic Stress, 22*(2), 106–112.

Cluver, L., & Gardner, F. (2007). The mental health of children orphaned by AIDS: A review of international and southern African research. *Journal of Child and Adolescent Mental Health, 19*(1), 1–17.

Conner, D. B., & Cross, D. R. (2003). Longitudinal analysis of the presence, efficacy and stability of maternal scaffolding during informal problem-solving interactions. *British Journal of Developmental Psychology, 21*(3), 315–334.

Copple, C., & Bredekamp, S. (2009). *Developmentally appropriate practice in early childhood programs: Serving children from birth through age 8*. Washington, DC: National Association for the Education of Young Children.

Costin, A. F. (2015). Negotiating in cross-cultural contexts. *International Conference Knowledge-Based Organization, 21*(1), 185–191.

Cramer, M. E., Lazoritz, S., Shaffer, K., Palm, D., & Ford, A. L. (2018). Community advisory board members' perspectives regarding opportunities and challenges of research collaboration. *Western Journal of Nursing Research, 40*(7), 1032–1048.

Davies, D. (1991). Schools reaching out: Family, school, and community partnerships for student success. *PhiDelta Kappan, 72*(5), 376–382.

Davis, H., Day, C., & Bidmead, C. (2002). *Working in partnership with parents: The parent adviser model.* London: Psychological Corp.

Davis, H., & Meltzer, L. (2007). *Working in partnership through early support: Distance learning text: Working with parents in partnership (book chapter).* Washington, DC: Department of Health.

Despres, L. A., Banton, M., Bennett, J. W., Cohen, R., Edmonson, M. S., Fojtik, K., & Whitten Jr., N. E. (1968). Anthropological theory, cultural pluralism, and the study of complex societies [and Comments and Reply]. *Current Anthropology, 9*(1), 3–26.

Donnelly, J. (1984). Cultural relativism and universal human rights. *Human Rights Quarterly, 6,* 400–419.

Ember, C. R., & Ember, M. (2014). *Cultural anthropology.* New York: Pearson.

Eriksen, T. H. (2001). *Small places, large issues: An introduction to social and cultural anthropology.* London: Pluto Press.

Eriksen, T. H. (2015). Towards a global conversation. *Glocal Times, 22/23.*

Flinders, B. A., Nicholson, L., Carlascio, A., & Gilb, K. (2013). The partnership model for service-learning programs: A step-by-step approach. *American Journal of Health Sciences, 4*(2), 67–78.

Forester, J. (2013). On the theory and practice of critical pragmatism: Deliberative practice and creative negotiations. *Planning Theory, 12*(1), 5–22.

Green, L. W., & Mercer, S. L. (2001). Can public health researchers and agencies reconcile the push from funding bodies and the pull from communities? *American Journal of Public Health, 91*(12), 1926–1929.

Harry, B., Klingner, J. K., & Hart, J. (2005). African American families under fire: Ethnographic views of family strengths. *Remedial and Special Education, 26*(2), 101–112.

Haviland, W. A., Prins, H. E., & McBride, B. (2013). *Anthropology: The human challenge.* Boston, MA: Cengage Learning.

Hewlett, B. S., Lamb, M. E., Shannon, D., Leyendecker, B., & Schölmerich, A. (1998). Culture and early infancy among central African foragers and farmers. *Developmental Psychology, 34*(4), 653.

Hoekstra, F., Mrklas, K. J., Khan, M., McKay, R. C., Vis-Dunbar, M., Sibley, K. M., . . . Gainforth, H. L. (2020). A review of reviews on principles, strategies, outcomes and impacts of research partnerships approaches: A first step in synthesising the research partnership literature. *Health Research Policy and Systems, 18,* 1–23.

Hofstede, G. (1980). *Culture's consequences: International differences in work-related values.* Beverly Hills, CA: Sage.

Ife, J. W. (2013). *Community development in an uncertain world: Vision, analysis and practice.* Cambridge: Cambridge University Press.

Israel, B. A., Schulz, A. J., Parker, E. A., & Becker, A. B. (1998). Review of community-based research: Assessing partnership approaches to improve public health. *Annual Review of Public Health, 19*(1), 173–202.

Jeynes, W. H. (2005). A meta-analysis of the relation of parental involvement to urban elementary school student academic achievement. *Urban Education, 40*(3), 237–269.

Kimme Hea, A. C., & Wendler Shah, R. (2016). Silent partners: Developing a critical understanding of community partners in technical communication service-learning pedagogies. *Technical Communication Quarterly, 25*(1), 48–66.

Klein, P. (1996). *Early intervention: Cross-cultural experiences with a mediational approach.* New York: Garland.

Klein, P., & Rye, H. (2004). Interaction-oriented early intervention in Ethiopia: The MISC approach. *Infants and Young Children, 17*(4), 340–354.

Klein, P., Shohet, C., & Givon, D. (2017). A mediational intervention for sensitising caregivers (MISC): A cross-cultural early intervention. In A. Abubakar & F. van de Vijver (Eds.), *Handbook of applied developmental science in sub-Saharan Africa* (pp. 291–312). New York: Springer.

Klein, P., Wieder, S., & Greenspan, S. (1987). A theoretical overview and empirical study of mediated learning experience: Prediction of preschool performance from mother-infant interaction patterns. *Infant Mental Health Journal, 8*(2), 110–129.

Knox, M., Mok, M., & Parmenter, T. R. (2000). Working with the experts: Collaborative research with people with an intellectual disability. *Disability & Society, 15*(1), 49–61.

Kochanska, G., & Aksan, N. (2004). Development of mutual responsiveness between parents and their young children. *Child Development, 75*(6), 1657–1676.

Marais, L., Sharp, C., Pappin, M., Rani, K., Skinner, D., Lenka, M., & Serekoane, J. (2014). Community-based mental health support for orphans and vulnerable children in South Africa: A triangulation study. *Vulnerable Children and Youth Studies, 9*(2), 151–158.

Matthews, A. K., Newman, S., Anderson, E. E., Castillo, A., Willis, M., & Choure, W. (2018). Development, implementation, and evaluation of a community engagement advisory board: Strategies for maximizing success. *Journal of Clinical and Translational Science, 2*(1), 8–13.

Minkler, M., Vásquez, V. B., Warner, J. R., Steussey, H., & Facente, S. (2006). Sowing the seeds for sustainable change: A community-based participatory research partnership for health promotion in Indiana, USA and its aftermath. *Health Promotion International, 21*(4), 293–300.

Mitchell, T. (2008). Traditional vs. critical service-learning: Engaging the literature to differentiate two models. *Michigan Journal of Community Service Learning, 14*(2), 50–65.

Mott, L., Crawford, E., & NIMH Multisite HIV/STD Prevention Trial for African American Couples Group. (2008). The role of community advisory boards in project Eban. *Journal of Acquired Immune Deficiency Syndromes, 49* (Suppl 1), S68.

National Technical Assistance and Evaluation Center for Systems of Care (NTAECSC). (2008). *An individualized, strengths-based approach in public child welfare driven systems of care.* Fairfax, VA: NTAECSC.

Nduna, N. J. (2007). The community voice on service-learning: A good practice guide for higher education. *Education as Change, 11*(3), 69–78.

Neale, D., & Whitebread, D. (2019). Maternal scaffolding during play with 12- to 24-month-old infants: Stability over time and relations with emerging effortful control. *Metacognition and Learning, 14*(3), 265–289.

Nel, P. J. (2005). Indigenous knowledge systems: Contestation, rhetorics and space. *Indilinga African Journal of Indigenous Knowledge Systems, 4*(1), 2–14.

Nel, R. (2016). "Children must be seen and heard"—Doing postcolonial theology with children in a (southern) African Reformed church. *HTS Theological Studies, 72*(1), 1–7.

Newman, S. D., Andrews, J. O., Magwood, G. S., Jenkins, C., Cox, M. J., & Williamson, D. C. (2011). Peer-reviewed: Community advisory boards in community-based participatory research: A synthesis of best processes. *Preventing Chronic Disease, 8*(3), 1–12.

Oldfield, S. (2008). Who's serving whom? Partners, process, and products in service-learning projects. *South African Urban Geography, 32*(2), 269–285.

Ortega, S., McAlvain, M. S., Briant, K. J., Hohl, S., & Thompson, B. (2018). Perspectives of community advisory board members in a community-academic partnership. *Journal of Health Care for the Poor and Underserved, 29*(4), 1529–1543.

Parker, R. S., Haytko, D. L., & Hermans, C. M. (2009). Individualism and collectivism: Reconsidering old assumptions. *Journal of International Business Research, 8*(1), 127.

Quinn, S. C. (2004). Ethics in public health research: Protecting human subjects: The role of community advisory boards. *American Journal of Public Health, 94*(6), 918–922.

Rani, K., Marais, L., Sharp, C., Cloete, J., Serekoane, M., Lenka, M., . . . Phakisi, T. (under review). The acceptability and feasibility of MISC in a low resource setting in South Africa. *International Journal of Child Care and Educational Policy.*

Reddy, P., Buchanan, D., Sifunda, S., James, S., & Naidoo, N. (2010). The role of community advisory boards in health research: Divergent views in the South African experience. *SAHARA-J: Journal of Social Aspects of HIV/AIDS, 7*(3), 1–8.

Robertson, J., Jepson, R., Macvean, A., & Gray, S. (2016). Understanding the importance of context: A qualitative study of a location-based exergame to enhance school children's physical activity. *PloS One, 11*(8).

Rosanbalm, K. D., & Murray, D. W. (2017). *Promoting self-regulation in the first five years: A practice brief.* OPRE Brief 2017–79. Washington, DC: Administration for Children & Families.

Shalowitz, M. U., Isacco, A., Barquin, N., Clark-Kauffman, E., Delger, P., Nelson, D., . . . Wagenaar, K. A. (2009). Community-based participatory research: A review of the literature with strategies for community engagement. *Journal of Developmental & Behavioral Pediatrics, 30*(4), 350–361.

Sharp, C., Shohet, C., Givon, D., Marais, L., Rani, K., Lenka, M., & Boivin, M. (2018). Early childhood development interventions: A focus on responsive caregiving. In M. Tomlinson (Ed.), *Child and adolescent development: An expanded focus for public health* (pp. 245–270). The Netherlands: Springer.

Shohet, C., & Jaegermann, N. (2012). Integrating infant mental health into primary health care and early childhood education settings in Israel. *Zero to Three, 33*(2), 55–58.

Stith, S., Pruitt, I., Dees, J., Fronce, M., Green, N., Som, A., & Linkh, D. (2006). Implementing community-based prevention programming: A review of the literature. *Journal of Primary Prevention, 27*(6), 599–617.

Strauss, R. P., Sengupta, S., Quinn, S. C., Goeppinger, J., Spaulding, C., Kegeles, S. M., & Millett, G. (2001). The role of community advisory boards: Involving communities in the informed consent process. *American Journal of Public Health, 91*(12), 1938–1943.

Vygotsky, L. (1978). Mind in society: The development of higher psychological processes. Cambridge, MA: Harvard University Press.

Index

Page numbers in *italic* indicate a figure and page numbers in **bold** indicate a table.

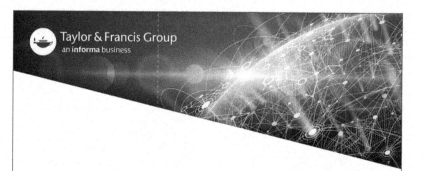